ncw
3.10

MANAGING IN HEALTH AND SOCIAL CARE

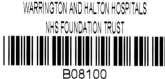

Managing in Health and Social Care is about developing skills age and improve health and social care services. The focus thr is on the role that a manager can play in ensuring effective de high-quality services. Examples from social care and health are used to illustrate techniques for managing le, resources, information, projects and change.

This new edition has been extensively revised and includes many new case studies and examples, as well as a new chapter on motivation. It covers topics such as:

- interorganisational and interprofessional working
- leadership
- responding to the needs of service users
- the service environment
- accountability and risk
- working with a budget
- standards and quality
- managing change.

The authors explore how managers can make a real and positive difference to the work of organisations providing health and social care. They consider what effectiveness means in managing care services, the values that underpin the services, the roles of leaders and managers in developing high-quality service provision, and the necessary skills and systems to enable service users to contribute to planning and evaluation.

Managing in Health and Social Care is a practical textbook for students of management in health and social care, whether at under-graduate or postgraduate level. It includes case studies with textual commentary to reinforce learning, activities, key references and clear explanations of essential management tools and concepts.

The first edition of this book was published in association with The Open University for the Managing Education Scheme by Open Learning (MESOL).

Vivien Martin works in management and professional development at the University of Brighton Business School, UK. **Julie Charlesworth** is Lecturer in Public Management at The Open University, UK. **Euan Henderson** was formerly Professor of Educational Technology in The Open University Business School. He is currently a non-executive director of a primary care trust.

MANAGING IN HEALTH AND SOCIAL CARE

Second edition

Vivien Martin, Julie Charlesworth
and Euan Henderson

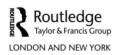
Routledge
Taylor & Francis Group

LONDON AND NEW YORK

First published 2001

Reprinted 2003, 2004, 2005, 2006, 2007

This edition published 2010
by Routledge
2 Park Square, Milton Park, Abingdon, Oxon, OX14 4RN

Simultaneously published in the USA and Canada
by Routledge
270 Madison Avenue, New York, NY 10016

Routledge is an imprint of the Taylor & Francis Group, an informa business

Typeset in Sabon and Futura by
Keystroke, Tettenhall, Wolverhampton

Printed and bound in Great Britain by
TJ International Ltd, Padstow, Cornwall

British Library Cataloguing in Publication Data
A catalogue record for this book is available from the British Library

Library of Congress Cataloging in Publication Data
Martin, Vivien, 1947–
Managing in health and social care / Vivien Martin, Julie Charlesworth
and Euan Henderson. – 2nd ed.
p. cm.
Includes index.
1. Human services–Management. 2. Health services administration
I. Charlesworth, Julie, 1964– II. Henderson, Euan S. III. Title.
HV41.M286 2010
362.068--dc22
2009034897

ISBN10: 0–415–49388–9 (hbk)
ISBN10: 0–415–49389–7 (pbk)
ISBN10: 0–203–85693–7 (ebk)

ISBN13: 978–0–415–49388–8 (hbk)
ISBN13: 978–0–415–49389–5 (pbk)
ISBN13: 978–0–203–85693–2 (ebk)

CONTENTS

List of illustrations   ix
Acknowledgements   xi

Introduction   1
Overview of the chapters   2

PART 1   THE MANAGER AND THE TEAM   5

1   **Your job as a manager in health and social care**   7
     A manager in action   7
     The nature of your job   17

2   **Improving your effectiveness as a manager**   20
     Reviewing what you need to do to be effective   20
     Determining your priorities in terms of objectives   28

3   **Management and leadership**   35
     Managing and leading   35
     Developing your style   45
     Managing with style   51

4   **Understanding motivation**   58
     What is motivation?   59
     Theories of motivation   62
     The impact of external initiatives on motivation   66
     Diversity and motivation   67

5   **Values and vision**   71
     Values   71
     Managing interorganisational values and vision   86

PART 2 MANAGING FOR SERVICE USERS   **91**

6   **What do your service users want?**   **93**
Different kinds of customer   93
Service users' requirements   103
Getting feedback from service users   107
Handling complaints   111

7   **Mapping the service environment**   **115**
Components of the service environment   115
Stakeholders and their interests   119
Influencing the near environment   124
Needs and demands   126
Working with your environmental map   131

8   **Engaging with service users**   **133**
Service user participation   133
The nature of evidence   138
Planning an investigation   140
What kind of information do you need?   144

9   **Managing outcomes with service users**   **153**
Purpose and outcomes   153
Working across boundaries   157

PART 3 MANAGING SERVICES   **169**

10   **Managing processes**   **171**
Defining and mapping processes   172
Process mapping   178
Designing process improvements   185

11   **Working with a budget**   **190**
Setting budgets   190
Approaches to budgeting   194
Timetabling and preparing the ground   198
Negotiating the budget   201
Target-setting, motivation and communication   205

12   **Service planning, accountability and risk**   **207**
Planning health and social care services   208
Accountability   212
Assessing and managing risk   218

PART 4 MANAGING IMPROVEMENT   **225**

13   **Quality in services**   **227**
What does 'quality' mean?   227

Perspectives on quality | 233
Why is quality important? | 236
Do you have a quality problem? | 238
Dimensions of quality | 239
Analysing the causes of quality problems | 242

14 Working with standards | **249**
What is a standard? | 250
Developing a standard | 254
Structure, process, outcome | 259
Frameworks of standards | 265
Monitoring standards | 268

15 Management control | **273**
Why control? | 273
The control loop | 275
Measuring and comparing | 279
Taking control as a manager | 284
Taking corrective action | 291

16 Developing effective performance | **295**
Team working in health and social care | 296
Planning systematically to meet training and
    development needs | 302
Dealing with poor performance | 310

17 Managing change | **316**
Diagnosis | 317
Planning for change | 330

18 Planning and managing projects | **338**
Planning a project | 339
Managing people and change | 346
Keeping on track | 347
Problems with planning | 353

Index | 359

ILLUSTRATIONS

FIGURES

2.1	The ladder approach to the analysis of objectives	26
3.1	Possible relationships between leadership and management	35
3.2	The leading role	39
3.3	A style grid for leaders in health and social care	49
4.1	Maslow's hierarchy of needs	62
4.2	Hygiene factors and motivators	63
4.3	Expectancy theory	64
5.1	Interactions between values held at different levels	72
6.1	Players and their roles in the Horizon House clubhouse project	97
6.2	Customer chains	100
6.3	A chain of benefit	101
7.1	The three environments	116
7.2	A stakeholder map for an organisation providing health or social care services	121
8.1	The service user participation continuum	134
8.2	Examples of services for people with disabilities	135
8.3	A bureaucratic service	136
8.4	A responsive service	136
8.5	An empowering service	137
8.6	The quality control loop: two kinds of involvement and consultation	144
10.1	A transformation process	174
10.2	Flow of transformation processes	174
12.1	Lines of accountability in a housing association's building and maintenance department	216
13.1	The quality chain	232
13.2	Quality means different things to different people	235
13.3	Basic fishbone diagram	242
13.4	Example of a fishbone diagram	244

14.1   Quality 'ball on the hill'   251
14.2   Monitoring standards   268
15.1   The control loop   276
15.2   The systems process   277
15.3   A feedback loop   278
15.4   The systems loop   279
17.1   The Nadler and Tushman diagnostic model   319
17.2   A mind map representation of the Dunford diagnosis   326
17.3   Driving and restraining forces   331
17.4   Dunford force field analysis   334
18.1   Logic diagram for the production of a directory   348
18.2   Gantt chart for extending 'shared action planning'   349
18.3   Multistage approach   354
18.4   Cyclical approach   355
18.5   Iterative approach   356

TABLES

7.1   Advantages and disadvantages of in-house provision
         and outsourcing   118
9.1   Customer assessment of quality   159
10.1   The patient's pathway   177
11.1   Budget statement   191
11.2   Budget statement for a day-care centre   195
11.3   An approach to the budget plan   196
11.4   A master timetable for budget preparation   199
11.5   An individual budget preparation timetable   200
13.1   Different perspectives on quality   234
13.2   Quality problems   239
13.3   Dimensions of quality in care services   240
14.1   Proceeding in steps   258
14.2   Quality standards for the provision of a cervical
         cytology screening programme   260
14.3   Standards for the occupational therapy service of Fife
         Health Board   263
14.4   Core and developmental standards for the 'safety'
         domain   267
14.5   Monitoring form for an occupational therapy service   269
14.6   Example of monitoring arrangements for patient safety 270
15.1   Levels of control in the treatment room of a general
         practice   293
16.1   Types of tasks   297
17.1   A commitment plan for Dunford   335
18.1   A key events plan for the opening of a hospice   352
18.2   Part of a milestone plan   353

ACKNOWLEDGEMENTS

We are indebted to the many individuals who have contributed to the development of the MESOL programme 'Managing in Health and Social Care' from which the material for this book is drawn, and also those individuals who have contributed to the current edition.

Alison Baker
Bob Baker
Sue Balderson
Sheila Begley
Lawrence Benson
Jennifer Bernard
Ceridwyn Bessant
Stanley Bonthron
Diane Bowler
Margaret Brand
Alex Bush
Chris Butler
Peter Byrne
Sheila Cameron
Miriam Catterall
John Charles
Andrew Clapperton
Steve Cooke
David Cottam
Sue Cox
Sally Cray
Nigel Crisp
Mark Cutler
Mel Daniels
Kathy Darby
Salle Dare
Anne Davey
Rachel Dickinson

Rob Dixon
Charlotte Douglass
Mervyn Eastwood
Toni Fisher
John Frith
Alan Garland
Neil Garret-Harris
Lynda Gatecliffe
Ken Giles
Bruce Gillam
Val Glenny
Jim Green
Nigel Grinstead
Liz Haggard
Charles Handy
Ann Harrison
Steve Harrison
Joyce Healy
Pat Heath
Nicki Hedge
Pat Honeyset
John Houlston
Phil Ingamells
Mark Isaac
Ken Jarrold
Alan Johnston
Judith Johnston
Peter Key

Gill Kitching
Judith Knight
Jacky Korer
Christa Laird
Hilary Lance
Carole Lawrence-Parr
Penny Lawson
Paul Lewis
Penny Lewis
Beryl Little
Brian Lund
Stuart Maguire
Mike Marchmont
Gill Marsden
Philip Marsh
Kathy Martin
Gill McDougall
Ian Moore
Elaine Mottram
Peter Munro
Geraldine Murrison
Steve Oliver
Alice Olliver
Helen Orme
Heather Paisley
Andrew Paterson
Marion Pearce
Sue Pearce
Clare Perry
Kay Phillips

Ann Plested
Christopher Pollitt
Lynne Quinney
Sally Ravenhall
Cathy Reilly
Colin Robinson
John Robinson
Julia Ross
Derek Rowntree
Jill Sandford
Brenda Sawyer
Paul Shanahan
Jill Sharp
Gillian Smith
Joan Smith
Tony Stapleton
Geoff Stevenson
Anne Tofts
Jill Turner
Trevor Walker
Vanessa Walker
Joe Walsh
Teresa Waring
Harry Watkins
Alan Watson
Maxwell Wide
Jo Williams
Norman Woods
Heather Worsley
Jennifer Yates

Further acknowledgements are included here for permission to use:

Figure 4.1 reprinted from Maslow, A. H., Frager, M. and Fadiman, J. (1987) *Motivation and Personality*, Pearson. Adapted by permission of Pearson Education, Incl., Upper Saddle River, New Jersey.

Table 9.1 reprinted from Berry, L., Zeithaml, V. and Parasuranam, A. (1985) *A Practical Approach to Quality*, Joiner Associates Inc., materials are copyrighted by Oriel Incorporated, formerly Joiner Associates Inc. and are used here with permission.

Table 13.3 reprinted from Maxwell, R. (1984) 'Quality assessment in heath' *British Medical Journal*, vol. 13, pp. 31–4, with permission from the BMJ Publishing Group.

Figures 14.1 and 14.2 reprinted from Koch, H. (1991) *Total Quality Management in Health Care*, Churchill Livingstone/Elsevier. By permission of Elsevier Limited.

Table 14.3 reprinted from Kitson, A. 'Rest Assured', *Nursing Times*, 27 August 1986, pp. 28–31.

Table 14.6 adapted from 'Terms and conditions for the provision of community health services', Milton Keynes Primary Care Trust (2008).

Figure 17.1 reprinted from Nadler, D. A. and Tushman, M. L. (1980) 'A model for diagnosing organizational behavior', *Organizational Dynamics*, vol. 9, no. 2, pp 35–51. By permission of Elsevier Limited.

Crown Copyright material is reproduced with the permission of the Controller of HMSO and the Queen's Printer for Scotland.

Every effort has been made to contact and acknowledge copyright owners, but the authors and publisher would be pleased to have any errors or omissions brought to their attention so that corrections may be published at a later printing.

INTRODUCTION

This book should be of value to all those with management responsibilities for health and social care – whether as departmental managers, team leaders or project managers. It is not only for those who are full-time managers, but also for those who have management roles alongside their professional roles.

Its focus is on practical approaches to management and leadership in the particular context of the need to continue to modernise health and social care services. The emphasis is on ensuring that services are responsive to the needs of service users, integrated across traditional professional and organisational boundaries, effective in achieving the outcomes that both individual service users and society as a whole are seeking, and inclusive in identifying and meeting the needs of disadvantaged groups.

This requires understanding what effective management and leadership mean, developing shared values with service users and other stakeholders, and managing performance by setting quality standards, monitoring progress against them and leading the drive to seek service improvements. It includes managing teams, managing projects and managing change. It also includes making the best use of available resources – people, money, facilities and information.

We use the term 'service users' throughout the book as an inclusive term for patients, carers and everyone who uses health and social care services. All the chapters are drawn from learning materials prepared for the Management Education Scheme by Open Learning (MESOL), a project that involved close collaboration between the National Health Service, the former Social Services Inspectorate, the Institute of Healthcare Management and the Open University Business School. Since they first appeared in 1990, the MESOL materials have been frequently redeveloped and updated by a broadly based team of practising managers and management developers (see the list of contributors on pp. xi–xiii) to meet the changing needs of health and social care services.

Over the past twenty years, over 25,000 managers in the United Kingdom have benefited from studying courses based on the MESOL learning materials – some in open-learning sets within their workplaces, others through supported distance learning with the Open University, and yet others in programmes offered by local universities, colleges and training organisations. The MESOL materials have also been extensively used overseas, adapted and translated where necessary – in Hong Kong, Australia, Malaysia, the Cayman Islands, Slovakia, Russia, South Africa, Namibia and Egypt. The materials continue to be studied and are now managed by The Institute of Healthcare Management.

Although the chapters have been designed to follow a logical sequence, management learning is not a linear process, and each chapter can be studied as a free-standing topic. Effective management learning is also a reflective process, and each chapter includes activities to encourage the reader to pause and consider the implications for his or her work as a manager.

OVERVIEW OF THE CHAPTERS

Part 1: The manager and the team

Chapter 1 – Your job as a manager in health and social care – focuses on what managers do. It offers some examples of how managers in health and social care work, and invites you to compare your work with theirs. You are invited to analyse the main roles you play as a manager and consider the demands these make on you.

Chapter 2 – Improving your effectiveness as a manager – sets you thinking about managerial effectiveness and how managers in health and social care today achieve effective results. You are asked to consider what effectiveness means for you in your job and to set or review your key objectives.

Chapter 3 – Management and leadership – considers what is meant by leadership and the extent to which managers are expected to show leadership. We discuss some ways in which you can develop your management style to improve your effectiveness as a leader.

Chapter 4 – Understanding motivation – explores the importance of some of the theories of motivation, which place different emphasis on needs, goals and rewards. We also explore how the context of working in health and social care impacts on the relevance and application of these theories. We also consider the role of diversity in these debates.

Chapter 5 – Values and vision – discusses the values that shape your organisation and influence the ways in which services are delivered. The complexity of managing values and vision in an inter-organisational context is also considered.

Part 2: Managing for service users

Chapter 6 – What do your service users want? – focuses on the ultimate customers of health and social care – the service users. It distinguishes between what the end-users of services *need* and what they *want*, as well as what their expectations are. It examines how you can collect feedback from the users of your service, as a basis for making service improvements. It considers your role in handling complaints, and how these can be another useful source of feedback.

Chapter 7 – Mapping the service environment – sets out to map the service environment by dividing it into the 'internal environment', the 'near environment' and the 'far environment'. It explores the boundaries of the internal environment and the stakeholders that comprise the near environment. We consider how organisations can influence their near environment and how health and social care services respond to needs and demand.

Chapter 8 – Engaging with service users – explores how to involve service users in the planning of services. It also considers the nature of evidence and focuses on how investigations can be carried out to collect evidence to support decision making. We introduce some basic research approaches in the context of planning a consultation with service users.

Chapter 9 – Managing outcomes with service users – stresses the importance of being clear about the purpose of the services for which you are responsible and their intended outcomes. We explore the need for collaborative working to ensure that services are effectively integrated for the benefit of service users. This involves you, as a manager, focusing on the boundaries between your service and other related services, within and outside of your organisation.

Part 3: Managing services

Chapter 10 – Managing processes – considers the importance of managing the service delivery processes that are part of your everyday work. Once you are able to map the flow of the processes in your work area, you will be able to identify potential areas for improvement.

Chapter 11 – Working with a budget – discusses the different ways of setting budgets and the implications for budget holders within health and care services. We give some suggestions for approaches to negotiating a budget and for making a proposal for funding.

Chapter 12 – Service planning, accountability and risk – reviews the planning frameworks within which health and social care organisations plan their activities and describes the process of business planning. This leads us to consider the concept of accountability in health and social care and how managers are accountable for themselves, for their staff and for their area of work. We examine the responsibility that you have as a manager for assessing and managing risk.

Part 4: Managing improvement

Chapter 13 – Quality in services – sets out to help you to identify what quality means to managers in health and social care and to those who use health and social care services – both for services in general and for your area of work in particular. It also helps you to identify the sources of quality problems.

Chapter 14 – Working with standards – is about quality standards. We discuss what standards are and how they can be developed, and invite you to think about how you can develop standards for your own area of work.

Chapter 15 – Management control – is about controlling quality. Once you have established standards for your area of work, you can monitor progress against each standard and take action if standards are not met. This is the process of management control.

Chapter 16 – Developing effective performance – considers how effective groups and teams work and how their performance can be improved. We consider multidisciplinary and multi-agency working and some of the tensions that can emerge. We discuss how you can plan systematically to meet training and development needs and some ways in which you can manage poor performance.

Chapter 17 – Managing change – examines the stages of the change process. We consider diagnosis, the change process and some approaches that can be helpful in ensuring that you understand the current situation fully enough to implement a change. We invite you to consider using these approaches to manage a change in your area of work and we demonstrate the application of several useful techniques in a case study of a change process.

Chapter 18 – Planning and managing projects – introduces some of the techniques available to you in planning and managing projects. Using these techniques will help you to ensure that outcomes are achieved within the time-scales and budgets available.

PART 1

THE MANAGER AND THE TEAM

CHAPTER 1

YOUR JOB AS A MANAGER IN HEALTH AND SOCIAL CARE

In this chapter we consider the nature of a manager's work. We begin by inviting you to compare your work with that of other managers in health and social care settings and to consider the extent to which your activities are similar to or different from theirs. This will help you to identify your activities and roles as a manager, and thus to gain a better understanding of the job of a manager in health or social care. Whatever your area of work, it is essential to understand the contribution that you can make as a manager, so that you can contribute more effectively to the delivery of high-quality health or social care for service users.

A MANAGER IN ACTION

There are many different types of manager in health and social care. Not all of them have the title of 'manager', but they include people who manage service provision, who manage delivery teams and who manage the various support systems for service delivery. Although management responsibilities may be very different in different types of work and in different types of organisation, the focus of the work is the same for any manager in health and social care – the delivery of high-quality services to those who need them. The activities which managers undertake to carry out their work have many similarities, although the contexts in which they work may be very different.

Let's begin by looking at a manager in action. We asked some managers in health and social care to describe their work. Each of their reports illustrates the wide range of activities that managers undertake and the correspondingly wide range of skills and knowledge that they use. Second, they show that a lot of these skills are common to many management jobs, irrespective of the level or functional special-isation involved. Third, they illustrate how the various skills and competences described may complement each other to produce an effective managerial approach.

ACTIVITY 1.1

What, exactly, does a manager do? The following passages are descriptions of the work of three different managers in health and social care:

- Case Study A: an intermediate care services manager
- Case Study B: a practice manager
- Case Study C: manager of a resource centre for children with disabilities.

Glance through all of them and choose one to read carefully – you might like to choose someone who works in a context similar to your own or to focus on the work of a manager in a very different setting.

As you read the description, consider what the manager did and how he or she achieved outcomes. You may like to highlight the activities or to make brief notes.

Case Study A: intermediate care services manager

For the last five years, I've been a manager of intermediate care services – a joint appointment between a unitary council and a primary care trust. Initially I spent a year as a project co-ordinator and that was about looking at how the service needed to change and engaging people. The task the next year was to integrate the services. I was then appointed as the service manager.

You learn a lot about being a manager in a different organisation. I think it was a real opportunity. If I was just a manager for the PCT I would just have learned about PCT management. The biggest challenge, though, is personnel management. We had about 150 staff of various different grades.

The interesting thing is that, when you start in a new job, you start with a blank computer, empty desk and blank diary. The first hard thing is being clear what the job is and what the parameters are. There's a tendency to take on everything that comes your way in those first few months, and fill the diary. There should be a process of being able to stop and to reflect and plan, start making contacts and going out with the individual service teams and really find out what they do on the ground, talk to some of the service users and find out what the experience is like for them. So the first thing was to gather information and the next thing was to start working with some of the key stakeholders and a lot of that was working with the other service managers.

So we set up a project team and it was very action-focused. We often worked with flip charts, doing process mapping and SWOT analysis and then gradually building up a picture of how the service needed to look. Some of that was around a single point of access and a lot of work was done on that. Once there was a clear picture, we developed a draft strategy for the next five years and consulted on it. It was clear that when you are merging services together, roles will change and potentially that was the most difficult thing. It was about getting HR support with that and making sure the process was done properly.

One thing I've learned is that you should never start a project unless you're very clear what your budget is going to be. It affects everything, for example what staffing you can afford. The budgets for intermediate care weren't going to change, what we had was the amalgamated budgets from the services. The objective of projects to redesign services is often to reduce costs but with this one, it was to increase activity and capacity.

The difficult thing was not planning the project or implementing it, it was when it started to affect people – that's when the problems started. As a manager it was probably one of the most traumatic experiences of my life, I lost a huge amount of weight, I was exhausted and I couldn't sleep at night. When you're leading a project it's a very isolating job. Our project group had all the service managers on it, including those who would be directly affected. While people were very supportive up to that point, then they became a little bit blocking and it felt extremely difficult to get things moving.

What I did at that point was to identify somebody who was really influential in the organisation and that person worked alongside me to support me especially at group meetings and that was so important. I think the only reason we got through that project was because I had got somebody who was important to provide that support to me. The problem was that, as a project co-ordinator, I wasn't actually managing the budget or managing the staff. I didn't have any influence. All I had was persuasion and if people don't want to be persuaded to do something, they're not going to do it. So it was about getting somebody who had got that power and that influence. Through her support, we managed to get the services integrated and changed.

There was a lot of resistance from other managers. It was manifested mostly through negativity. I felt that people were going away from our group meetings where things were agreed and saying to staff 'this is going to happen, you're not going to like it'. We tried to counter that by holding lots of face-to-face meetings with staff to give them the opportunity to say what they wanted the service to look like and how they felt the service could be structured, as well as meetings with individuals to talk about preferences for rotas.

We were aware there were certain people who were dominant at group meetings and that can be useful, because sometimes they say things other people don't want to say. But we also wanted to make sure that people who had got a view but were too intimidated to speak up or didn't like speaking in a group had the opportunity to say what was important to them as well.

At the end, we went to one meeting where someone said we've been talking about this for ages, can't we just get on and do it and see what it feels like. When we got to that stage we knew we'd probably done enough.

We got the carers from both organisations together at a team-building event. That was quite important as it meant that the other service managers and I could actually sit with the other staff as part of the groups to listen to what they had to say and discuss things with them. That was really helpful and it raised a lot of issues about how people felt about the other team. In general, the health teams felt they had got more status: they worked alongside nurses and they felt they were going to lose that. They felt the social care teams didn't have as much status as they were managed by social care staff who weren't qualified. We knew we wouldn't get over that in a workshop but we felt it was a useful forum for actually raising these issues in front of each other and, while you can't address a lot of them, knowing about them was a first step.

The next big thing which we knew would make a difference was getting joint accommodation. People were scattered across the city, so an awful lot of effort went into getting people together as a team. We thought it would be a good thing and it was: it was key to integrating the services. Since we've got into the joint accommodation, the teams have really gelled. Now you can't tell who was health and who was social care. They're a good team and really supportive of each other and all get on really well now.

What I've learned from change like this, people shouldn't be disheartened, it is really hard work but the thing is to make sure you've got some key support for yourself as a manager. Any change like that takes at least two years before you start seeing what you've been working for. People have got cultural issues they need to leave behind and that's really difficult and painful and I think it's a mistake to rush people.

There was a formal process of service user involvement. We organised some focus groups in the evenings and service users and the general public were invited. They didn't turn up in huge numbers. The people who turned up were those who had a particular view or were interested enough to want more information. Since integration, everybody who uses the service is encouraged to fill out comments forms and they can be anonymous. Last year we did a focus group as well, around dignity and privacy. I think it's important to keep your eye on who your customer is.

The philosophy I always try to get into the service is that I know that we've been through a big change and we have to remember that the change is never complete so you'll never get to a point where you think it's all done. What our service users need will change, what our organisation needs from us will change, our budgets will get altered and the training that staff can do will change. As part of continually improving what we provide, we need always to be aware we're never ever there. That's quite a useful philosophy to get through to staff: if they realise that change isn't just now, it carries on all the time.

We suggested that you tried to identify the activities that this manager carried out and we think that these include the following list. The intermediate care services manager:

- collected data
- managed a budget
- made plans
- arranged and led meetings
- consulted service users
- consulted and communicated with staff
- motivated others
- monitored the progress of her project
- kept her staff informed
- promoted the service.

Case Study B: practice manager

I'm the practice manager here. My responsibilities are for the bricks and mortar, the buildings, the staff, safety for all the staff and patients. I make sure everyone is up to date. I keep an eye on all the new things that come through, for example the NICE guidance, and opportunities for continuing education. We run journal clubs, focusing on new journal and government papers and change our practice accordingly. All staff attend those including the reception team. Everyone is treated equally in this practice.

I make sure this place runs smoothly. Finances are important, for example, trying to make sure we can provide enhanced services at the price they're paying us. We run a cardiology service under practice-based commissioning (PCB). I'm always looking at different opportunities out there under PCB. It pays for the staff I have here. It's not about making tons of money – we have to pay the bills. We want to provide our patients with the best quality service. I do use PCB to help finance that – it improves the quality of care we have here. It enhances the experience for our patients and because all the other surgeries refer patients to us, it brings income to us.

In terms of our role as a lead practice, my responsibilities include nit-picking through the information, looking at courses I want to send members of the team on and working out logistically how to do it. So I make lots of phone calls, talk to other practices, arrange meetings. You have to make it happen, you have to carry the team along with you, with enthusiasm. You have to come in with a smile on your face. The hardest thing I've been dealing with recently is that we put in for planning permission for a new building and we were turned down at first and we'd all been carried along on this wave of 'we're moving' and then suddenly we weren't, and it was a case of well, we didn't get it, how are we going to motivate everyone?

The key staff are the senior receptionist, who supervises all the reception staff, an assistant practice manager, who is first line for all the administration, and the lead practice nurse who manages all the nursing staff. I am the next tier. Staff sometimes need to be able to move problems up a level. For complaints, also, they're mostly dealt with by front-line staff, but it does sometimes help that patients can bring it up a level. Now I'm not so directly involved with the patients, they can come to me knowing that their care will not be compromised in the future.

We're very passionate about patient participation. We were one of the first surgeries to start up a patient group and it brought some great improvements to services. When we make decisions about the surgery, we take the patients' views on board.

We have to be strong for the future. Another surgery nearby will be open 8–8. Patients will vote with their feet. We want more patients. We're doing extended hours – we were one of the first, not because there's more money but because our patients wanted it. Now everyone's doing it because there's money to help cover the costs. At the moment, we do three early mornings but that will change. That's going to be every day. It's hard to manage that change. The GPs find that quite difficult – they see themselves in a professional service and it's hard to get across to them that actually the patient has the power now. We're having to change to give people what they want. The patients are aware of what they can have, what their rights are. People move into the area and look around at the different websites to choose which practice they want to attend.

The fact that we're moving and will expand is very unsettling for the doctors and the staff. It's like we've been stuck in a box and now the doors are opening and everyone's grabbing and wanting, fighting for the future. But the GPs' visions are all different. One says 'I like being a traditional doctor, I just want to care for my patients,' which doesn't cut it with 'we've got to pay the bills'. Another says 'I want to bring in the latest technology, the latest medicine and the trainers who want to educate the doctors for the future'. They all want completely different things. I have to manage these aspirations – I try to make everyone understand that we all want to go on the same journey, get them to respect others' visions, get them to share and bring it altogether. The training has to continue: we do want to keep up to date with medical developments, but with the realisation we have to pay for it.

The partners take turns to chair strategy meetings. That's brilliant for me – it's a pleasure to go to a meeting I'm not chairing. Chairing a meeting is one of the skills a manager needs, bringing people in, shutting people up! Good planning is needed beforehand. I always sort the agenda for the partners' meetings. There's relevant material to get together, for example on appraisals, salaries, etc. You don't want to force a decision, but it can go disastrously wrong, if you haven't given them the information.

We noted the following activities carried out by the practice manager who:

- managed budgets
- managed the building
- collected data
- negotiated with GPs
- motivated staff
- solved problems
- arranged and chaired meetings
- involved service users
- communicated with staff
- managed change.

Case Study C: manager of a resource centre for children with disabilities

I manage the Wood House Resource Centre for children with disabilities. We are based in a converted bungalow in a small Midlands town, and we provide a range of services to 40 children and their families. Some of the children have profound and multiple disabilities and/or severe learning difficulties, some have sensory impairments, and some have very disturbed behaviours which are very hard for families to cope with at home.

Our service was moved to the bungalow about seven years ago by the County Council. We're about 25 miles from the nearest city, where my line manager is based, and where the senior managers are grouped together in County Hall.

We provide:

- short-term residential care;
- outreach – offering time-limited support in the child's home to help parents and children to establish sleep, feeding and play patterns;
- staffing for a youth club for 14–18-year-olds once a week in a local youth centre;
- a fortnightly session with 9–12-year-olds, offering opportunities for social interaction and working together;
- a range of day care from three hours to whole days;
- support to families – siblings' days, pre-school work, training for parents in lifting and handling.

Each child has personalised care. We visit the family home and find out how they are cared for, their likes and dislikes, and special diets and equipment. Our aim is to make sure that they are treated as individuals when they come to us. I have to ensure that their needs are properly assessed and that each has a care plan. I match the staff and the children, and ensure that we have sufficient staff available, with appropriate skills, for the children who are with us.

We have to be very careful that the living environment we provide is both homely and safe and hygienic for the children and the staff. A large part of my job therefore involves ensuring that these requirements are met – that the kitchen is properly run and that all the equipment (including hoists and wheelchairs) is properly maintained so that, as far as possible, we protect staff from injury. I delegate as much of this work as possible to my senior staff.

Some of the children have great difficulties expressing themselves and their behaviour can be very difficult and sometimes aggressive. All our staff are trained both in the techniques of physical care for children and in ways of handling them to keep aggression to a minimum and to protect themselves and other children from harm. The senior staff carry out a risk assessment each day, looking at the children who are with us and their needs, and checking that we have the skilled staff available to meet them. We normally have one staff member for each child, and occasionally two.

A large part of my job involves liaison with other people, especially parents. Our role is to share the care of the children to reduce the strain on parents and siblings. We see parents every time they bring their children to us and we listen to how things are going at home, as well as making sure we keep them informed of what is happening at Wood House. We keep in regular touch with the children's care managers, with the medical staff who work with the children and with the special schools that they attend. We are part of a county-wide service to children with disabilities, and I meet regularly with the managers of the four other centres in the county to keep up to date with changes and developments and to make sure that we all provide a consistently good service.

Each member of staff has a regular meeting with his or her line manager, at which they discuss the care of the children they are responsible for, deal with any problems arising in practice or care, and plan training and development. We call this 'supervision'. I supervise the four senior members of staff and they each supervise other members of staff.

My deputy prepares the staff rotas, always making sure that there is a senior member of staff on duty. All the senior staff take a turn at 'sleeping in' – providing cover on the spot at night in case of emergencies.

I am responsible for Wood House's budget. I have some freedom in how I use it to maintain staffing levels, although restrictions are sometimes imposed centrally when there are county-wide budget problems. The County Council has been under severe financial pressure for some years, and this has meant that our budget has been progressively reduced, leading to reductions in the services we provide. This year, the financial crisis is severe, with proposals for reductions of services of all kinds across the county. One proposal is to close three of the five resource centres for disabled children unless a suitable arrangement can be made for independent financing of the services we provide. At the moment, we don't know which three would close if no rescue plan is forthcoming.

We have always had a strong parents' group, who have elected representatives to speak on their behalf in relation to matters affecting the centre. This group has been particularly active over the past three years. I support them and the county-wide parents' group by providing clerical help, a meeting place and any other support I can. They have recognised the threat to the service that is posed by budget problems. Two years ago we took a 16 per cent cut in budget, which meant that we had to choose between reducing the number of children we could take at any one time or closing for one day a week. We asked the parents to help in making this decision, and they opted for closing for one day a week. Over the past two years, the parents' group has lobbied local and national politicians, worked with the local press and made a very moving *Newsnight* programme. The county has no wish to close Wood House or reduce our services, but has to make cuts or go into the red. Senior managers are happy to support our activities by bringing the needs of these children and their families to the attention of opinion formers and people who may be able to offer financial support.

Managing the resource centre in these times presents major problems. Stress is taking its toll on parents and staff alike, and we have several staff on long-term sick leave, all with stress-related problems. I have permission to recruit more staff, but qualified staff are hard to find and potential recruits are not attracted to a job without a firm future. It is easier to recruit temporary staff, but they need more support and training and cannot take the same level of responsibility. The summer is always a difficult time because of staff holidays, but this summer has been particularly difficult, and I have sometimes had to withdraw services because of having insufficient staff. I recently had to send all the children home over the weekend because we did not have sufficient staff to meet their needs safely. Each time we have to reduce our services, parents have to reorganise their lives to accommodate the change. This can involve complicated arrangements for the transport and care of their children, adding to the stress of their lives.

Sustaining morale is hard in these times of uncertainty. We do not know whether we are preparing to close or preparing to be taken over by a new organisation. My mood – and that of my staff – swings from optimism to pessimism and back again, with occasional bouts of exhaustion. I try to offer the staff as much choice as possible in how they work so that they do not feel too pressured. However, with staff in short supply, much of my time is spent in keeping the basics going.

The good thing is the sense of common cause between staff and parents. We are all committed to providing an effective service. We will fight hard to keep Wood House open because we know how much it is needed.

We noted the following activities carried out by the resource centre manager who:

■ ensured that needs were assessed and care plans made
■ delegated tasks to others
■ ensured that risk assessments were carried out

- listened to and informed parents
- liaised with those providing related services
- supervised staff
- planned staff training and development
- managed a budget
- recruited staff
- maintained staff morale
- promoted the service.

An impressive number of activities were carried out by the manager in each of these studies. A manager's work often appears very busy and muddled because many of the activities are interrupted and progress is made on several issues in parallel rather than in a neat and logical sequence. Reading between the lines, we might deduce many other things that all three of these managers must have done, which are only implicit in the case studies. They must certainly have:

- built and developed their teams
- developed a network of contacts
- consulted and persuaded other decision makers
- made some deals
- listened to people's complaints and worries
- sorted out innumerable problems
- made many decisions
- compromised on occasion
- written papers and letters
- written reports
- studied other people's reports.

ACTIVITY 1.2

Now use a highlighting pen to mark every activity on our summary lists that these managers undertook which you also carry out at some time in your own work as a manager.

It would be surprising if your activities were exactly the same as the ones in these examples. It would be equally surprising if you did not find a significant number of similarities between your activities and those described by these managers (though the similarities are more likely to occur in *how* they did their work than in *what* they did). For example, most managers, whatever the context of their work, do some planning and some monitoring or supervision of the work of others, and all communicate in a variety of different ways. These are some of the skills and activities that are the very essence of management, and you probably find yourself doing them day after day.

One likely difference is that your work as a manager might seem to be more of a jumble of events concerned simply with keeping your department running. The list of activities and skills involved in your daily tasks may seem to be endless. In the remainder of this chapter, we encourage you to search for coherent patterns among the things that you do. This should help you to gain a better understanding of the nature of your job and this, in turn, will open the way towards improving your effectiveness as a manager. To be more effective, you need to understand the purpose of your job and to be able to achieve the outcomes required in a way that is appropriate to the setting in which you work.

THE NATURE OF YOUR JOB

What are the things that you do – and what should you be doing – to make sure that you are an effective manager? Your chances of doing the job effectively will certainly be improved if you have a good understanding of what you should be doing. There are several different ways of looking at your job, and each provides its own particular insights.

Many researchers have attempted to identify the elements of management work. Colin Hales (2001) identified elements of 'what managers do' from examining 50 years of published research into this field. Although he found that there were variations, he summarised the similar elements which had been found in all these different studies.

ACTIVITY 1.3

The elements Hales identified are listed below. Consider whether each one is something that you do as part of your work as a manager and tick the ones that you can recognise to some extent in your own work.

1 Acting as a figurehead or leader of a work unit, representing it and acting as a point of contact ❐
2 Monitoring and disseminating information ❐
3 Networking ❐
4 Negotiating with staff at different levels ❐
5 Planning and scheduling work ❐
6 Allocating resources to different work activities ❐
7 Directing and monitoring the work of other staff ❐
8 Fulfilling specific human resource management activities ❐
9 Problem-solving and handling disturbances to work flow ❐
10 Innovating processes and products ❐
11 Doing technical work relating to the manager's professional or functional specialisation ❐

Many of these characteristics indicate that the work that managers do is complex and involves a great deal of interaction with other people. The skills required for achieving chartered manager status (from the Chartered Management Institute) cover the wide range of work that a manager is now expected to do:

- leading people
- managing change
- managing information and knowledge
- managing projects, processes and resources
- managing yourself.

Not every manager has all of these responsibilities: it depends a great deal on the context in which he or she works. It would also be unusual for all of the activities to be equally important: a manager's work depends on the purpose of the organisation in which he or she works.

There are also differences in how managers are expected to work. In some settings a manager will be expected to look smart and behave in a formal way; in others informal dress is expected and behaviour may be similarly informal. Many other expectations reflect the 'culture' of the organisation. However, some features are typical of any manager's work. They flow from the responsibility held by managers for work processes and for the people who perform the processes. Hales recognised that much of the research into how a manager works demonstrates frenetic activity.

ACTIVITY 1.4

Here is the list Hales made from his research into the activities that are typical of how a manager works. Think about whether any of these descriptions remind you of your own work and tick those which apply to your work.

- Fragmented – short, interrupted activities ☐
- Reactive – responding to, rather than initiating, events and requests ☐
- Concerned with *ad hoc*, day-to-day matters ☐
- Embedding of activities within others ☐
- High level of verbal interaction with others (face-to-face, phone, email) ☐
- Degree of pressure, tension and conflict in juggling demands ☐
- Considerable choice and negotiation over the nature and boundaries of the job and how it is done. ☐

All these features indicate responsiveness – noticing what is happening around you and responding to people and events. Much of a manager's work involves responding to other people and to situations. However, a manager is expected to do more than just respond to day-to-day issues and manage routine work. Managers are also expected to make progress towards particular objectives. It is all too easy for a manager to be very busy but not necessarily to have achieved what he or she had intended. This may mean that progress is not being made towards achieving key objectives. If you ticked most of the boxes in the previous Activity, you will need to manage your time well to be effective.

If you work in a setting where there is frequent change – and most people do these days – it is unlikely that you will be effective unless you take enough control over your time to make sure that you are able to achieve your key objectives. This is not to suggest that your time is more important than that of the people you manage. However, if you can demonstrate that you manage your time in a way that helps you to be effective, it will help others to respect and value their time as well as yours.

REFERENCES

Chartered Management Institute, <www.managers.org.uk> (accessed 28/05/09).

Hales, C. (2001) 'Does it matter what managers do?', *Business Strategy Review*, vo. 12, no. 2, pp. 50–8.

CHAPTER 2

IMPROVING YOUR EFFECTIVENESS AS A MANAGER

Working in health and social services, you will undoubtedly be accustomed to the language of objectives, targets, ratings, indicators and performance assessment. If you have just moved into a managerial position, clarifying your own objectives and the means of achieving them will inevitably be one of your first concerns. It doesn't make a great deal of sense to contemplate how you will set about doing a job if you are not clear about what it is you are trying to achieve. If you have been a manager for some time, you should not overlook the importance of reviewing your objectives. Objectives can be used to clarify the purpose of your management activities, and they can also help to identify the processes through which you will make progress.

Setting clear objectives and planning how they will be achieved are fundamental to managing effectively. But you will usually need to allow for some flexibility in how objectives are pursued so that you can accommodate other people's views and adjust to changes in circumstances.

A sense of direction and purpose is critical to effectiveness. In this chapter we discuss what is meant by effective management and the factors upon which effectiveness depends. We consider the needs to which you and your organisation respond and the priorities between them. This leads to identifying main objectives to ensure that you address these priorities. We examine the process of setting objectives in three stages: reviewing what you need to do to be effective, determining your priorities in terms of objectives, and planning how you will achieve your objectives.

REVIEWING WHAT YOU NEED TO DO TO BE EFFECTIVE

You may already have some idea of what being an effective manager means, even though we have not yet precisely defined 'effectiveness'.

Before proceeding further, we'll attempt to define it now. Managerial effectiveness is a measure of the extent to which the results one sets out to achieve are achieved. However, just achieving what you have set as targets is not enough in itself. It is very important that the targets that you set are ones that will really add value to the area of work for which you are responsible. The quality of your objectives is as important as the fact that you set objectives at all. There are two important stages in achieving your planned results. The first is to set clear objectives so that you know what you are trying to achieve; the second is to review your progress against these objectives so that you know how you are doing and can take action to keep on track if necessary.

But setting and reviewing objectives are not as straightforward as they might appear at first glance. Even in a well regulated manufacturing process, many factors make this procedure difficult to apply. In health and care services, the variables are numerous and situations are often in a state of frequent change. If we are to judge the performance of an individual, a team, a department or a whole organisation, we must know against what criteria the judgement is to be made.

ACTIVITY 2.1

Let's say that effective management is performance measured against intentions. Using this definition, tick the boxes which show how accurately you are currently able to assess managerial effectiveness for:

	Accurately	*Loosely*	*Not at all*
Yourself	❏	❏	❏
Your team	❏	❏	❏
Your service area	❏	❏	❏
Is this satisfactory for effective management?	*Yes* ❏	*No* ❏	*Partially* ❏

It would be unusual if you found that the current approach to evaluation of effectiveness is entirely satisfactory. You might feel that having a loose definition of managerial effectiveness has its advantages. However, if people are to be judged on the extent to which they achieve the outcomes that are expected of them, it is important to have a common understanding of what these outcomes include. Your answer to the final question might suggest that you need to set some clearer objectives for yourself or for your team to ensure that everyone has a similar understanding of what is expected.

It is also interesting to consider whether service users would be entirely happy with your current approach to reviewing effectiveness. Staff may all be working very hard, but are they achieving the high quality of service delivery that everyone would like to be part of? Effectiveness is not easy to pin down because it has to be considered in relation to the ever-changing needs and expectations of service users.

However, you should now have a clearer picture of what we mean by effective management. You are also probably aware from your own experience that, to be effective, managers need a very wide repertoire of skills and competences to carry out the many different tasks that they are asked to do. However, important as these skills are, effective management does not come automatically from having the right skills. The reality is much more complex than that.

A number of factors influence your effectiveness as a manager, not all of which are under your control. Let's consider five such factors.

In the first place, *you* are a factor. You are unique. You bring a unique blend of knowledge, skills, attitudes, values and experience to your job, and these influence your effectiveness to some extent.

Then there is *your job*. It will have many features in common with other management jobs but, just as you are unique, so your job is likely to be unique both in its detailed features and in the unique demands it makes upon you. The match between your skills and the demands made on them by your job shapes your potential effectiveness.

The resources you have to work with exert a major influence on how effective you can be as a manager. The most important of these resources is people – your staff. You may have come across such definitions as 'a manager is a person who gets work done through other people' or 'managers are people with so much work to do that they must get other people to do it' or 'a manager is the person who works out what needs doing and gets someone else to do it'. Some of these definitions are a bit tongue in cheek, but nevertheless get close to the truth with their emphasis on the importance of other people in the achievement of a manager's work. One measure of your effectiveness as a manager is the extent to which you can motivate your staff and co-ordinate their efforts to achieve optimum performance. However, you do not control people in the way that you can control the other resources – such as finance and information – that are needed to get work done.

Your organisation is another major factor in determining how effective you can be. Both the structure and the culture of the organisation, whether it is large or small, place limits on what you are able to achieve as a manager. The structure, and your position in it, make an impact on the nature of your authority and your responsibilities and impose constraints on what you are able to achieve. Similarly, the culture of the organisation – its norms and standards, its written and unwritten rules, and its style of working – also has a direct bearing on your ability to be effective as a manager.

Finally, your work can be affected by influences from *the world outside your organisation*: by social trends, changes in technology, the state of the economy, and in general by the people and other organisations with whom your organisation must interact. Health and social care services are delivered by many different types of organisation. To improve the integration and quality of services for service users will require more co-operative working and the formation of partnerships, many of which require their own jointly agreed objectives and targets.

So effective management does not come just from learning a few skills and techniques. Skills and techniques are important and necessary, but effective management is more complex than that. It depends on you, the job you do, the people you work with, the other resources you have at your disposal, the organisation you work in, and the wider world with which your organisation must interact.

ACTIVITY 2.2

This activity will help you to identify some of the factors upon which effectiveness depends.

Think about a piece of work you recently carried out as a manager. This might have been an improvement in your area of work or an occasional, but more routine, activity. Choose something that was fairly complex, something that you had to think about and plan to some extent and something that involved other people. Answer the following questions about the activity.

- To what extent was the outcome influenced by your own level of competence?
- Did you bring particular skills or knowledge to the situation?
- To what extent were your actions influenced by personal or professional values?
- What contribution did your staff, colleagues and line manager make to the outcome, positively or negatively?
- How critical were the abilities and attitudes that others brought to the situation?
- Did you have the influence in your organisation that was required to achieve the task?
- Do you feel that your job allows all your abilities to be brought into play?
- Does it make demands that you feel unable to respond to?

All these questions refer to aspects of work that you can think about before taking action. Preparation for a complex task can be, to some extent, a rehearsal for the real thing. If you start a major task by considering what is involved and what you are trying to achieve, this will clarify the direction and purpose of your work. It is then possible to consider how the desired outcomes will be achieved – what steps are needed to achieve each of the outcomes. This is the planning stage.

A simple recommendation for effective management is:

- plan
- do
- review.

Once these steps are expressed as separate tasks, you have created an agenda for action. You can then think about who should carry out each of the tasks. Your planning at this stage will include consideration of who has the necessary skills and experience or who could be supported to develop the necessary skills with appropriate supervision. In health and social care settings you will also have to consider who has the appropriate professional or clinical background and qualifications for some of the activities, and this may raise the question of your ability to bring people from different backgrounds together to work effectively. You might also need to have sufficient influence in your organisation to secure other necessary resources. All this may seem daunting, but much of your effectiveness as a manager will result from your ability to plan and co-ordinate the work of other people.

When you have reached the stage of carrying out activities, there is still a further stage – review. This is crucial in making sure that your actions are leading in the direction you intended. The simple sequence of plan, do, review is a useful way to remember these stages.

One approach to becoming effective as a manager is to set objectives and to review them to make sure that you are progressing in the right direction and at the right speed to achieve them. However, it is never quite this easy because other people are always involved. There is a stage before planning which involves making sure that you understand the situation well enough to inform your planning. You may think that you know what is needed, but deciding what needs to be done is not simply a matter of indicating your perception of those needs. You must also give careful consideration to other people's views about what needs to be done (which may mean the perceptions of service users, your team, your manager, other managers, people in collaborating organisations).

Your perception of what needs to be done

If you are to be effective as a manager you will be concerned to ensure that you clearly identify what you see as the needs of those you are serving – your target groups. If you are the manager of an Age Concern day centre, for example, the needs of your service users will be crucial, but so will those of your management committee and of the staff of the local authority's adult care department to whom they are contracted to provide this service. If you are a nurse or therapist, your patients will be an important target group, but so will be the doctors and consultants with whom you are working. If you are a finance officer, your target group may be the staff for whose pay cheques you are responsible, or senior management to whom you are providing budgetary information. If you have line management responsibility for other staff, these staff will be an additional target group. You will find it useful to devise a system for identifying needs, and Activity 2.3 suggests one possible approach.

ACTIVITY 2.3

Consider *one* of the target groups of the service for which you are responsible. Identify and list the different types of needs to which you try to respond.

If your chosen target group is your service users, your list might well include their physical, emotional and social needs. Remember that, as a manager, you also provide a service to your staff, so you could choose your staff as your target group.

You have probably drawn up an impressive list of the needs of this target group that you try to meet in your work. Your knowledge and experience and that of your team allow you to understand and attend to the detail of your day-to-day service provision.

Identification of needs is more difficult if you are a manager new to an area of service provision or if you have responsibility for areas of work with which you are unfamiliar. It is also sometimes difficult for those supporting direct service providers to see how they contribute to the quality of service to the service users. Managers and staff in finance, personnel, audit and all the other support areas have other staff in the organisation as their target groups and do not always find it easy to recognise the importance of providing them with a good service to enable them to deliver services to service users.

In health and social care nowadays, the boundaries around service areas are changing. Many managers have responsibilities for broad service areas or for multiprofessional teams and it is inevitable that they will be more familiar with the service areas in which they gained their own experience. Few managers of complex services will have had wide enough experience to understand fully all of the detailed work carried out by members of their teams. If you are in this position, it is important to spend time with each different area of service provision to understand more about why they deliver their part of the service as they do and how they perceive the needs of the users of their service.

One of the reasons why more multidisciplinary teams have been formed is that, in the past, some services were very good at one part of health or social care but did not link with the next stage needed by the user. For example, people could be treated in hospital and become well enough to go home, but would be sent home without provision being made to ensure that they had adequate support and help to stay well. Your service may be excellent at achieving its immediate results, but less effective in ensuring that the overall purpose of the intervention is achieved.

Other people's perceptions of what needs to be done

The needs you identified for your service users are likely to be only part of the work of your organisation. Organisations often deliver a number of services and, unless you are a manager in a very small organisation, there will be other considerations to take account of. Before you begin to identify what you believe ought to be done in response to the needs you have identified, you must take careful note of other points of view. An efficient organisation will normally have gone through a similar process of identifying needs of target groups in developing its policies. It will have identified the needs that it perceives to be important, and will have developed statements about what the organisation ought to do to respond to them. These are likely to be in the form of corporate objectives – often referred to as aims or goals.

It is the responsibility of senior management to communicate their corporate objectives to the people whose responsibility it is to achieve them. In large organisations with several layers of management, each level of management bears the responsibility for communicating the objectives, strategies and implementation plans that apply at their level to those below so that they, in turn, can plan accordingly. This 'cascade' process is illustrated in the ladder diagram (Figure 2.1). Each rung on the ladder represents a separate level of objectives, the number and nature of the levels reflecting the site and structure of the organisation.

At the corporate level, objectives are likely to be identified in very broad terms, but as they are transmitted down through the hierarchy they will be translated by departments and units into increasingly

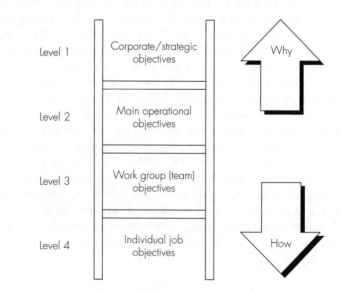

Figure 2.1 The ladder approach to the analysis of objectives

specific terms. You must study any statements of objectives that come down to you, for they may determine to a large extent both what you can do and what you can't. In some organisations, they may simply provide you with broad guidelines within which you have great freedom to think for yourself. In others, the guidance provided might be much more specific.

At the level of your work group or team there may be clear overall objectives for your team to meet, or you may need to develop your own objectives from a broad statement of the purpose of your team's work. The guidelines you are expected to work within may require your objectives to meet some of the following requirements:

- contribute to the overall strategy of the department or organisation;
- be within the constraints of the budget;
- be at an acceptable level of risk (to be defined);
- make use of, or reinforce, organisational strengths;
- meet a major need that has been identified as a local priority;
- avoid, reduce or mitigate major threats or hazards;
- be consistent with other major strategies;
- be capable of implementation.

Not all organisations are as organised or directive as this. Some may not even explicitly identify their corporate objectives. Nevertheless, they will have philosophies which guide their direction and their objectives will be implicit in what they do or try to do. Unless your organisation is completely adrift, it will have some objectives at a strategic level, but these may be implicit rather than explicit. Given the emphasis on regulation and inspection, few public sector organisations will be without departmental and organisational objectives and targets.

ACTIVITY 2.4

Think about the objectives of your organisation (or your part of the organisation).

Do you know the objectives of your organisation?	Yes/No
If not, do you believe that they exist?	Yes/No
Are they in writing?	Yes/No
Do you know where to find them?	Yes/No
Do you know who determined them?	Yes/No
Do you know the arrangements for reviewing them?	Yes/No
Did you (or will you) help to formulate (or review) them?	Yes/No

---

If you answered 'no' to several of these questions, you should try to find out more from your line manager or colleagues. Part of your effectiveness as a manager is determined by the extent to which you are seen to be contributing towards achieving the objectives of your wider service or organisation. This will inevitably be difficult to do if you are not sure what they are!

Objectives almost certainly do exist in some form or another within your organisation, even if only as ill-defined and unarticulated ideas inside the heads of the senior management group. Your service may have a strategic plan in which the main objectives will be stated. A smaller or less formal organisation might produce an annual report in which the aims and objectives are outlined. If your organisation is large and provides many different services (both itself and in partnership with others), you may only need to know about the objectives for your service area (for example, if you work in learning difficulty services, you may not need to know the objectives for the services for older people).

DETERMINING YOUR PRIORITIES IN TERMS OF OBJECTIVES

Once you have a list of important needs categorised in a meaningful manner (for example, according to different types of needs and with regard to different target groups), you can start to convert this list of perceived needs into statements indicating what you might aim to achieve in response to each need.

ACTIVITY 2.5

Convert the list of needs you made in Activity 2.3 into statements of what you intend to do to respond to them. For example, you might have determined that one of your groups of service users needs information about your service. Your aim might be 'to give accurate information about the service'. Use your previous list to write a few more statements of aims.

But identifying your aims is not enough. The aim 'to give accurate information about the service' describes what you want to achieve in relation to a particular need – it sets out your direction – but it does not indicate how you are going to achieve it, when you are going to do it, or how you will know that you have been successful in doing it. So you need to convert the *aims* into *objectives*. Objectives need to be as precise as possible if they are going to help you to become more effective. This means that they should have some particular characteristics. An easy way to remember these characteristics is to think of them as 'SMART'. They must be:

- *Specific* – clear about what is to be achieved;
- *Measurable* – state how success will be measured;
- *Agreed* – ideally with the person who will carry out the objective and with anyone who will be affected by the result;
- *Realistic* – achievable within the constraints of the situation and in alignment with other objectives;
- *Timed* – target time set for achieving objectives.

For example, the aim 'to give accurate information about the service' might be rewritten as a SMART objective as:

To give accurate information about the service by producing 1,000 copies of a leaflet, using our team experience to design them and our clerical resources to copy them, so that they are on display for use on 1 September.

This is now a specific objective: you know how you will measure success, it is realistic, and there is a time limit. However, there is another dimension. Although an objective like this could be put into action and the degree of success could be measured, is it an action worth carrying out? It is very important that objectives lead to a worthwhile result. Effectiveness is not only about doing things well (efficiency) but also about doing the right things.

If we look again at this example of an objective, it would be of little use if the leaflet could not be read or understood by the service users. A draft of the leaflet needs to be tested, perhaps with some willing members of the potential readership. There may be problems with size of print or layout or over the language used: it is easy to make assumptions when you are writing about something that is very familiar to you. There may also be problems about different ways of seeing things – perhaps different values – which might mean that the way in which you present information is less acceptable to particular groups of people. You may even discover in trying out the draft that using leaflets is an unhelpful way of presenting information to some communities and that you have to find an alternative approach. You might then amend your SMART objective to:

To give accurate information about the service by producing sufficient copies of a leaflet (or something similar) that fully meets the needs of service users, using our team experience and resources to produce the information ready for use on 1 September.

Achieving this objective might not be quite as easy to measure: the emphasis is on finding out what would meet the needs of service users and then providing the information in an appropriate way. Success will be measured against the criteria that have been identified in terms of what service users need, as well as in terms of both quality and quantity. If it turns out that users want information in leaflets, this objective will be helpful in reminding the manager responsible to pilot drafts of the leaflet to make sure that it fully meets users' needs, and also to find out how many leaflets will be required. If it is found that users of the service would prefer a poster or access to information via email or the internet, a different approach can be taken and money will not be wasted on leaflets. Whether you can frame your objectives in very precise terms depends on how much you know about the situation or whether you need to allow for more research before deciding exactly what action to take.

ACTIVITY 2.6

Rewrite three of the aims you drafted earlier so that they meet all the SMART criteria and provide a guide for meaningful action.

Long-term and short-term objectives

If you systematically develop a list of aims and objectives from your and your organisation's perceptions of the needs of your different target groups, your list will probably contain far more objectives than you can hope to achieve in the near future. You will have to establish priorities. One way of doing this is to review your list to identify what has to be done urgently and what can be planned to be achieved later.

You might begin by asking yourself what it is that you want to achieve in the long term, and what you might realistically achieve in the short term. Your long-term objectives are likely to emerge in response to such fundamental questions as 'What is our real purpose?', 'Where are we going?' and 'Where do we want the service to be in five years' time?' Your short-term objectives should be a first step on the way towards achieving your longer-term objectives, and are likely to be identified in response to much more basic questions such as 'To what extent can we reduce our waiting lists over the next twelve months?' or 'In what ways might we improve our services over the next twelve months?' As your thoughts begin to clarify, create two lists – one of objectives to be achieved in the long term (say, over three years) and the other of those to be achieved in the short term (say, over one year).

Having produced separate lists of long- and short-term objectives you might then review each of these in turn, asking yourself which of the objectives are absolutely essential and which are simply desirable.

If determining priorities is an effort involving several people – as it usually is – it is almost inevitable that you will encounter conflicting points of view from time to time. Different people are likely to have different perceptions of what needs to be achieved in the short or long term and to have different views about what is essential as opposed to desirable. Value judgements are involved. It is up to those concerned to make their views explicit, and for you to ensure that an agreed view is established.

However, these are not the only conflicts that might arise. Whenever a multiplicity of aims or objectives is identified, there is always a possibility of some being in conflict. For example, one of your aims might be 'to provide the best possible conditions for the care of service users' while another might be 'to maximise throughput of service users in order to reduce waiting times'. There may be a conflict between these, and it is up to you and your team to determine an appropriate balance between them. It is sometimes helpful to look at each objective and to ask, 'How will this improve the experience of service users?' as a way of deciding how to set priorities. There may, for example, be ways in which the conditions for care could be improved quickly (making appointments to reduce the need for long waiting times, providing more chairs, making refreshments available). The other objective of maximising throughput might be a longer-term objective needing more research and wider co-operation (including the co-operation of service users or partner organisations) to achieve success.

> The government seems to equate good management practice in the private sector with the achievement of objectives through clear, precise targets. But this is to ignore the unique features of public sector management. . . . The unrelenting concentration on objectives can distort because the problem of balancing objectives, values and interests is neglected. This balancing act lies at the heart of management in the public sector. Setting objectives is easy, balancing them less so.
>
> (*Hunter, 1999*)

ACTIVITY 2.7

Think of an example of two conflicting aims or objectives which your own organisation is seeking to fulfil.

What is the nature of the conflict? Is there a possible compromise? How can you, as a manager, help your team to achieve your objectives with as little conflict as possible?

Now that you have some clear objectives, you can set about achieving them.

Achieving your objectives

As a manager, your objectives are not only your own concern: they are also your team's concern. Your objectives probably include some that involve the work of the whole team. If you involve your team in agreeing how these objectives will be achieved, this will help to develop a shared understanding.

Once you have determined your priorities, you should ensure that your objectives are expressed in terms that ensure that your team can determine for themselves whether or not their contributions to them have been achieved. You will need to work with your team to identify the sequence of activities that needs to be completed to achieve each objective and the measures that will demonstrate that each has been achieved. It is helpful to agree a process for the whole team to review progress. This provides an opportunity to correct things if they are not working as planned. It is particularly helpful if you plan early review dates, so that if things are going wrong there is time to rethink your plans. If review dates are too late to allow plans to be revised, there is often a tendency to look for someone to blame for the lack of success rather than to think positively about how to achieve success in a different way.

It is important to bear in mind the distinction between *key objectives* and *key activities*, since you want to be sure that, at the end of the day, you are measuring what you achieved rather than simply what you did. The key activities might be expressed as sub-objectives, the smaller tasks that have to be completed in order to achieve a key objective. For example, the objective:

> *To give accurate information about the service by producing sufficient copies of a leaflet (or something similar) that fully meets the needs of service users, using our team experience and resources to produce the information ready for use on 1 September.*

could be subdivided into the tasks:

1 Check what information is most often required by service users.
2 Draft the answers you and your team usually give and agree their accuracy with your team.
3 Research with service users how they prefer to access information.
4 Design a leaflet (or poster or information service) to meet the needs identified.
5 Agree the design of the leaflet (or other approach) with your team.
6 If you are proposing an alternative approach rather than the leaflets that were anticipated, confirm with your manager that this is acceptable.
7 Try out the draft leaflet (or other approach) with a few service users to make sure that it meets their needs.
8 Revise if necessary and secure final agreement from your team (and other managers if necessary).
9 Ensure that there are sufficient resources to go ahead within the time-scale.
10 Ensure that the information is available for use from 1 September.

Each of these tasks needs a time-scale attached to it to ensure that the whole job will be completed by the target date. Each task will also need to be allocated to someone who will take responsibility for completing it on time. You will need to have a way of keeping an eye on overall progress to make sure that it goes to plan. You should also arrange to review the extent to which the leaflet or other approach has achieved its purpose and whether you need to make any changes after a few months.

Setting clear objectives makes it much easier to identify the tasks involved in achieving results and to review progress using both your list of tasks and your objectives. You can be very busy but find that you achieve very little unless you are clear about what you are aiming to do and when you expect to achieve your outcomes. In addition, of course, the staff who carry out the tasks will need to be motivated and co-ordinated through effective leadership and management.

Now try this Activity, which will enable you to apply these ideas in your workplace.

ACTIVITY 2.8

Prepare up to five draft key objectives for your department or section. Write these in SMART format so that they provide a framework from which key activities could be derived for you and your team.

Discuss them with your line manager to ensure that you have captured the essential aspects of the work expected of you.

Once this has been agreed, discuss the objectives with your team and agree how each will be achieved. This would be a useful team-building exercise, as well as helping to develop clarity of purpose. It is important to recognise that your team might not agree with your proposals and to be ready to listen to their ideas and accept some of their suggestions. This approach would demonstrate to your team how you intend to be effective as a manager and how you expect them to be able to demonstrate their individual and team effectiveness.

This chapter has focused on one of the most fundamental skills that managers need. We have stressed that if you want to be an effective manager you must be clear about what you want to achieve and how you intend to go about it. In particular, we have stressed the importance of giving careful consideration to:

- the needs which you and people in other parts of your organisation perceive to be important;
- the priorities to which you intend to respond;
- the main objectives you intend to achieve;
- the main activities through which you will achieve your objectives;
- the main results which will indicate whether or not you have achieved the objectives.

You should now be able to identify the factors upon which managerial effectiveness depends, to clarify your own objectives and to plan means by which your objectives can be effectively achieved.

REFERENCE

Hunter, D. (1999) 'Dangers of target practice', *Health Service Journal*, 24 June, pp. 16–17.

CHAPTER 3

MANAGEMENT AND LEADERSHIP

In this chapter, we take a look at some of the different theories that informed our understanding of leadership in the past and that continue to be influential because they have helped to shape current thinking. We also consider how these ideas might help managers and leaders in health and social care working in the complex interprofessional and inter-agency context. We conclude by inviting you to think about your personal preferred style and the extent to which you can vary it to meet the needs of different situations.

MANAGING AND LEADING

Both managing and leading are practical activities. There are three frequently discussed ways of 'seeing' the relationship between leadership and management. These are represented in Figure 3.1.

View A implies that management and leadership are broadly the same thing and that the words can be used interchangeably. This used to be a very common view in health and social care. In recent years, however, the term 'leader' is frequently used to describe someone in a professional or medical role with both management and leadership responsibilities. As managers in health and care services are often expected to take leadership roles in some aspects of their work, there appears to be some confusion. View B implies that there is a difference between the two words and that management is one of the components of leadership. For people who take this view, leadership somehow

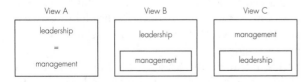

Figure 3.1 Possible relationships between leadership and management

subsumes management and may appear more highly valued. View C also implies that there is a difference, but leadership is perceived as one of the components of management, possibly a function of management. The confusion is deep-seated and the words often continue to be used interchangeably.

One way of using the word 'leadership' is to describe the way in which senior managers and directors set out a strategy for the work of an organisation. For example, the leaders of political parties are expected to provide the vision and the inspiration, but the party managers look after the day-to-day running of party business. In commerce and industry the same is often true, with many (although not all) top executives taking a high profile and leading the way. From this perspective, managing might appear to be something that supports the leaders of an organisation. Could it be that those people who rise to the top specialise in just a few of the functions of management, such as setting goals and inspiring people to work towards them? The more routine functions of management, such as planning, resourcing and organising, then become the responsibility of managers further down the line. However, these managers also have to lead their teams – to motivate them and to plan and co-ordinate each area of work. In health and social care it is common to find people who are nominated as team leaders. The qualifications for appointment as a team leader are often connected with expertise and experience, particularly the experience of supervising and developing other people.

Management roles have traditionally required managers to organise and control work – to plan, implement and review the effectiveness of work. Leaders are usually concerned with change, so might develop new systems and structures, new frameworks and directions. Therefore, although leaders do not have to be managers, managers are now often expected to demonstrate some leadership ability. Kotter (1990) distinguished between management as being concerned with *transactions* and leadership as being concerned with *transformation*. So management roles involve planning, budgeting, organising, staffing, controlling and problem solving, to create a degree of predictablity and order. Leadership roles are more concerned with establishing vision and direction, communicating the direction and aligning people, inspiring and motivating them and producing change.

Another way of thinking about the relationship between managers and leaders is to think of both of these roles as being 'added' to other roles. For example, a social worker, nurse, doctor, allied health professional, accountant, administrator or technician might all take on an additional role as a manager. Each of these might also take a leading role in progressing an improvement or change. Each might also be a member of several teams in which they take roles related to their expertise, experience or interests.

Traditional ideas about leaders and leadership are often based on a military model in which the leader decides, directs and commands. However, in a modern organisational setting, few of us are willing to follow a leader with absolute trust that their view of what action should be taken is always right. Most of us want to contribute something from our own perspective and want our experience, knowledge and skills to be acknowledged as colleagues rather than as followers.

Behavioural theories of leadership

Ideas about leadership in the early part of the twentieth century were based on the belief that leaders were born to the role. Traits that were consistently found included high energy levels, tolerance of stress, integrity, self-confidence and emotional maturity. The situation in which leadership was demonstrated was important, because in some situations it was not possible to lead unless you were an experienced practitioner and able to command the respect of the group.

Early trait theory was rejected partly because of the impracticability of reviewing the range of characteristics proposed, but also because of the implication that if leadership was only a result of birth it was the birthright of some privileged people and not of others. This belief implied that leaders could not be developed. Adair (1983) discussed trait theory as including a need to have a distinct personality and proposed that an important aspect of this would be integrity. He described integrity as 'wholeness', 'the type of person who adheres to some code of moral, artistic or other values'. Studies found that the situation in which a leader was operating was also important and that successful leaders often needed to balance one trait against another to accommodate the issues in the situation (van Maurik, 2001).

When trait theories seemed not to be providing acceptable answers about how effective leaders were produced, researchers began to study the behaviour exhibited by leaders. Behavioural theories are based on the idea that leadership is largely a matter of learning to display appropriate behaviour. Tannenbaum and Schmidt (1958) suggested that a person could choose a leadership style from a continuum that ranged from 'manager-controlled' leadership through to 'subordinate-centred' leadership. This continuum demonstrates the tension between use of authority by a manager and the freedom of action allowed to subordinates.

Tannenbaum and Schmidt's leadership styles

Tannenbaum and Schmidt studied leadership styles in the 1950s. They expressed their results as a continuum ranging from manager-centred leadership (where authority was based in a traditional line management system) to the degree of freedom allowed to subordinates in this system. continued

continued   Seven positions were identified, broadly described as:

1. Tell (announce a decision and expect everyone to act accordingly).
2. Sell (explain the decision but do not invite discussion).
3. Discuss (present the decision and invite questions).
4. Negotiate (present a tentative decision subject to change after discussion).
5. Consult (present problem for discussion and sharing of ideas before the leader makes the decision).
6. Delegate (leader defines limits to enable decisions to be made by team members).
7. Collaborate (shared decision making and monitoring of progress).

(Adapted from van Maurick, 2001)

Contingency theories

One of the main criticisms of behavioural theories was that they failed to acknowledge the importance of differences in situations. Contingency theories of leadership focused on the flexibility of a leader to choose and adapt an approach in response to different situations – contingencies. One of the earliest theorists was Fiedler (1967) who argued that both task- and people-oriented styles might be appropriate in different circumstances and that the effective leader chooses an appropriate style according to the demands of the situation. He identified three elements that indicate whether the situation is favourable to the leader:

■ whether the leader is liked and trusted by group members;
■ whether the task is clearly defined and well structured;
■ the power the leader has to reward and punish subordinates.

He found that a situation is very favourable to the leader when all three of these elements are strong. He also found that task-oriented leaders performed best in situations that were either very favourable or very unfavourable. Leaders whose style was more people-oriented performed better when situations were moderately favourable. Importantly, his work emphasised that the performance of the leader depends as much on the situation as on the style of the leader.

Fiedler thought that it was difficult for a person to change his or her leadership style but that it was possible to change the favourableness of a situation. This might be possible by, for example, increasing the authority and power of the leader or improving the structure and clarity of the task. Hersey and Blanchard (1988) disagreed with this idea and proposed that effective leaders should change their styles and should be able to adapt to the situation as they find it.

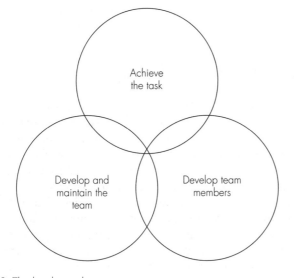

Figure 3.2 The leading role
(Source: adapted from Adair, 1983)

John Adair has been very influential in his contributions to thinking about both management and leadership. One of his key ideas was that a leader has to consider three sets of needs in approaching a task. These are the needs of the task itself, the needs of the group or team that are working on the task and the needs of the individuals that make up that group. His simple diagram of three focal areas in a leading role (Figure 3.2) has been very helpful for people seeking a way of structuring their approach to a new situation.

His model focuses on what a leader has to do in relation to the needs of each of these three areas. The first area, achieving the task, requires a clear understanding of the task and what success will mean. There will also be issues associated with the nature of the task, including need for information and maybe materials and equipment. The development of the team will normally include forming, developing and maintaining the team. The development of individual team members will include ensuring that individuals feel able to perform in the team and development in relation to the context and task. Adair gives a full discussion of the issues in each of these circles and suggests that the relationship a leader might take to each circle is to be 'half in and half-out'.

Both behavioural and contingency theories have limitations. Most of them equate leadership with management and assume that this one senior person has power and authority over a number of subordinates. As organisations become less hierarchical, these theories offer little to help us think about leadership among colleagues and in groups where roles frequently change. These theories are also focused more on the behaviour of leaders and the activities involved in completing tasks than on the strategic direction and sense of purpose needed to achieve goals. Even the use of the term 'goal' is revealing as some of our ideas about leadership have emerged from sports coaching.

Transformational leadership

Earlier thinking about leadership – trait, behaviourist and contingency – was all about actions and transactions. The next wave of thinking was more about the nature of change and leadership became considered as the ability to achieve a transformation. This is why we now associate leadership with change. Warren Bennis (discussed fully in van Maurik, 2001) was one of the earlier writers who associated learning with leadership. He thought that leadership could be learned and that because learning is about taking control of your own life, learning is key to making transformations. In his view, the individual who can learn through reflection and who is able to make personal transformations is well equipped to translate this into achieving action and results in a wider context.

The main focus in ideas about transformational leadership is on people, and change as something achieved by people. Peter Senge (1990) proposed that there are five essential disciplines that underpin organisations that are successful in learning from experience and transforming themselves to be effective in changing situations. These disciplines are:

- *systems thinking* (concerned with the ways in which an organisation achieves its purposes and the extent to which each component part makes a contribution);
- *personal mastery* (the abilities of individuals to manage themselves and their self-development);
- *mental models* (our conceptual view of the world that might need to be revised as the world changes);
- *building shared visions* (the ability to develop collective imagination);
- *team learning* (learning as a team from shared experience).

These ideas imply that leadership and management are necessary at all levels within an organisation.

The linking of leaders to change has challenged ideas that leadership can be objectively analysed and defined, because there is so great an emphasis on people and the reactions of people to other people. As Grint observed:

> *it is not that leaders are those who identify the wave and ride it; rather, leaders are those who persuade us a wave is coming, who go out of their way to appear the most visible surfers to onlookers, and whose actions are taken by the onlookers as actions appropriate for leaders to take.*
>
> (Grint, 1997)

Transformational leadership implies being able to inspire people to lift their attention above everyday affairs (although these must still be carried out efficiently and effectively). It is concerned with sharing values and developing a sense of doing something purposeful. The focus is more on the purpose and excellence of work than the power or personality of the leader. The essence of transformational leadership is that leaders transform the way their staff see themselves and the organisation:

- They make staff aware of the importance of their role to the success of the organisation, and of how dependent organisational achievements are on their individual achievements.
- Because the skills of staff are so crucial, they encourage people to manage their own personal development and performance.
- They motivate staff to work both for their own personal goals and for the goals of the organisation.

These principles are uncontentious, but they have significant implications for the behaviour of leaders. Transformational leadership depends to a considerable extent on the personal power of the leader: he or she is expected to communicate a clear and achievable vision, and to do so with an enthusiasm that inspires staff. If staff are to be encouraged to engage with and 'own' organisational issues, and to use their intellects in group problem solving, the leader must focus on the development of their capabilities. The use of symbols is important – the leader manages meetings, ceremonies and appearances in a way that communicates to staff his or her vision of how the organisation should function, thus 'binding' them into this vision.

The NHS Confederation view

A consultation document from the NHS Confederation (1999) said:

> Leadership is largely about a relationship between the leader and those who follow . . . transformational leadership . . . embodies the notion of leaders as having a responsibility to serve those who follow them, to engage their commitment and develop their potential.
>
> This in no way undervalues the contribution of managers. Indeed, at present, 95% of those who lead healthcare organisations as chief executives have a managerial background and it is of the utmost importance that they are developed as individuals to assume these leadership roles effectively. To do so, they also need to be developed in their professional roles as managers . . .
>
> The concept of transformational leadership . . . refers to the process of influencing followers or staff by inspiring them or pulling them towards the vision of some future state. Transformational leaders exhibit some or all of the following four characteristics:

continued

---

continued

- **charisma**: provides vision and a sense of mission, instils pride, gains respect and trust
- **inspiration**: communicates high expectations, expresses important purposes in simple ways
- *intellectual stimulation*: encourages followers to question basic assumptions, and to consider problems from new and unique perspectives
- individual consideration: gives personal attention, treats each employee individually, coaches, advises . . .

There is also interest in the ways in which others perceive the behaviour of leaders as this may shed light on what behaviours are considered successful in health and care services.

Beverly Alimo-Metcalfe and Robert Alban-Metcalfe carried out a large-scale research study to identify the constructs that people in public and private services held about people that they considered to be leaders (Alimo-Metcalfe, 2002). Constructs are mental models that people use to differentiate one leader from another, so express what people consider to be important characteristics of leaders in public services. Some key factors of successful leaders were identified:

- concern for others
- approachability
- encouraging questioning and promoting change
- integrity
- charisma
- intellectual ability
- ability to communicate, set direction, unify and manage change.

Interviews with people in the public sector cited integrity much more often than those in private organisations. Sensitivity to the organisation's various stakeholders was also mentioned much more frequently by those in public services.

Many of the values of health and social care are about empowering others. A report to the Local Government Management Board gives an example:

Competence and disposition in transformational leaders

Transformational leadership is not simply the result of performing certain competences, though these are no doubt essential prerequisites for the credibility of a manager. It is also reflected in fundamental personal dispositions. These include empathy, openness to criticism and the ideas of others, a degree of selflessness, and some judicious risk-taking in empowering others.

It is also about enthusiasm, articulating a clear vision and showing a determination to achieve it, and involving others so that they take on ownership of the vision. Transformational leaders are perceived as individuals of high integrity and self-confidence. They not only maintain a close relationship with and accessibility to staff within their organisations, they are also very sensitive to the concerns of elected councillors and develop a wide network of external relationships.

They are highly skilled both in internal organisational politics, and in relating effectively to external politics that impact on their organisation and service.

Transformational leaders also have the intellectual capacity to think broadly – even divergently at times – but also to adopt rational modes of analysis and to see some of the detail in an issue or problem.

(Adapted from Alimo-Metcalfe, 1998)

Gone are the days when managers had subordinates whom they could 'command'. Going are the days when people readily accept that the role of a manager in normal circumstances is to 'direct'. The majority of people in the democratic and high-tech world of today are highly educated and highly trained. Commanding them or directing them is unlikely to gain their willing collaboration and their commitment.

Leading as a social process

Leaders cannot exist without others, those who follow the lead. Following a leader implies more than simply doing what is asked because leaders are asking people to commit to making changes that will, potentially, have individual and collective impact. Once people agree to follow a lead, they become central to the process. Grint (1995) comments:

> If we argue, then, that leaders are those who in some way embody, articulate, channel and construct the values and direction that the followers think they ought to be going in, then we dispense with the leader as isolated hero and return to the leader as the embodiment of the collective.

If we follow this thought we realise that for a leader to be at all influential or effective, there must be a collective view of the direction of change. This requires an increasing emphasis on development in our organisations of an egalitarian social model that demonstrates social inclusion and intercultural approaches.

There are some important implications from the process view of leadership: a leader influences how people think about issues but they do not necessarily have formal power within an organisation. Therefore a group can have more than one leader – all members of a group can make leadership contributions. In 'dispersed' leadership different people may demonstrate leadership in different areas. For example, different leadership abilities are required to develop strategy, develop team commitment and morale and to progress detailed tasks.

If everyone is to be involved in committing to change, everyone needs to know something about the impact of forces in the wider environment surrounding our organisations and our work and understand why change is necessary to respond to these forces. We need to consider development of all employees as potential leaders. In public services, we may also be concerned to involve service users in our teams as we develop our understanding of the need to change and commit to implementing it.

Those who have been working in health and care services are sometimes sceptical about the contribution that leaders can make in achieving improvements to service provision. In writing about nurses as leaders Colleen Wedderburn Tate (1999) comments:

> As the 21st century comes tip-toeing into life, the debate about leaders and leadership becomes more intense. But with all this talk, who has time to lead? The trouble is, leaders make us feel uneasy. After all, they are lauded, rewarded, and accorded all kinds of powers. We 'ordinary people' who like nothing better than to see the powerful get their comeuppance, make suitably disgusted noises, while firmly denying that we have a hand in the events we so roundly criticize . . . every healthcare worker has a responsibility to lead and exercise leadership. The fact that we may choose not to do so does not lessen our responsibility.

This challenging view was earlier adopted by Kouzes and Posner (1987), whose approach identified key elements that characterise newer, social process models of leadership, including:

- challenging the status quo
- inspiring a shared vision
- enabling others to act
- modelling the way
- encouraging the heart.

These elements acknowledge the need to challenge existing practice to ensure that improvements are made where they are needed and the importance of not only developing a vision of a better and inspiring future but of doing this in a way that inspires all those who need to contribute if it is to be achieved. Once people are inspired and willing to act, they will often need to be enabled by supporting and empowering them to take leading roles at all levels within the organisation. Those who are in senior positions can provide leadership by demonstrating ways of empowering others, modelling the ways in which leadership can be shared. Importantly, this social process approach also recognises that there is an emotional aspect to be considered and that people who take on the responsibility of contributing to leadership need to be supported and encouraged.

If leaders are to be encouraged to emerge from all levels and all areas of health and care organisations we must develop ways to identify and support the ideas that people propose. Teams will need to be open to leadership from those who can inspire confidence to take action over a particular initiative rather than those in the most senior posts. We might expect our values to be frequently challenged and sometimes to be revised or re-interpreted to be more inclusive of the concerns of increasingly diverse groups and teams. The thinking and actions of team workers and leaders will need to fit the context, both the organisational environment and the culture. Power, responsibility and decision making will not be invested in one person but shared within a group. Leadership will be increasingly understood to be a dynamic process that includes and impacts upon people and progresses with a particular purpose.

Hartley and Allison (2000) grouped the themes and elements of leadership in public services as:

- persons (characteristics, behaviours, skills and styles of leaders);
- positions (both formal authority and those perceived to be influential);
- processes (between individuals, groups and organisations, and partnerships).

Health and care services increasingly work across traditional organ-isational boundaries to find better ways of responding to the needs of service users. Rogers and Reynolds (2003) added another P – Purpose – to this list, suggesting that it is a focus on purpose that brings a reason for changing things, that builds on underlying values and helps in developing vision and strategy. Although each individual organisation has its purpose as a primary task, the purpose of the joint initiative brings the rationale for collaboration between organisations, which, when working together, can provide improvements for service users.

DEVELOPING YOUR STYLE

Whether you are primarily a leader or a manager, you can influence people to do the things that must be done by the way you do things, your personal style. As Handy (1989) commented:

> The modern leader lives vicariously, getting kicks out of other people's successes – as teachers have always done. Authority [in new-style organisations] does not come automatically with the title; it has to be earned. The authority you need is not based on being able to do the job better yourself but on your ability to help others do the job better – by developing their skills, by

liaising with the rest of the organisation, by helping them to make the most of their resources, by continual encouragement and example. The job of the leader is a mixture of teacher, consultant and trouble-shooter. Some say it is not a job for mere mortals. It isn't, unless you have been trained and developed for it. Then it can be a most exciting way to work.

You can go a long way towards inspiring people and winning their willing commitment if you carry out your managerial functions and exercise your authority in a style that suits the circumstances of your job and your organisation and is acceptable to the people you are managing. If you can find the style to match the circumstances, you will gain respect as a manager, your personal standing will rise, your confidence and authority will increase, and you will be accepted as a leader. By learning to carry out your managerial functions in a competent, professional, understanding, compassionate and appropriate way, you can improve your leadership abilities.

There are, however, limitations. The way in which you prefer to do things (in other words your preferred or natural style) is primarily a reflection of *you* – your fundamental nature, your values and your beliefs. Some managers prefer to adopt a high profile and to lead from the front assertively. Others prefer to manage quite differently, fulfilling the functions of management in a less forceful way, leading from the side rather than from the front. Others may prefer to push from the back.

But the style that you adopt should not only be a reflection of you and your preferences. To be successful, it must be appropriate to the *situation*. In times of crisis and emergency, for example, most people look for a leader who can confidently point the way and inspire people to follow it, and who can act as a focus and rallying point. This decisive – even authoritarian – style of leadership may also be the most appropriate when a member of staff fails to perform to the appropriate quality or safety standards. You might also lead from the front when a decision has been made that is non-negotiable and must be implemented, for example, actions that must conform to legislative, financial or service constraints.

The *setting* is also important. Different organisations, and different departments within them, need different styles to match their particular circumstances. Virtually every organisation, whether it be a railway or an electronics company, a residential home or a general practice, requires its management to fulfil broadly the same functions. The managerial functions – of setting objectives, planning, providing resources, and so on – remain the same. The thing that varies from one to the other is the way in which these managerial functions are carried out. Each organisation, indeed each department within an organisation, is in a different situation and requires a different kind of leadership. Each organisation probably has a different view about the kind of leadership that it needs, and it selects its managers to provide that kind of leadership. Its view about the kind of leadership it needs is influenced by the traditions and experience of the organisation and by the prevailing values of the people running it.

Some kinds of leader could never hope to survive in some kinds of organisation – they would not be tolerated. However, situations change and organisations (and departments) must change with them. What happens to the organisation whose management style is not changing as quickly as the situation? What happens when the organisation's traditions and values cannot tolerate the kind of thrusting, dynamic, entrepreneurial leader who is needed because other factors in the situation require a new and different kind of leadership? They need someone to carry out the same functions of management as before, but they need someone who can carry them out in a different way. They need a different style of management, one in which the leadership element matches the changed circumstances.

Most organisations tend to select and develop managers who are capable of managing in a style that is suited to the culture of the organisation and the circumstances in which it has operated in the past. If the management cannot change its style to provide the leadership that is needed, it may have to be replaced. Successful managers are those who can develop a leadership style that is appropriate to the circumstances. We shall now consider some of the choices you have about your actions as a manager and a leader.

ACTIVITY 3.1

Go through the checklist below and tick each item that you, as the leader of a group, have done in the past six months. Then go through the list again, this time thinking of yourself as a member of a different group, and tick the items that the leader of the group has done in the past six months.

	You as a leader	*You as a member of a group*
1 a Set the task of the team	❏	❏
b Put it across with enthusiasm	❏	❏
c Remind people of it often	❏	❏
2 a Plan the work	❏	❏
b Pace its progress	❏	❏
c Design jobs to encourage the commitment of individuals and teams	❏	❏
3 a Set individual targets after consultation	❏	❏
b Discuss progress with each person regularly	❏	❏

		You as a leader	You as a member of a group
4 a	Delegate decisions to individuals	☐	☐
b	Consult those affected	☐	☐
5 a	Communicate the importance of each person's job	☐	☐
b	Explain decisions to help people to implement them	☐	☐
c	Brief the team regularly on progress	☐	☐
6 a	Train and develop people	☐	☐
b	Gain support for rules and procedures	☐	☐
c	Set an example	☐	☐
d	'Have a go' at those who break the rules	☐	☐
7 a	Care about the well-being of people in the team	☐	☐
b	Improve working conditions	☐	☐
c	Deal with grievances	☐	☐
d	Attend functions	☐	☐
8 a	Monitor action	☐	☐
b	Learn from successes and mistakes	☐	☐
c	Regularly walk round each person's place of work, observe, listen and praise	☐	☐

Were you aware of a difference in your experience of leadership when you considered the things that you did yourself as a leader and the way that you felt as team member without the leadership role? Once you have been in a leadership position you might feel frustrated as a team member if the team leader does not carry out most of the actions mentioned above. If you feel that you are achieving something as a team member, you are likely to want to continue to work productively. However, if you feel that your team is not being helped to perform well by its leader, you might be critical of the leadership. This view of leadership sees it as a facilitative role.

A different approach to choice of styles was taken by Blake and Mouton in their model of the Management Grid in 1962. Their work developed the emerging idea that leadership styles varied in two important dimensions, concern for people and concern for achievement of the task. People-oriented leadership styles concentrated on good working relationships and the well-being of staff. Task-oriented leadership styles focused on setting goals and planning activities to ensure that the task was successfully completed.

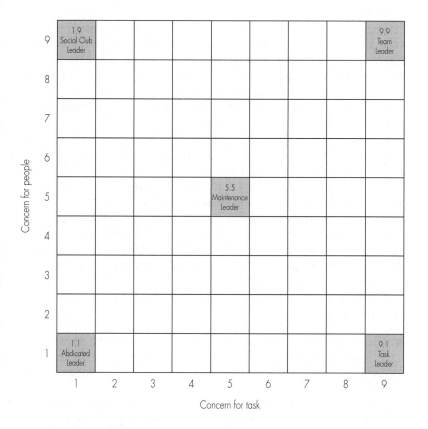

Figure 3.3 A style grid for leaders in health and social care
(Source: Martin, 2003)

ACTIVITY 3.2

On a scale of 1 (low) to 10 (high) what scores would you give to the
following for concern for the task and concern for people?

	Concern for the task	*Concern for people*
Yourself	❑	❑
Your boss	❑	❑
Your boss's boss?	❑	❑
What scores do you think your colleagues would give you?	❑	❑
What scores do you think your boss would give himself or herself?	❑	❑

The scores in Activity 3.2 do not tell you your style: they merely indicate your sense of values as between task and people. Nevertheless, they probably give a hint of the kind of style that you would naturally fall into if you did not give careful thought to the style that is best suited to the particular circumstances in your section or department.

But there are other personal values that also affect the management style you prefer. We each have our own sense of the 'proper' way to behave. Many people feel that a manager has to assume responsibility, and should not share it with those who are more junior. Such an attitude would belong to the directive end of the scale. Others feel exactly the opposite, believing that the leader is the voice of the group, and as such should always consult the members of the group and expect them to participate in decision making. Such beliefs belong to the more consultative end of the scale. Some enjoy telling others what to do, others hate it. None of these attitudes is right or wrong, but they do restrict your range of operation. It is wise to be honest with yourself about your instinctive preference.

Besides your personal values, a number of other factors may influence your style:

- *Your confidence in your staff.* Your staff may be thoroughly competent, but if you are not entirely convinced of their abilities, you are unlikely to let them participate in deciding what to do or how to do it.
- *Your need for certainty.* An open style or approach involves handing over some control to others. There is a positive gain in that, but there is also some risk, as there always is when you relinquish control. If you have a low tolerance for uncertainty, do not like risks or do not think that the situation justifies it, you will prefer to lead in a more directive way.
- *Your personal contribution.* Your need for certainty is affected by your estimate of what you can contribute. If you believe that you know what is the right thing to do, you will not want to treat the problem as an open one, and will tend to want to tell others what to do. Managers who have done every job in their departments tend to be more directive, although this may be inappropriate.
- *Stress.* The pressure of work and events can produce a sense of overload, worry and pressure which, in excess, can lead to stress. Stress usually pushes people to one or other end of the style continuum. They either become very directive, in an attempt to reassert control over the situation, or they abandon control altogether and become apathetic.

ACTIVITY 3.3

Many factors influence the extent to which we can choose to be directive or consultative. Which way does each of these factors tend to push you? Place a cross on the scale below to mark where you are now in your present job. Place a tick where you think you would like to be.

	Directive	*Consultative*
Personal value system		
Confidence in subordinates		
Need for certainty		
Personal contribution		
Stress		

Many people lie further towards the directive end of the scale than they would like to be. This is not to say that it is always wrong to be at that end of the scale: it is not. However, to be locked into that end because of factors in you, rather than because of the situation, is to limit your flexibility and your potential effectiveness as a leader.

Leadership is a facet of management – the facet that reflects the style in which the manager carries out management functions and uses power and authority. You may not be a born leader, but if you ensure that all these functions are fulfilled in a way that satisfies the needs of your team and meets with their approval, the likelihood is that they will willingly accord you the status of leader. They will give you the authority to lead.

MANAGING WITH STYLE

We are taking the view that leadership is a reflection of the way in which you carry out your managerial functions. How, then, can you do this in ways that will provide the kind of leadership that is needed in health and care services? Leadership is mainly concerned with winning and sustaining the enthusiasm and willing commitment of staff. You cannot *direct* people to devote their efforts and energies willingly, but you can *lead* them to do so by managing them in an appropriate style. Within the complex blend of behaviour that makes up management style are five forms of behaviour that are often associated with being an effective leader:

- setting an example
- developing your 'image'
- projecting self-confidence
- influencing others
- establishing personal authority.

Let's look at each of these in turn.

Setting an example

No doubt you expect that the people who work for you will do their work. However, you probably hope for something more from them than that they should merely come to work and do the job in a disgruntled or, at best, an uncommitted way. You probably seek their enthusiasm, energy, effort, commitment, high standards, professionalism and perhaps many other things. Is it likely that your team will provide these very desirable qualities if they fail to detect the same qualities in you? Are you, in carrying out your managerial work, setting the sorts of examples that will influence your team to act in the ways that you want?

As a manager, you emit signals continuously that are received and interpreted by your staff. Your style, your manner, your tone, your attitudes and your values are all assessed and determine how your staff react to you as their manager and leader. If they detect in you someone who shows little enthusiasm for the job or the organisation, are they likely to feel enthusiastic themselves? If they do not feel enthusiastic, your job as a manager will be more difficult. Your staff might not follow you in the classical sense but, whether you like it or not, they will almost certainly follow your example.

Developing your 'image'

Like it or not, you have an image. It is the way that you are viewed by your colleagues, your staff and your service users. It is what people perceive as being true that represents the truth for them, even if you see things totally differently. It is in your interest, therefore, to work on your image to make it more professional and positive. Some people might find this idea distasteful, but there is nothing wrong with projecting the best image that you can in a conscious, considered way. It is important to take account of what is expected of you as a manager in your organisation. If you present yourself in a way that is very different from the expectations, it may be more difficult for people to respect you and to listen to you as a manager. We constantly suppress our personal feelings to act in ways that are appropriate at work rather than in ways that we might personally prefer. There is an opportunity for you, as a manager, consciously to seek to project an image of yourself that will help you to manage better and to provide the leadership that is needed.

You have opportunities to improve your image in everything you do as a manager. You can work energetically, plan enthusiastically, show commitment to your job, your staff and your service users and carry out all your managerial duties with high standards of thoroughness and attention to detail – exactly the standards that you would aim to achieve in your professional duties if you moved into management from a professional role.

I have learned the difference between my own view of myself and that of others. I thought I was perhaps too democratic, whereas others see me as somewhat autocratic. This was quite a shock.

(Comments of a young health service manager, quoted in Stewart, 1989)

Make a point of congratulating people who do a particularly good job and make sure that your team recognises and shares a sense of success whenever this is appropriate.

It is not just the way you *do* things as a manager, it is also the way you *say* things. You are communicating much of the time, gathering and disseminating information, checking progress, explaining plans and policies, counselling and advising, criticising or praising. The manner in which you do this 'speaks volumes'.

Unfortunately, it is often when you are feeling most pressed yourself that revealing it to your staff can increase your problems rather than reduce them. However, it can often be helpful to share information about your workload and deadlines and to expect co-operation at particularly busy times. As always, this works both ways and your staff will reasonably expect you to recognise their particularly busy times too.

Projecting self-confidence

There is an unwritten contract that exists between managers and their staff. Your staff expect things from you just as surely as you expect things from them. Your staff will look to you to point the way, not necessarily to have a new and exciting vision of the future, but rather to make clear – and keep clear – what their objectives are and how they are going to achieve them.

To achieve this implies that you must project self-confidence. Your manner, your style, your voice, your appearance and your posture all send out messages about your self-confidence. You may not feel very confident but you can suppress signals that suggest nervousness and lack of confidence. Better still, you can emphasise signals that imply self-confidence.

It is a long-term undertaking to transform yourself 'on the inside' from being an under-confident person to becoming self-assured. However, to transform yourself 'on the outside' is not so difficult. You can learn to hide any lack of confidence and to project a self-assured image. Many experienced managers would privately admit to suffering from 'butterflies in the tummy', amounting almost to panic, every time that they have to speak at a formal meeting or address a large group. Many of them, however, have learned the techniques of suppressing or hiding the give-away signs. These techniques include consciously standing (or sitting) still, imagining that you are speaking to just one person – a close friend – in the comfort of your home, and holding on to something so that your arms do not wave around or your hands scratch nervously at your nose and ears. Many managers find that learning presentation skills boosts their confidence in other situations.

You need to learn the art of acting, of appearing confident even if inside you are scared . . . most important is learning to be confident.

(Manager, quoted in Stewart, 1989)

Influencing others

Your ability to influence others is a crucial management skill. It is particularly important in settings where there are complex power relationships and many different types of teams working together to provide a service. In order to clear the way for action you may need to negotiate or influence, particularly in joint working situations where you have no formal authority other than in your own area of work. How you influence others – your staff, your service users, your peers and senior managers – is very much a matter of style.

Your staff will develop trust in you if you are consistent and fair. You need to be prepared to explain your decisions to make sure that they understand why you think that they are fair. You might have to reconsider a decision if your staff put a point of view that you had not been aware of.

You can be supportive in helping staff to assess their development needs and in providing training. You can support staff to explore tasks and projects that are new to them. You can win trust by making sure that those who have completed difficult tasks or who come up with good ideas are given the credit for doing so.

Your service users will see you as representing your organisation and area of work and will expect you to demonstrate confidence and to be approachable. Your influence can be important in helping a service user to feel confident that they are receiving a high quality service, particularly if they approach you with a question, comment or complaint. The way in which you listen, respond and take action if required, will all make a direct impact on that service user's experience.

Influencing your peers can be more difficult. However, there are very few areas of work in health or social care in which a high-quality service can be provided to service users without the co-operation of a number of complementary service areas. Influence is often about co-operating in ways that allow both parties to benefit and maintain high quality.

It is unlikely, however, that it will be quite as easy to do this as it is to describe it. If you do not already have an open relationship with your peers, you may have to be prepared to share some of the problems you face and to be open to discussion of alternative ways of addressing issues. You will also need to listen to the problems others want to discuss and to share your ideas about how they might address problems in their areas of work. Influencing your manager and other senior managers is often called 'managing upwards'. You may think that this is not something for which you should take any responsibility, but senior managers do not have access to the detailed operations of the organisation in the way that you do as an operational manager or team leader. There may be times when you are aware of something that it would help them to know about or that they should be warned about. You are in a position to provide feedback to them about how their actions and behaviour affect your staff and service users. Your manager and other senior managers have objectives to achieve and will welcome your contribution to furthering them.

Establishing personal authority

Your staff expect you to show authority. Every manager needs to establish and maintain personal authority. Possibly we need to distinguish between being an authority and being in authority. Most managers need to be both. It helps to have the facts at your fingertips. This means thorough preparation for meetings, thorough attention to detail, thorough mastery of techniques and procedures, a detailed awareness of what is going on. Some people amass information and detail easily. Others need to work at it. Few managers can afford to be exposed as being ignorant of the facts or unaware of what is going on.

Being *in* authority is rather different. It might be a matter of confidence that helps you to present an authoritative air and style.

One aspect of conveying an image of authority is to seem in control and to be able to cope with situations that arise unexpectedly as well as those that had been anticipated. Managing time is an important aspect of appearing to be calm. The managers who create the best impression and who inspire most confidence in their staff are those who can give the impression of being in control. Inside, they might feel jumpy, anxious, irritable. They might feel snowed under and be wondering to themselves how they are ever going to get through the workload. Yet somehow they manage to suppress the signals that would reveal their anxiety and that might disconcert their staff. One way in which you can give the impression of being in control of yourself and in control of events is by setting aside enough time to see people and discuss their problems in a relaxed way.

Managers cannot hope to be accepted as leaders unless they carry out their managerial functions with an appropriate style. Some people can do this naturally. Others, possibly most, need to do it in a conscious, considered way.

You have power because of your position as a manager. Power is necessary to manage resources and to ensure that they are used to meet the goals of the organisation. Some people are frightened to think of themselves as having power because it is sometimes considered that power is corrupting. But power is not good or bad in itself: it is the way in which you use your power that is important. To use your power for personal gain would be abusing the trust that your organisation places in you. However, failing to use your power can mean failing to contribute as fully as you can to the work of your organisation. You are expected to use the power of your position to do your best to achieve the goals of your work area. Using your power does not mean that you have the adopt a directive style so that everyone can see that you have power. You can choose to delegate some tasks and resources

People have looked to me as a leader so I have had to do things even if I am quaking inside. I always think I look calm on the outside: serene as a swan on the outside, yet underneath I am paddling like hell.

(Hospital manager, quoted in Stewart, 1989)

I know my preferred style. I am a benevolent autocrat at heart. I tend to reach conclusions much more quickly than most people, and I get impatient with their endless discussions in search of the answer. Experience also tells me that my solutions are usually right – so my natural tendency is to impose them if I possibly can. Fortunately, perhaps, I recognise that I must be a pain to work for. So generally I try to curb my natural preferences, and manage in a way that is better suited to the very experienced and well-qualified people who report to me.

(Confessions of a senior manager)

to your staff and you can choose to share decision making with them in a consultative style when it is appropriate.

Some managers might feel that a consultative style is expected by their staff and that nothing else would be acceptable. In health and social care, staff are usually highly intelligent, highly qualified and highly motivated people who could usefully contribute to making managerial decisions – if not to decisions about 'what to do', at least to those about 'how to do it'. It is widely believed that staff who participate in decision making will have some 'ownership' of the outcome and will co-operate to take the action that is decided upon. However, it is not always appropriate to adopt a consultative style, even if this is your preferred approach. In emergency situations, or when a decision is needed very quickly, you must take the responsibility. And at the other extreme, your staff would very soon tire of participating if they were involved in making all the repetitive and trivial decisions that are necessary in any work area.

So should you just rely on your preferred style because that is the one which you are most comfortable with? Or should you consciously push yourself to the consultative end of the scale? Or should you become tougher and consciously move towards the directive end? Is there a right style to use? There is often a need for different management styles within a single managerial job. Consider your job, for example. You may have several different tasks within that job, which will require you to adopt different management styles with the same group of people. The routine activities may well be suited to a directive style because they are well defined and need to be carefully monitored. You should not need to consult your team about them once they have been defined. Your job is to see that the duties are done.

There are likely to be other aspects of your job that require you to take initiatives or develop new opportunities. Tackling these challenges will probably require a different style of management. You will need the commitment and the creative ideas of your team. When you step into the unknown it is best not to do it alone, although the inspiration, the energy and, ultimately, the responsibility remain with you. A shift towards the consultative end of the scale may well be needed for this part of your job.

To be effective in their jobs, let alone between different jobs, all managers need to vary their management styles to suit the particular circumstances. However, this raises the question of whether managers are capable of varying their styles of management. Research shows that few managers are able to change their preferred styles. The reasons for preferring particular styles are as deep-seated as those underlying their very personalities, and nobody can be expected to change personality at the drop of a hat. Fortunately, however, most managers have a range of styles on either side of their preferred style within which they can operate without discomfort and within which they can maintain credibility. For some managers, that range is quite extensive. The effective manager knows that the style that he or she would prefer to adopt is not likely to be appropriate in all circumstances, and that the ability (and willingness) to adjust his or her management style, within the available limits, is a fundamentally important managerial competence.

REFERENCES

Adair, J. (1983) *Effective Leadership*, Pan Books.

Alimo-Metcalfe, B. (1998) *Effective Leadership*. Local Government Management Board.

Alimo-Metcalfe, B. and Alban-Metcalfe, J. (2002) 'Half the Battle', *Health Service Journal*, 7 March .

Blake, R. R. and Mouton, J. S. (1962) *The Managerial Grid*, Advanced Management Office Executive, vol. 1, no. 9.

Fiedler, F. E. (1967) *A Theory of Leadership Effectiveness*, McGraw-Hill.

Grint, K. (1995) *Management: A Sociological Introduction*, Polity Press.

Grint, K. (ed.)(1997) *Leadership: Classical, Contemporary and Critical Approaches*, Oxford University Press.

Handy, C. (1989) *The Age of Unreason*, Hutchinson.

Hartley, J. F. and Allison, M. (2000) 'The role of leadership in the modernisation and improvement of public services', *Public Money and Management*, vol. 20, pp. 35–40.

Hersey, P. and Blanchard, K. H. (1988) *Management of Organisational Behaviour*, 5th edn, Prentice-Hall.

Kotter (1990) *A Force for Change*, Free Press.

Kouzes, J. M. and Posner, B. Z. (1987) *The Leadership Challenge: How to Get Extraordinary Things Done in Organizations*, Jossey-Bass.

Martin, V. (2003) *Leading Change in Health and Social Care*, Routledge.

NHS Confederation (1999) *Consultation: The Modern Values of Leadership and Management in the NHS*, NHS Confederation.

Rogers, A. and Reynolds, J. (2003) 'Leadership and vision', in Seden, J. and Reynolds, J. (eds) *Managing Care in Practice*, Routledge.

Senge, P. (1990) *The Fifth Discipline*, Century Business, Random House.

Stewart, R. (1989) *Leading in the NHS: A Practical Guide*, Macmillan.

Tannenbaum, R. and Schmidt, W. H. (1958) 'How to choose a leadership pattern', *Harvard Business Review*, March–April, vol. 36, pp. 95–102.

Van Maurik, J. (2001) *Writers on Leadership*, Penguin Books.

Wedderburn Tate, C. (1999) *Leadership in Nursing*, Harcourt Publishers.

CHAPTER 4

UNDERSTANDING MOTIVATION

This chapter explores working with others – whether colleagues, volunteers, professionals or managers in partner organisations – in the context of understanding people's behaviour and motivation at work. Why do people choose to work (paid or unpaid) in a particular profession, job or organisation? Why is there a difference in the quantity and quality of the work people do?

People's behaviour at work is complex, governed by an interaction of their interests, background, previous experience, goals, expectations, values and beliefs. Yet behaviour and motivation is not purely a result of individual factors: often the individual is influenced by the organisation in which he or she is working. Organisations have formal rules and procedures and also exert indirect influences on what are perceived to be accepted ways to behave at work.

Not all managers have studied psychology, however, so cannot be expected to have an in-depth understanding of colleagues' behaviour. But as an essential part of working well together – especially in increasingly complex partnership and commissioning arrangements – it is useful to understand what influences behaviour and motivation. As a manager, you have considerable influence over some of the circumstances that can affect people's motivation, not least by organising their jobs in ways that make them more satisfying.

We begin by considering what we mean by motivation and why it is important, both for individuals and for the organisations they work in. We then look at some of the theories of motivation, which place different emphasis on needs, goals and rewards. We also explore how the context of working in health and social care impacts on the relevance of these theories. We conclude with a consideration of the role of diversity in these debates.

WHAT IS MOTIVATION?

Motivation can be defined as the psychological or emotional drivers that cause people to behave in a particular way. It has three aspects:

■ the direction of people's behaviour – what they try to do
■ the effort they exert – how hard they try
■ their persistence – their behaviour in the face of adversity.

(Smith and Smith, 2005)

Part of a manager's role is to encourage others to work effectively. People increasingly expect to be treated well by their managers and colleagues and achieve some fulfilment from their work. Most people expect some degree of autonomy and empowerment and do not expect simply to be told what to do. But managers can legitimately expect their team to be working towards the same goals – those of the service, organisation and possibly partnership organisation – and that people will co-operate with decisions. Theories about motivation are usually based on the experiences of paid workers but in many areas of health and social care, volunteers provide key services and work alongside paid members of staff. We therefore also need to consider how appropriate motivation theories are that focus on financial rewards as a means of motivating team members.

Motivation at work

Some years ago I was appointed as a senior researcher for a large project involving an interprofessional team of clinicians and social scientists. I was really pleased to get the job and felt that it would be an interesting departure from my previous work. Although nervous about moving to a new town and into a new role, I felt it was the right career decision. According to the job description, my responsibilities included organising the work of junior members of the team, contacting other researchers, dealing with technical enquiries and writing papers associated with the project. The work was so different from what I was used to that, at first, I did not always understand what all the members of the team were doing. But I persevered and got to grips with the role.

After a few months the team manager went on maternity leave and, although not formally asked to do so, I gradually took over her role. The organisation of the office had always been very haphazard with an inadequate filing system. Scraps of paper with important information on them were frequently lost, and the manager had always kept a lot of decisions and knowledge to herself. Taking over her role was a real challenge but I worked hard at it, organised the office more effectively and kept the team well informed about progress and decisions. It was very busy but we all felt we were doing a good job. We even organised a major conference. The atmosphere was much more relaxed and all the team were making progress in their work.

Then the team manager came back to work. She felt excluded from the changes and decisions we had made and decided to reassert her authority. She took over the high-level organisation of the conference (although she still expected me to do the routine work for it) and went back to excluding me from decisions. She also began interfering in my work, arguing that it was not part of my role to be so involved in the research. I was left with tasks which I felt did not utilise my skills and knowledge. Morale among the junior members of staff declined and people were reluctant to work extra hours in the busy time leading up the conference. The team were making mistakes following up enquiries and processing data and I was usually left to deal with them.

I started to feel unhappy in work and at home, so I decided to look for another job. I assumed that nothing would ever change or improve in the team's working relationship.

This example demonstrates how people can feel different levels of motivation, depending on their surroundings.

ACTIVITY 4.1

Write down both the motivating and the demotivating factors that you feel affected the researcher's motivation.

It would be easy to make assumptions about the person in this case study. For example, did you think the researcher was male or female? (She was actually female.) Did this influence how you saw the issues affecting her motivation? Did you have strong ideas about how she should have dealt with the situation or what her manager should have done to improve team morale and working relationships?

We all make assumptions about what motivates our colleagues. If we sense they are not working well, we want to take action. What we decide to do will be influenced by what we think makes people perform well or perform poorly. Most of us have ideas about this even before we study motivation as part of management theory.

ACTIVITY 4.2

Think about a time in your working life when you felt motivated and were performing well and also another time when you were demotivated and performing less well. Write down the reasons why you think you felt this way on these occasions.

Compare your notes on Activity 4.2 with the box below, which summarises the results of some research into motivating factors for NHS staff.

Emotional motivators within the NHS

Patients

- Making people's lives better
- Improving people's quality of life
- Saving lives
- Giving back to the community
- Serving society

Colleagues

- Teamwork
- Social networking
- Mutual support and regard
- Sense of overcoming challenges collectively

Profession

- Status, prestige and respect

Organisation

- Ability to input into management decisions
- Opportunities to use initiative
- Relationship with direct manager
- Feeling valued, involved and recognised
- Management competence
- Opportunities for training, development and progression

(Ipsos MORI, 2008)

We now discuss some different theoretical approaches to motivation, all of which have had some impact on the development of management thought.

THEORIES OF MOTIVATION

One traditional approach to motivation is Maslow's growth motivation theory (1987). Although he developed his theory over 60 years ago, and his work has subsequently been heavily criticised, his idea of a 'hierarchy of needs' is still part of the language of managers. Maslow proposed that everyone has the same needs or desires that must be satisfied. If managers appreciated the nature of these needs and goals and organised work to meet them, workers would be satisfied and more productive.

Maslow presented these needs as a hierarchy (Figure 4.1). From the basic level upwards, they are:

■ physiological needs – food, drink and shelter;
■ safety needs – protection against physical and emotional threat or harm, desire for predictability;
■ social needs – love, affection and acceptance as part of a social group;
■ esteem needs – to have high self-esteem and the respect of others;
■ 'self-actualisation' needs – to fulfil our potential to become what we believe we are capable of becoming.

He suggested that if such needs are unsatisfied then we become pre-occupied with them and other needs are marginalised. Furthermore, as one level of needs is met, then higher needs emerge and dominate our thoughts. The previous – and now satisfied – need no longer motivates us.

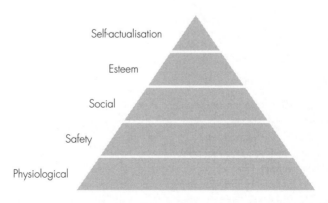

Figure 4.1 Maslow's hierarchy of needs
(Source: Maslow, 1987)

ACTIVITY 4.3

Think of occasions when each of the different needs – physiological, safety, social, esteem and self-actualisation – have been dominant in your thinking and note down how you felt about them.

For each set of needs, briefly list what could be done by colleagues and managers to meet those needs.

The needs identified by Maslow probably do play a part in people's behaviour. One key problem highlighted with Maslow's theory, however, is that the concept of self-actualisation is unlikely to be realised by the majority of people through their work. Furthermore, the concept of levels assumes a linear progression, and people's behaviour is not as simple as that.

Frederick Herzberg also worked with the concept of needs in his 'motivation hygiene theory'. This was based on research in organisations and had a particular focus on job satisfaction and dissatisfaction. His team discovered that the factors causing dissatisfaction were entirely different from those causing satisfaction. In other words, satisfaction and dissatisfaction are not clear opposites on a scale as one might have expected (Figure 4.2). For example, one person might cite low pay as causing dissatisfaction but would not list high pay as a factor in job satisfaction. Therefore, 'the opposite of job satisfaction is not job dissatisfaction but, rather, *no* job satisfaction' (Herzberg 2003).

Herzberg described 'motivator' factors as intrinsic to the job, for example, achievement, recognition, the work itself, responsibility, or advancement. He perceived 'hygiene' factors as extrinsic to the job, for example organisational policy, supervision, interpersonal relationships, working conditions, salary, status and security: these could reduce dissatisfaction but not necessarily increase job satisfaction and motivation.

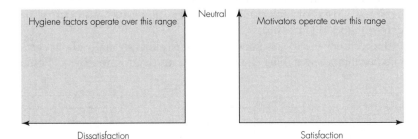

Figure 4.2 Hygiene factors and motivators

ACTIVITY 4.4

How does Herzberg's theory fit with your experience? Which of the factors described as motivators (intrinsic) motivate you and how much?

Now consider the hygiene (or extrinsic) factors. Which of these do not necessarily motivate you but could easily demotivate you?

Herzberg's approach has been criticised as focusing too much on satisfaction rather than motivation – these are not interchangeable concepts – and as being too simplistic. It also ignores the fact that people's behaviour can change over time.

Expectancy theory

A further, and perhaps better regarded, approach to motivation is 'expectancy theory', developed by Vroom (1964), which is based on outcomes rather than needs. Vroom highlighted the level of effort that people put into their work and how this relates to their prior experience at work. His approach accepts that people are not just driven by needs but are able to make sense of their experiences and change their effort accordingly. Vroom also suggested that the link between effort and reward is crucial in motivation. Many people are paid irrespective of the effort they expend but, in some cases, rewards are linked in a probabilistic way to effort: for a person to be motivated by reward and to decide to work hard, that person must strongly believe that their effort will result in the reward.

Vroom focused on the issue of performance: when a reward is given, it is usually based on the results or outcomes of the effort rather than the effort itself. The effort needs to be measurable (as in performance-related pay). If targets are not met, there might be costs (punishment) instead of rewards. The focus of Vroom's theory is on the link between performance and effort: if the link is strong, then rewards and the personal costs of achieving them are powerful motivators or demotivators (Figure 4.3).

Expectancy theory assumes that people think rationally about costs and benefits when making choices on how much effort to expend. Some

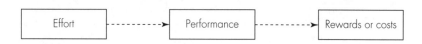

Figure 4.3 Expectancy theory

people may feel the stress and reduced leisure time of working hard far outweigh the benefits and instead seek a better work–life balance when considering additional responsibilities or promotion. Vroom's theory is more useful in thinking about how people reach more strategic decisions about their work and careers rather than in relation to more minor day-to-day decisions, when most people do not have time to speculate about what they are doing.

ACTIVITY 4.5

List five factors that reduce and five factors that increase the strength of the effort–performance link for you within your team.

The psychological contract

The concept of 'psychological contract' is a different approach to making sense of motivation and behaviour and is rooted in an understanding of organisational culture. It takes a broader perspective by considering the role of the organisation and relationships between individuals and organisations as a form of exchange. The psychological contract refers to expectations between the organisation and the individual employee in terms of obligations, privileges and rights which go beyond what is formally agreed in a written contract. It is based on expectations of what each will provide in the employment relationship. It is inevitably highly subjective and based on perceptions and beliefs about obligations.

Expectations are described as transactional (salary, working hours, safe working environment) and relational (confidence, stability, high commitment, sense of community, job security). If the organisation provides these then the individual exchanges them by giving loyalty, commitment and hard work. People working in the same organisation may have different psychological contracts.

If expectations are not met, however, the result may be a breach of the psychological contract which leads to conflict. For example, an employee may feel unsupported in taking on a new responsibility or upset if required to work longer hours.

This approach is useful in providing a framework for understanding problems in employees' behaviour and their reactions to change. It also highlights the importance of considering motivation beyond financial rewards and has been applied in studies of volunteers, for whom there are no financial incentives. Volunteers expect certain returns for their contribution to the organisation in terms of the extent to which their needs are met through, for example, organisational support, organisational success, the resources available, feedback, collegiality, identity and pride, perceived value of their contributions, and training opportunities (Taylor *et al.*, 2006).

ACTIVITY 4.6

1 Think about your current or a previous job (paid or unpaid).
2 Describe what the organisation expected of you.
3 What policies or practices did the organisation use to encourage these expectations?
4 What did you expect of the organisation?
5 How well did the organisation meet your expectations?
6 How did these expectations – and the degree to which they were met – affect your behaviour?

(based on Boddy, 2005)

THE IMPACT OF EXTERNAL INITIATIVES ON MOTIVATION

Theories about motivation are useful tools for managers in understanding individuals' motivation and the importance of factors beyond financial reward. However, these theories are inevitably fairly abstract and generic and we also need to consider the context of working in health and social care, in order to assess what other factors affect people's motivation and their ability to work together successfully in teams. A key contextual factor in health and social care is what impact *external* initiatives and policies have on people's motivation: people are working to meet their own and their organisations' needs and expectations, but linked to these is often a crucial element of 'public service motivation' based on altruism and wanting to serve the needs of the community of service users and citizens (Anderson, 2009). For some categories of staff there is also an established set of professional norms and values, which can influence motivation and behaviour.

One example of external influences was the introduction, in 2004, of the Quality and Outcomes Framework (QOF) for general practices in the UK which provided financial incentives to meet a range of quality indicators in clinical care (based on ten chronic conditions), practice organisation and patient satisfaction. The funding that a general practice receives is thus partially related to an assessment of the quality of care they provide.

Although there is growing interest internationally in the use of financial incentives to improve the quality of care, this approach does seem to contradict some aspects of the theories we have considered in this chapter about motivation: for example, the ideas contained within the notion of a psychological contract. Various commentators have highlighted the problems inherent in an externally driven approach involving financial rewards:

- The type of work that professionals carry out tends to be intrinsically motivating and is inherently satisfying and not necessarily linked to financial reward.
- Financial incentives can actually have negative effects on motivation and morale.
- The QOF is part of a general trend away from placing implicit trust in individuals towards an emphasis on performance management.
- Evidence on the use of financial incentives has shown an impact in some clinical conditions but this is contingent on the design and context of the incentive.
- Managerial incentives need to be aligned with GPs' professional values.
- External incentives can reduce internal motivation, thereby affecting behaviour and GPs' values, for example subordinating patient interests to financial gain.

(based on Roland *et al.*, 2006; McDonald *et al.*, 2007)

This list of problems seems very negative, but GPs were consulted during the design of the QOF, particularly about the measures to be used, and these have continued to be supported in practice (Roland *et al.*, 2006). It may be, therefore, that if teams are satisfied with what they are trying to achieve (in this case, improving the quality of care), and with the processes involved, the negative impacts on motivation may be reduced. There may be differences, however, between the different categories of staff involved; for example, the findings from one research study suggested that, although GPs were generally positive and experienced minimal threat to their internal motivation or core values, some nurses reported lower job satisfaction and decreased internal motivation, as well as concern about increased 'surveillance' of their work within general practices (McDonald *et al.*, 2007).

DIVERSITY AND MOTIVATION

Given the increasing diversity of the health and social care workforce in terms of age, ability, culture, ethnicity, gender, race, religion and sexual orientation, it is important to consider the impact of diversity on motivation. Factors such as feeling appreciated, earning a fair salary, and having access to promotion and training opportunities will be influenced by the extent to which staff feel that colleagues, managers, their own organisation and partner organisations understand diversity and treat the workforce equally. If employees do not get the rewards they expect due to inequalities and discrimination, then they are likely

to become demoralised and demotivated. Although there is legislation in place to protect the workforce from discrimination, there can
still be a mismatch in the assumptions and expectations held by
managers and employees.

Diversity studies as applied to management focus on transforming
diversity from being a 'problem' into becoming a 'resource' if managed
appropriately. One example is through perceiving the contribution
of diversity to providing customer service; if customers are diverse, it
is important to ensure that this diversity is reflected in the staff dealing
with them (Knights and Willmott, 2007).

**Addressing diversity and motivation in a social services department:
the aspiring managers' programme**

Fourteen staff completed the programme: 70 per cent were from ethnic
minorities, 60 per cent were women, and lesbian and gay staff were also
included. Within six months of completion, eight were in management posts,
including deputy and acting-up positions.

Participants spoke highly of the opportunity to share new experiences with
'like' colleagues in the workplace. What they valued most was a reported
increase in professional confidence linked to an increased responsibility. This
enriched their relationships with line managers, peer groups and service
users. Mentoring relationships were particularly useful and helped to develop
appreciation and respect for managers and the work they do.

Mentors found the experience rewarding on both personal and professional levels. They became more aware of their own practice and
experiences. Some mentors reported minor conflicts between the vision
and aims of the organisation and the day-to-day issues arising for staff on
the programme.

Development of management staff often takes place by sponsoring staff
on external programmes with set performance targets allowing senior
managers to get on with other priorities. This aspiring managers' programme
challenged these practices as the department had to sign up to it and deal
with the cultural issues that inevitably arise with positive action training
initiatives. Strategic ownership did not always permeate down through the
organisation. Changes in culture do not happen overnight.

Outcomes from such initiatives can be difficult to evaluate. As well as
numbers of staff completing, we were interested in the added benefits, such
as organisational learning and career opportunities for those involved – to
mention just a few. This points to the need for a longer-term evaluation.
The aspiring managers' programme had a positive effect on most participants who realised the importance of continuous learning and personal
development. Employees on the aspiring managers' programme reported
psychological rewards; they felt more valued by the organisation and were
encouraged to undertake more interesting and challenging work within it.

This is important in working towards a 'learning organisation' and motivating staff through change.

The organisation wanted to create a win-win scenario with a shared understanding of the skills, knowledge and competences desirable in managers. This was an experimental approach to developing management using traditional methods of management development, tailored to a group of potentially disadvantaged staff. It is important to use current resources and build on the potential and aspirations of people already working in the organisation.

(Edited from Hafford-Letchfield, 2005)

ACTIVITY 4.7

Use the case study above to consider how the issues raised and the type of initiative proposed compare with the experience of your team/department or organisation.

If you work in partnership with other organisations, can you identify any differences between your organisation and others in understanding and progressing diversity initiatives?

In this chapter, we have highlighted the complexity of people's motivation at work and explored some of the theories which have sought to explain motivation and how they continue to influence management thought and practice today. We have also considered the importance of thinking beyond abstract theories to incorporate issues affecting health and social care practice, including the impact of government policy on motivation, as well as the realities of diversity in influencing people's motivation and career progression.

REFERENCES

Anderson, L.B. (2009) 'What determines the behaviour and performance of health professionals? Public service motivation, professional norms and/or economic incentives', *International Review of Administrative Sciences*, vol. 75, no. 1, pp. 79–97.

Boddy, D. (2005) *Management. An Introduction*, 3rd edn, Prentice Hall/Pearson Education Ltd.

Hafford-Letchfield, T. (2005) 'On the up', <http://www.communitycare.co.uk>, 14 April (accessed 20/6/2009).

Herzberg, F. (2003) 'One more time: how do you motivate employees?', *Harvard Business Review on Motivating People*, Harvard Business School Press.

Ipsos MORI (2008) *What Matters to Staff in the NHS*, Research Study Conducted for the Department of Health, Department of Health.

Knights, D. and Willmott, H. (2007) 'Organization, structure and design', in Knights, D. and Willmott, H., *Introducing Organizational Behaviour and Management*, Thomson Learning.

Maslow, A.H. (1970) *Motivation and Personality*, Harper and Row.

Maslow, A. H., Frager, M. and Fadiman, J. (1987) *Motivation and Personality*, Pearson.

McDonald, R., Harrison, S., Checkland, K., Campbell, S. M. and Roland, M. (2007) 'Impact of financial incentives on clinical autonomy and internal motivation in primary care: ethnographic study', *BMJ Online First* (accessed 20/6/2009).

Roland, M., Campbell, S., Bailey, N., Whalley, D. and Sibbald, B. (2006) 'Financial incentives to improve the quality of primary care in the UK: predicting the consequences of change', *Primary Health Care Research and Development*, vol. 7, pp. 18–26.

Smith, M. and Smith, P. (2005) *Testing People at Work: Competencies in Psychometric Testing*, BPS Blackwell.

Taylor, T., Darcy, S., Hoye, R. and Cuskelly, G. (2006) 'Using psychological contract theory to explore issues in effective volunteer management', *European Sport Management Quarterly*, vol. 6, no. 2, pp. 123–47.

Vroom, V.H. (1964) *Work and Motivation*, Wiley.

CHAPTER 5

VALUES AND VISION

This chapter is designed to help you to identify some of the important values that underpin your work and to consider to what extent your own values are aligned with these. Managers sometime assume that the values of all the members of their team are at one with the prevalent organisational values. In practice, there are often differences that have not been recognised or understood. Assuming that values are held in common may bring difficulties because it implies that there is agreement about ways of doing things that are consistent with these values.

The values held within an organisation have an important influence on its goals and the ways in which it works. An organisation's vision is the picture of its goals – what it is trying to achieve. Vision and values are closely connected because a vision is inevitably coloured by values that view one set of goals as more desirable than another. The picture is made more complex, however, by partnership working and moving towards integrated services: there may be huge differences between organisations' values and vision.

VALUES

Values are deep-seated beliefs about what is right or wrong, and what is important and unimportant. An organisation's values are influenced both by values held in the wider world within which it functions, and also by values held by the people who work in it and who use its services. In thinking about values, it is helpful to consider these different levels. A useful mnemonic is SOGI:

■ Societal values
■ Organisational values
■ Group/team values
■ Individual values.

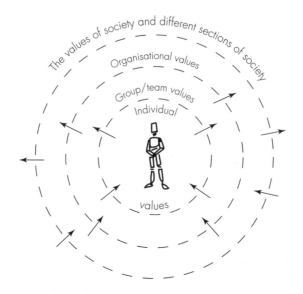

Figure 5.1 Interactions between values held at different levels

The interactions between the levels at which values are held are illustrated in Figure 5.1. The values of a society influence organisations and an organisation's values influence the values of teams and individuals within it. But the influence does not only pass downwards: individuals also influence their groups, their organisations and the society in which they live.

Societal values

Values vary enormously in different countries, communities and cultures. In Western cultures, for example, time is thought of as linear and progressing in one direction, whereas in Bali it is thought of as cyclical and in Japan as ephemeral. Darwin proposed that there is competition in the natural world between and within species; the Navaho think of the universe as a mutualism between human beings, nature, spirits, animals and ghosts. Different religions have different explanations for how the world was created, and may have one God or many. Societies are organised in different ways: democracies accept majority rule, whereas Inuit and Navajo societies are organised without hierarchies.

Modern industrial societies are complex: they include communities with very different values, living and working together in ways regulated by society as a whole. Frequently there are tensions between different societal values. In the United Kingdom, for example, there has traditionally been a tension between the extent to which a 'free market' is allowed to shape the ways in which people live and work, and the extent to which public services are funded by taxpayers to provide essential services. A mixed economy of provision based on both competition and collaboration and involving a range of public, private and voluntary service providers has gradually developed in health and social care since the 1980s. Partnership has become central to planning and delivering public services and involves working across traditional organisational boundaries as well as with communities, citizens and service users.

Public services are shaped by societal and government values. Over the past few decades, the dominant influences on health and social care have included:

- Social model of health – this holistic approach emphasises the social and psychological dimensions of health, stressing 'health' over 'sickness'. It also acknowledges that the causes of poor health are often connected to wider social and economic issues, such as poverty and deprivation, housing, employment, crime and the environment.
- Rights and responsibilities – the language of rights and responsibilities is now a key component of citizenship in the UK. The idea of a 'contract' between the individual and society is about awarding rights and opportunities but in return expecting obligations and responsibility. According to the contract, 'healthy citizens' are better able to work and make an economic contribution to the state. Clearly, this is not possible for all members of society.
- Choice and meeting service users' needs – the emphasis is on meeting individuals' particular needs and offering them choice about the services available to them.
- Working in partnership – a wider range of organisations is expected to work with the government in delivering services. Service users, citizens and communities are expected to take a greater role in planning and decision making as part of 'active citizenship' and empowerment.

In recent years, the tensions between professionals, service users and the public have been exacerbated by concerns that those who were entrusted with responsibility for public funds have not always put the interests of the public before their personal interests. Lord Nolan was asked to convene a committee to consider and report on the expectations that the public might reasonably have of those holding public office. The Nolan Committee was particularly concerned with setting principles for those who hold senior and influential positions in public life, but the values expressed in these principles might be considered appropriate for anyone with any level of responsibility in public service. The Committee reported its findings in 1996 and its principles continue to influence codes of practice (for example, that of the Institute of Healthcare Management).

Selflessness

Holders of public office should act solely in the public interest. They should not gain financial or other material benefits for themselves, their family or their friends.

Integrity

Holders of public office should not place themselves under any financial or other obligation to outside individuals or organisations that might seek to influence them in the performance of their official duties.

Objectivity

Holders of public office should make choices on merit in carrying out public business, including making public appointments, awarding contracts or recommending individuals for rewards and benefits.

Accountability

Holders of public office are accountable to the public for their decisions and actions. They must submit themselves to whatever scrutiny is appropriate to their office.

Openness

Holders of public office should be as open as possible about all the decisions and actions that they take. They should give reasons for their decisions and restrict information only when the wider public interest clearly demands it.

Honesty

Holders of public office have a duty to declare any private interests relating to their public duties and to take steps to resolve any conflicts that may arise in a way that protects the public interest.

Leadership

Holders of public office should promote and support these principles by leadership and example.

(Nolan Committee, 1996)

This statement of principles is helpful in making the notion of a 'public service ethic' more explicit. You may have personal experience of feeling compromised by the expectations of others. For example, you may have been offered a free lunch by a sales representative who hoped to be rewarded by your support for a decision to purchase their drugs or equipment. You may have been offered some benefit for giving someone preferential treatment or you may have been asked to help someone to jump the queue for a service. It is more difficult to be selfless in a situation like the last one if you see a member of your own family in pain and waiting for an operation. If you have been involved in appointing staff or in contracting for services provided by other organisations, you will recognise the importance of objectivity, openness and accountability.

If you are managing in an organisation in the voluntary or private sector, your service users are also likely to expect you and your organisation to demonstrate values similar to those expressed by the Nolan Committee's principles. They will also expect selflessness, integrity, objectivity, accountability, openness, honesty and leadership to be evident. Within society as a whole, people who work in various professions and occupations often have their own sets of values which, though drawing on broader societal values, have their own particular characteristics. These are often expressed in the form of codes of ethics or statements of values or standards. The multi-occupational nature of health and social care means that different sets of values can be seen within a single organisation, or between organisations that are working collaboratively to deliver a coherent service to patients or service users. Here are three examples.

British Association of Social Workers

Social work is committed to five basic values:

- human dignity and worth
- social justice
- service to humanity
- integrity
- competence.

Social work practice should both promote respect for human dignity and pursue social justice, through service to humanity, integrity and competence.

Institute of Healthcare Management

The IHM have based their code of conduct on the Nolan Committee principles:

- integrity: members should act in such a way as to generate and maintain the trust and confidence of the patients and clients at all times. This includes the rejection of any gifts and hospitality which might be interpreted as seeking to extend influence.

continued

continued

■ honesty and openness: members should be open and honest about the decisions and actions they take.

■ probity: implies using resources responsibly and showing loyalty at all times to the employing or contracting organisation but embraces the right to challenge decisions and actions that are believed to be against the patient's or client's interests.

■ accountability: ensuring that members are able to justify their actions, or lack of action, under political or public scrutiny.

■ respect: respecting others by giving one's best at all times and keeping up to date with best practice.

In addition every member has a responsibility towards:

■ the environment: to have awareness of energy and environment conservation and that decisions for eliminating waste and recycling are made in partnership with the community as a whole, and beyond the minimum requirements of the law.

■ society: respecting and understanding the impact of one's actions, not only on the immediately surrounding society in which they live and work, but also within the community with whom they may negotiate and purchase.

General Medical Council

Patients must be able to trust doctors with their lives and health. To justify that trust you must show respect for human life and you must:

■ make the care of your patient your first concern
■ protect and promote the health of patients and the public
■ provide a good standard of practice and care
■ treat patients as individuals and respect their dignity
■ work in partnership with patients
■ be honest and open and act with integrity.

You are personally accountable for your professional practice and must always be prepared to justify your decisions and actions.

ACTIVITY 5.1

If you were the manager of a service in which doctors contribute to its delivery, are there any aspects of doctors' values that could potentially conflict with values held by other members of your team?

There is little in the General Medical Council's statement about efficiency, choice, democracy or universality. It focuses primarily on the relationship of the doctor with the individual patient rather than the relationship with the general public. Thus, for example, keeping to appointment times in clinics may be seen by doctors as less important than taking enough time to give full attention to the patient in front of them. The focus on the individual patient may also sometimes lead to a tension between delivery of a service to one person and delivery of that service to many people.

Organisational values

Organisations develop values and beliefs about how staff should behave and how work and staff are managed. Values embedded in an organisation's culture could include dress codes at work, behaviour at meetings (are people confrontational or supportive?), the importance of meeting deadlines and time-keeping, whether staff are encouraged to use their initiative or follow the rules, and the importance of social occasions organised through work. In recruiting new staff, some organisations may use personality tests in addition to interviews in order to assess the 'fit' of candidates both against their organisational values and culture, as well as their perceptions of the values required of the candidate for that particular post.

Organisations in the health and social care sector are guided by values expressed at a national level. Here are some examples drawn from the health service that reflect the influence of government policy.

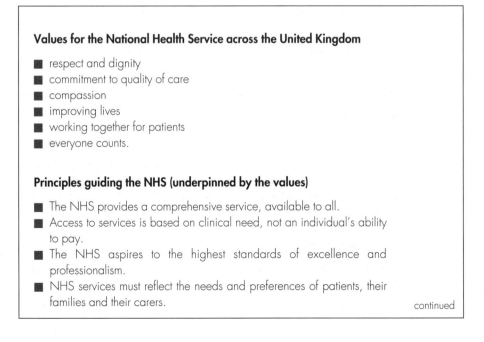

Values for the National Health Service across the United Kingdom

- respect and dignity
- commitment to quality of care
- compassion
- improving lives
- working together for patients
- everyone counts.

Principles guiding the NHS (underpinned by the values)

- The NHS provides a comprehensive service, available to all.
- Access to services is based on clinical need, not an individual's ability to pay.
- The NHS aspires to the highest standards of excellence and professionalism.
- NHS services must reflect the needs and preferences of patients, their families and their carers.

continued

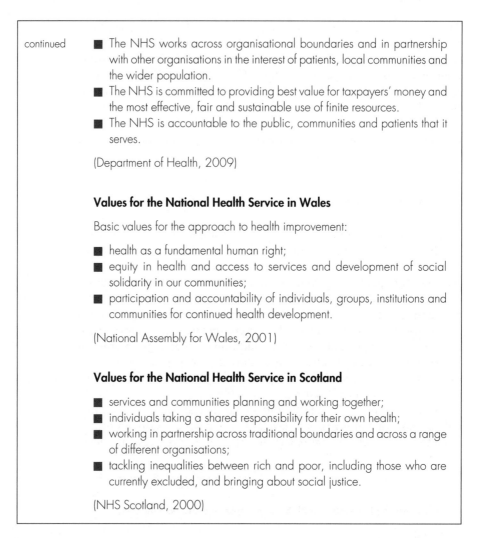

continued

■ The NHS works across organisational boundaries and in partnership with other organisations in the interest of patients, local communities and the wider population.

■ The NHS is committed to providing best value for taxpayers' money and the most effective, fair and sustainable use of finite resources.

■ The NHS is accountable to the public, communities and patients that it serves.

(Department of Health, 2009)

Values for the National Health Service in Wales

Basic values for the approach to health improvement:

■ health as a fundamental human right;

■ equity in health and access to services and development of social solidarity in our communities;

■ participation and accountability of individuals, groups, institutions and communities for continued health development.

(National Assembly for Wales, 2001)

Values for the National Health Service in Scotland

■ services and communities planning and working together;

■ individuals taking a shared responsibility for their own health;

■ working in partnership across traditional boundaries and across a range of different organisations;

■ tackling inequalities between rich and poor, including those who are currently excluded, and bringing about social justice.

(NHS Scotland, 2000)

ACTIVITY 5.2

The statements of values in the box are taken from government documents in the United Kingdom in general and in Wales and Scotland. Many of the themes will be familiar to you whether you work in health or social care and whether you work in one of the countries in the examples or elsewhere – the emphasis on reforming public services is international. Some of them will be relevant even if you work in the private or voluntary sectors.

Identify any values from these examples that you recognise as concerns within your area of work.

All the statements have an emphasis on partnership working across organisational boundaries and with local communities. The values for the UK as a whole and Wales highlight equity and equal access, which were founding principles of the NHS. Participation by service users/and or communities is mentioned in all three sets of values.

The Scottish values bring a different perspective by highlighting broader influences on people's health such as social inequalities and social justice. These values fit well with the notion of a social model of health. The Scottish values also specify shared responsibility for health (fitting with notions of citizenship and rights and responsibilities) and the UK-wide values bring in the importance of addressing needs and preferences of service users.

The UK-wide statement refers to standards of excellence and providing best value for taxpayers' money and efficiency in using resources.

All these themes are related to reforming services in ways that fit more closely with public expectations as well as meeting national and local needs. Although the examples were drawn from health services, the themes that emerge are relevant to all areas of public services and are central to the aim of providing integrated services rather than separate specialist services. People who are working in health services, for example, are increasingly working with people in social care, housing and education. There is an emphasis on making sure that services are integrated or streamlined and do not leave patients and service users with their needs only partially met.

The Institute for Public Policy Research (1999) attempted to identify eight values that provide a national health service with its 'moral base':

- good health – a commitment to improving the nation's health;
- efficiency in the use of public resources – treatments should provide high value relative to opportunity costs;
- equity – with recognition that this is a major issue given the climate of priority-setting and rationing;
- choice – the state should allow some degree of personal choice for individuals;
- democracy – public accountability for the quality of service provision;
- respect for human dignity – the relationship between the provider and the receiver of health care should reflect this;
- public service – includes some of the above but also covers 'altruism rather than profit' and the notion that health service staff should work for the common good;
- universality – a service for all, paid for by everyone via taxation, is essential to provide security and reassurance to the population and to foster social cohesion.

The Institute's report acknowledged that some of these values conflict: for example, patient choice may conflict with efficiency. The public may place a much higher value on access to a local hospital threatened with closure than on (possibly) higher-quality outcomes for a small group of patients with a particular condition.

This list of values relates to a national health service as a whole, but you will probably be able to identify organisational values in relation to the unit or department in which you work. However, within a large organisation like a hospital or a social services department, the extent to which staff are aware of and influenced by organisational values can vary enormously. A junior doctor or social worker may be completely unaware of the hospital's or department's values and may identify far more readily with the values of his or her medical college or professional association. It is therefore unlikely that a large, complex organisation has a single unified culture and set of values.

In addition, there is sometimes inconsistency between the values that an organisation tries to uphold and those that it demonstrates in its actions. This is sometimes referred to as the difference between an organisation's *espoused* values and its *enacted* values.

Group/team values

Within health and social care organisations, there is usually a complex array of staff teams comprising people from many occupational areas and, increasingly, people from other organisations brought into an integrated service. This could result in several possibly competing or conflicting sets of values. Teams that work together regularly often adopt common values that focus on the purpose of their work, and recognise the contribution made by team members who bring particular and different skills. In addition to these teams, as we said earlier, an increasing number of groups within the community have their own sets of values. These groups seek to influence the values of organisations, teams and individuals that are responsible for health and social care. Their values are often expressed in codes of practice directed towards the behaviour they expect of health and social care professionals. Here is an example that focuses on empowering users of services for people with mental illness.

Here a service user proposes some dos and don'ts for staff wanting to relate to individual service users in ways which are empowering:

1   DO let us know what our rights are. Often we feel we have none, and are treated as if we have none. Let us know about our rights to refuse treatment, leave, make a complaint, or be represented at a mental health tribunal. It helps to be told more than once, and also to be given the information in writing.

2 DON'T hide behind a mask of professionalism. Don't use words we don't understand. Don't pretend you know more than you do. Mental health work is full of uncertainty, confusion, controversy and contradictions. Honesty is empowering.

3 DO ask us what we want. You may not be able to provide it. You may disagree. But do ask us. Potentially at least, we are the experts on our own needs.

4 DON'T dismiss our complaints and worries as symptoms of our 'mental illness'. Too often people's physical illnesses have been disregarded, women sexually molested in hospitals and hostels have not been believed, and genuine grievances have not been taken seriously.

5 DO recognise our talents, capabilities and potential. Support us in trying new activities, taking on responsibilities and finding outlets for our creativity.

6 DON'T panic when we express feelings. Often it is useful to sob, shout, scream, shake or shiver. We appreciate being listened to and encouraged. We want space to do that without disturbing other people.

7 DO tell us as much as you can about the drugs we are on, the diagnosis we have and the options open to us.

8 DON'T write us off. We are fed up with being told 'You will have to take these pills for the rest of your life' or 'There's no cure for manic depression'. Throwaway, negative or dismissive remarks may cause great hurt and be a source of pain to us for years. Many of us have overcome the most disabling distress, often despite the pessimistic predictions of so-called experts.

9 DO talk to us. Emotional distress is isolating. Help us break through it. Be friendly and treat us as equals. But don't try to force us to talk when we clearly don't want to.

10 DON'T forget that we live in a multicultural society, in which people have different beliefs and values. Learn all you can about the people who use your service, not least by asking them.

(Cited in Spear et al., 1994)

ACTIVITY 5.3

Read through these dos and don'ts again. How might service users for whom you are responsible feel? Make a note of anything that you could do or influence that might make the service better from the point of view of service users (or the people who use your services if you are in finance, administration, or another supporting or commissioning service).

This perspective might be one that you have not considered before, particularly if the setting in which you work puts more emphasis on the operational side of service delivery than on the experiences of service users. Could this code of practice be applied to any service?

Other managers may be more familiar with the need to consider values in delivery of services. For example, values are recognised as an important element of competence for those who practise in social care. The expectations are explicit in two of the standards set for vocational qualifications in care:

Promote people's equality, diversity and rights.

Develop, maintain and evaluate systems and structures to promote the rights, responsibilities and diversity of clients.

These values place a responsibility on managers in a care setting to do rather more than respect the equality, diversity and rights of other people. There is an explicit expectation that they should be proactive in promoting these values, and in developing systems and structures that demonstrate that these values are underpinning practice.

Many service teams have statements of their guiding principles which, although differing in detail, have much in common. Here are some examples.

Older people's team

To respect the dignity and choice of older people, and to enable them to enjoy the maximum independence possible, whether their choice is to live at home or in residential care.

Mental health team

Everyone experiences stress at times of crisis. This can sometimes trigger a mental illness. People with a mental illness should be treated with dignity and respect, and be given the chance to make informed choices about their care whenever possible. Support should be offered in the community to enable independent living and to minimise the need for institutional care.

Physical disability team

To base services on the recognition of individual needs; to help and enable people to live a lifestyle of their choice, as fully and as independently as possible, in their community.

Learning difficulties team

To enable people with learning difficulties to secure a normal way of life, living independently wherever possible; to support and consult families and carers about their needs; to enable people to develop their potential to the maximum; to recognise their ambitions and preferences, and to protect their legal and human rights.

(Adapted from Williams, 1989)

As public services are encouraged to develop more integrated provision and to work more closely together, the values underlying principles like these need to be more widely discussed and considered from a number of perspectives if they are to be implemented across services.

Individual values

If you were asked what your personal values are, would you find it easy to explain them? The next Activity might help you to clarify some of them.

ACTIVITY 5.4

Imagine that you are discussing your area of work with a close friend. What will you say? Complete the following sentences:

One of my greatest concerns is _____

One thing that I would really like to change is _____

If there was enough money I would _____

I get most angry about _____

I am most proud of _____

Now read through your sentences and try to identify what values underlie each statement. For example, if you said that one of your greatest concerns is the time that some service users have to wait before they can receive an important service, your values might be related to equal opportunities or quality of life.

Our personal values arise from the values of our social background, our religion (if we have one), our ethnic origin or subculture, our upbringing and education, and our experience of life and work. They continue to develop and change throughout our lives as we encounter new and contradictory situations, and as we reflect on our experiences. Our early values are based on the culture in which we grew up, often in the narrow confines of a family or social group. It is not until we experience unfamiliar settings that we encounter views and behaviours that surprise us or, sometimes, offend us. We then have opportunities to consider the values that we hold which cause us to respond as we do. Some people are very aware of their values and how they use them when making judgements, but others make judgements without questioning the value base that underpins them. We are all individuals and we are all different. No wonder that it is sometimes difficult for an individual to fit in with a group or an organisation!

ACTIVITY 5.5

How familiar are you with the values of your organisation or service? You might find statements of values in annual reports, staff handbooks or information leaflets for service users. Think about your personal values – particularly those that influence your choice of the work you do. Make a note of areas in which you are comfortable with the ways that you are able to work in your organisation or service. Then make a note of any aspects of your work that you feel do not fully fit with your personal values.

Individual values fit broadly into two types – those that are about how you think things should be done and those that are about goals. Values about how things should be done include working hard, and being honest, open-minded and forgiving. Values about goals include happiness, prosperity, accomplishments and self-respect. The challenge is to understand your own values and why you hold them, so that you can be more aware of how other people are driven by their values. If you can recognise the differences and tensions that arise from value conflicts, you are more likely to be able to help to resolve them. It is often possible to secure agreement over the core values of service delivery, and to work from that agreement to an understanding of how individuals and teams can contribute to the work of the organisation without feeling that their values are being compromised. If you challenge another person's values, you may appear to be challenging very personal issues – even the other person's identity.

As an individual, have you considered the values you hold with respect to other people's equality, diversity and rights? It is important for you to be aware of them if you are not to be prejudiced when you have to make judgements in delivering any aspect of a service. Prejudice is based on assumptions made about the world. It has no rational basis. It is often difficult to identify our own prejudices because they are often associated with assumptions that are central to our sense of personal security. When our assumptions are challenged, we feel uncomfortable and have to deal with our feelings as well as with the issues that have been raised. Managers in health and social care work in complex settings in which their personal values are sometimes challenged. The assumptions that they have been able to make in previous settings may no longer be appropriate. It is helpful to develop the ability to listen and to suspend judgement for a while, even to take time to check out an issue with a colleague if it is outside your experience.

ACTIVITY 5.6

O'Hagan (1996) suggested the following list of beliefs that underpin the values that an individual might hold in relation to child care. Tick those with which you agree.

I believe that:

- ☐ any child's welfare is of paramount importance
- ☐ children should be listened to and respected
- ☐ every child is a unique individual
- ☐ parents are individuals with their own needs
- ☐ parents have rights as well as responsibilities
- ☐ children should be raised in families
- ☐ child care services should be an expression of social justice and must be anti-discriminatory
- ☐ child care workers are individuals who have rights and feelings.

Depending on which of these beliefs you have ticked, you might have a problem when there is a conflict between the interests of a child and the interests of the parents. It might then be necessary for you to make judgements about the relevance and relative weighting of each value, and these could change according to the circumstances. If there is a situation in which a child may be at risk because of the behaviour of a parent, there is a tension between assisting the parent to gain control and to improve the quality of his or her life, and taking action to prevent harm to the child. However, there is legislation and policy within *Every Child Matters* (Department for Education and Skills, 2004) governing how public services must treat children and, in addition, your organisation may have set out key values to guide practice. These must override your personal values.

Anyone in a management role has to work within the values of their organisation and also has to be aware of their own values, the values held by the various individuals and teams in their area of work, and those held by patients, service users and carers.

MANAGING INTERORGANISATIONAL VALUES AND VISION

A vision can be created by an individual or by a group of people: it describes a desirable future in a way that conveys meaning and inspiration to others. Vision is therefore closely associated with values. The word 'desirable' carries a multitude of value implications, as each aspect of a desirable future implies a judgement about what is good and what is not. Vision has overtones of seeing something that is not clear to everyone, seeing details that others are not able to see and being able to convey to others a picture of an optimistic future that they have not imagined. One of the characteristics associated with leadership is the ability to identify a vision and convey it to others – the leader does not necessarily have to be the person who creates the vision.

Once there is a clear picture of the outcomes that an organisation is aiming to achieve, it is much easier to plan how the vision can be attained. By clarifying goals, a vision can give more meaning to the day-to-day activities that take the organisation into its future. Since all individuals can contribute to achieving the objectives of the organisation, they can also relate to the organisation's vision, and understand how their actions can help to shape its future.

Some organisations involve all their staff in developing their vision. This is probably the best way to ensure that everyone feels part of the outcome and is committed to the vision. However, it is more usual for the most senior leaders of an organisation to develop and communicate the vision, and for managers at lower levels to be involved in developing the strategies and plans that are needed to work towards achieving it. These managers thus have the opportunity to demonstrate their own leadership skills in interpreting the vision with their teams.

Vision is important because it offers a picture of the future state that an organisation or service wants to achieve. It is a picture of the outcome for which to aim. When a new integrated service or partnership organisation is established, developing a shared vision becomes crucial. Sharing a vision highlights that the different groups are working well together, and the statements contained within the vision give people (staff and service users) a clear idea of how the service can develop and lead to service improvement.

Yet the process of developing shared aims and vision is frequently reported as fraught with difficulties. As we saw earlier, tension may arise when different sets of values come together in a partnership arrangement. There can be historical differences between organisations or professions, assumptions about how things ought to be done and what needs to be accomplished and, even where the same values are shared, different people may highlight different priorities (Genefke, 2001). The history of partnership working in a locality can become part of the local culture, particularly where it includes negative experiences, and this legacy may continue to exert an influence on how well people work together (Charlesworth, 2001). Thus there are many factors influencing the process of developing and sustaining a shared vision in a new organisation or service.

Managers talk about new partnerships

Partnership is very hard work, you don't all just sit down, agree you're going to work together and everything's hunky-dory. It all starts falling apart at different points when you discover how different you are.

(PCT manager)

Previous joint working had been dominated by processes, attitudes and values that were locked into the public sector. We needed to find new ways of working in partnership; we needed to do it differently. So we rebadged it. It will have its own logo. It will have its own way it presents information, shares information. We will not be in the normal committee style. For me the hallmark of a good partnership is to do with process more than outcome and I think people look back with warm, glowing feelings about things they've done in partnership, but it tends to be because of that high level of co-operative working and trust which has developed round process and is almost incidental in terms of the outcome. So yes, they were united in terms of what they wanted to do, that was the vehicle, the target they wanted to get to, but actually it was the way they went about working together that taught them the lessons and gave them the trust and confidence to work together in other ways. But you need to get some decent co-working going, develop a confidence and that becomes trust and from that trust, you then start to get some serious changes. Both sides can understand each other and I think tribal behaviour will only be overcome once you've gone through that sort of evolution and then maybe one of the outcomes is you get away from some of the tribal badging and professional description of what people do into something more generic and more partnership focused.

(Director of partnerships)

The action plan was based on a wide ranging consultation and importantly set out the views of children and young people regarding service delivery. Children and young people were saying they wanted consistency from the people who supported them and did not want to have to tell their story several times. Placing the child at the

continued

continued   centre, rather than the service, reinforced the move to needs-led
services and created organisational and cultural challenges to services
which had their own developmental histories. The children's services
management team agreed to use 'How good is your team' [a self-
evaluation tool], seeing this as part of the wider picture of continuous
improvement and service development and reinforcing the ownership
of service development throughout the organisation.

(Strategic development officer, children's services)

ACTIVITY 5.7

From these examples of managers' experiences, highlight issues that
you have personally experienced in developing shared aims or vision,
or which you can envisage being problematic if you were to work more
closely with another organisation.

In this chapter, we have described the different sets of values that may
influence you and your work. These can be your personal values, as well
as those of your organisation and also wider societal and government
values. We concluded by highlighting the complex nature of managing
shared – and possibly conflicting – values in working in partnership
with other organisations or in developing an integrated service, and in
developing a shared vision.

REFERENCES

British Association of Social Workers <http://www.basw.co.uk> (accessed
20/6/2009).

Charlesworth, J. (2001) 'Negotiating and managing partnership in primary
care', *Health and Social Care in the Community*, vol. 9, no. 5, pp. 279–85.

Department for Education and Skills (2004) *Every Child Matters*, The
Stationery Office.

Department of Health (2009) *The NHS Constitution*, available online
<http://www.dh.gov.uk>.

Genefke, J. (2001) 'Joining two organisational units: managing cultural threats
and possibilities', in Genefke, J. and McDonald, F. (eds) *Effective
Collaboration: Managing the Obstacles to Success*, Palgrave.

General Medical Council <http://www.gmc-uk.org/guidance/good_medical_
practice/index.asp> (accessed 20/6/2009).

Institute of Healthcare Management <http://www.ihm.org.uk> (accessed
20/6/2009).

Institute for Public Policy Research (1999) *A Good Enough Service: Values, Trade-offs and the NHS*, IPPR.

National Assembly for Wales (2001) *Improving Health in Wales: A Plan for the NHS with its Partners*, National Assembly for Wales.

NHS Scotland (2000) *Our National Health. A Plan for Action, a Plan for Change*, Scottish Executive.

Nolan Committee (1996) *First Report of the Committee on Standards in Public Life*, The Stationery Office.

O'Hagan, K. (ed.) (1996) *Competence in Social Work Practice*, Jessica Kingsley Publishers.

Spear, R., Leonetti, A. and Thomas, A. (1994) *Third Sector Care*, Open University/Department of Trade and Industry.

Williams, F. (1989) *Social Policy: A Critical Introduction*, Polity Press.

PART 2

MANAGING FOR SERVICE USERS

CHAPTER 6

WHAT DO YOUR SERVICE USERS WANT?

Almost everyone who works in health and social care is, at one level or another, aware that their function is to deliver – or to support the delivery of – care to service users. However, there are a number of other types of 'customer' in health and social care services. For example, if you work in a home care service in the voluntary or private sector, the local social services or social work department is, in a rather different sense, also your customer. If you work in an out-patient physiotherapy department, local general practitioners (GPs) are also your customers. If you work in a payroll department, all the staff whose payslips you prepare are your customers. As a manager, you might also view the staff in your team as your customers.

So, given the size and complexity of many of the organisations that provide health and social care, among the critical issues for you as a manager are:

- identifying who your customers are
- understanding what it is that they require
- knowing how effectively you are meeting their requirements.

The aim of this chapter is to help you improve the responsiveness of your services to the needs, wants and expectations of your customers.

DIFFERENT KINDS OF CUSTOMER

The terms used to describe people who are the recipients of health and social care services have been and continue to be the basis of much discussion – and changing fashion. 'Patient' is still commonly used in the health service, 'client' has been a favourite word in social care and 'service user' is regarded by many as a more neutral term in both. Another important term in common use is 'carer', meaning some-one who provides a significant level of support to a person in need of health or social care (often a relative or partner, though not necessarily living with the person being cared for). Carers may also require services, and many have needs and views that differ from those of other service users.

The concepts of customer and consumer have added to the confusion for public service managers in recent years. As Clarke *et al.* (2007) highlight, some people would not see themselves as customers of a service such as the police or some areas of mental health services (i.e. they are not customers by choice). Their research further illustrated how, even in a private care home, a care worker found it difficult to think of her residents as customers since that implied a formal relationship with the organisation, and did not cover the personal relationship she had with residents.

For the moment, however, we are going to use the term 'customer' to describe all those who receive services from health and social care organisations – including service users and carers, and also including those who commission services on their behalf and those within organisations who receive, for example, financial, training and information management services. We are using the term 'customer' to emphasise a particular kind of relationship between those who provide a service and those who use it. Instead of seeing service users as people whose requirements are assessed by the provider and who are then offered a service that the provider defines and controls – we need to see them as people who have an understanding of their requirements and who can make choices about the nature of the service most likely to meet these requirements, which has resonance with the concept of the 'expert' or 'responsible' service user.

We are all customers: every day we buy and receive services from many different providers – banks, shops, transport operators, and so on. The success of each of these providers depends on them delivering what we, as customers, want, such as a reliable, convenient and friendly service and value for money. Satisfying customer requirements is a key element of providing a quality service.

As customers we are often not particularly concerned with *how* our requirements are met. The fact that buying a can of beans involves a complex network of suppliers is of little interest to us. However, managing that network is a critically important task for providers. They need to ensure that all the goods and services that allow them to provide what their customers require are available to the correct level of quality, where and when they are required.

The plethora of agencies involved with commissioning and providing health and social care creates a complex web of customer–supplier relationships. Even within a single organisation such as a hospital, there is a network of providers and customers. The pharmacy provides the barium meal for the radiologist-customer who provides the X-ray for the surgeon-customer who needs to perform a bowel operation on the patient-customer because the gastroenterologist-customer's diagnosis, requested by the local referring GP-customer, has proved correct. The subsequent successful operation is of great interest to the primary care trust-customer which has invested extra cash to help deal with waiting lists.

A helpful way of simplifying the complexity is to stick to the fundamental point: service users are the ultimate customers. They are at the centre of defining and delivering health and social care services. They are the reason that the services exist: the complex interlocking network of health and social care services is constructed to meet their needs. As a manager within a large organisation, however, it is easy to lose sight of what the job is really about and how you can ensure that the efforts of your department or service are contributing effectively. How easy it is to keep in touch with these things probably depends on your function and that of your team.

Whatever your job within health or social care, your most important customer is always the service user, though there will always be other departments or agencies inside or outside your organisation who are also your customers. If you are part of a team that has direct contact with service users, it will be clear that they are your customers. However, if you are providing a service that supports those who have direct contact with service users, you and your staff may rarely come into contact with them. You may offer services, for example the delivery of catering services, the maintenance of essential equipment or the payment of bills, directly to *internal customers*, other departments within your organisation. In these circumstances, knowing how much you contribute to meeting the needs of service users is more difficult to assess because of your remoteness from them.

ACTIVITY 6.1

Describe in a few words two services that you and your team provide and note the customer(s) for each. Keep your list – you will need it later.

A hospital trust provides services for patients in the district (and further afield), referred to the hospital by local GPs. Who is the hospital's customer – the patient, the GP or the primary care trust (to which it has a degree of accountability)? A community meals service provides services for a local authority's social services department on behalf of older and disabled people living at home who have been referred to the service by social workers and others. Who is this service's customer – the social services department, the person who receives the meals or the social worker? The answer in both cases is all three, but each one will have a different interest in the services being provided. Your customers may be various and, to meet the variety of their requirements, you have to be clear about what exactly each is seeking. What is needed is a way of thinking about the array of customers of (and in) health and social care. Let's look at two ways of approaching this – through the notions of *customer roles* and *customer chains*.

Customer roles

To introduce the concept of customer roles, have a look at the following account of a service and try to identify the customers.

A 'clubhouse' for Bromley

Horizon House is a 'clubhouse' run by Oxleas NHS Foundation Trust (a specialist mental health trust) for people recovering from mental illness and supporting them in their return to employment. The clubhouse concept is that people attending are club members rather than service users – with lifelong membership of the clubhouse. Members and staff work together to run all aspects of the clubhouse, such as running the reception desk, cooking and shopping, visiting other members, assisting other members to pursue their careers. Transitional employment placements are offered with employers, giving members the opportunity to use their newly acquired or recovered skills with security, resulting in a gain of personal confidence. This sometimes enables members to go on to obtain employment on the open market. Horizon House is accredited by The International Centre for Clubhouse Development (ICCD), which has developed a series of standards.

In the clubhouse project, the ultimate customers are the members who benefit from the service. So the first major customer role is that of *beneficiary*. However, there are a number of other 'customers' without whom the clubhouse would not exist. Oxleas NHS Foundation Trust specifies the clubhouse project as part of its strategy for mental health services. It is assisted in its role of *specifier* by the ICCD which sets the standards for the organisation's classification as a clubhouse. The costs of running the clubhouse fall to the Trust and thence to the Department of Health, who thus fulfil the role of *payer*. Day to day, however, the running of the clubhouse is carried out by its staff, including volunteers, and also by the members themselves. The members, then, as well as beneficiaries, play another customer role, that of *participants*. Figure 6.1 is a diagram of the players and their roles in the Horizon House clubhouse example.

To explore these roles further, you can try applying them to your own situation in the following Activity.

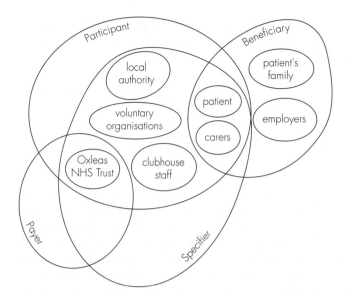

Figure 6.1 Players and their roles in the Horizon House clubhouse project

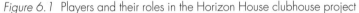

ACTIVITY 6.2

For one of the services you identified in your own area of work, either write down or illustrate with a diagram like Figure 6.1:

- who benefits from the service
- who specifies what is required
- who pays for that service
- who participates in the delivery of the service.

Although the four customer roles of beneficiary, specifier, payer and participant are distinct, you may have found that:

- One of the roles is played by more than one customer (for Bromley, there were several specifiers).
- One customer plays more than one role (Oxleas NHS Trust played both specifier and payer and even, arguably, beneficiary).
- One of the roles is not played at all (this is not the case in the Bromley example, but some voluntary services do not have a formal payer).
- Some roles are played by customers outside the system (in Bromley, members' families and employers have benefited from the clubhouse project, and some services – such as cervical screening – may be specified by national initiatives quite remote from local circumstances).

Despite these complications, identifying the four separate customer roles can be helpful. It may begin to suggest to you what influences or controls the delivery of the services for which you are responsible, and where you might want to intervene to make improvements.

However, if you have different people or agencies taking different customer roles, there are three reasons why you may have quite a challenging job on your hands:

■ Where there are several different customers, the volume of work in keeping them all happy may be a test of your time-management and organisational skills.
■ Tensions may arise from serving several customers with different roles at the same time. Many managers will appreciate what it is like 'changing gear' between service users, their representatives (such as advocacy groups or voluntary organisations) and the commissioners of the service, not to mention their own line management.
■ There may be potential for conflict in the different interests of the players of a single customer role. Conflicts are most likely around the specifier role: for example, clinical staff might want the most up-to-date treatment services which require expensive equipment, the Trust might want the most economic services, and patient representatives might want the services that give patients the most say in their own treatment. But other customer roles are also not without the potential for conflict: for example, the payer role for home care services is usually shared between a local authority social services department and service users, and some service users may find the scale of the charges difficult to meet.

In situations of potential conflict, your communication and negotiating skills will be tested: there are often no easy solutions to clashes of priorities between customers. Making judgements about the relative significance of conflicting requirements is part of your job as a manager and requires you to be:

■ clear in your objectives
■ consistent in setting priorities
■ forthright in communication
■ imaginative and flexible in planning.

Keeping the four customer roles in your mind as a framework should help you to define the relationship between your services and their various customers, and to set priorities between their requirements and your services.

In the case of a community meals service, for example, all the specifiers need some involvement in deciding what the purpose of the service is. Is it to do the following:

■ enable people to continue to live at home?
■ improve their quality of life?

- provide regular contact with the person delivering the food?
- keep the price of meals down to a level that is easily afforded by an older person on a state pension?
- facilitate the discharge of older people from hospital?
- avoid the costs of more expensive residential care?
- allow carers who normally provide hot meals to take a break?

The priority given to each of these purposes will determine what service is provided, how it is provided, and by whom. Arriving at a 'best fit' will involve resolving conflicts between the priorities of the different customers. For instance, improvements in food technology present a choice between delivering frozen meals in bulk or offering the regular daily contact of a person who delivers a hot meal.

Customer chains

We have highlighted some of the management complexities that derive from the variety of your customers and the various roles they play in the delivery of your services.

However, your services form only part of the complex network of health and social care. For the benefit of service users, the ultimate customers, all these services have to work in concert.

The key to coming to grips with sorting out relationships with customers is the notion of chains. A simple example is the manufacture of taxis. The taxi cab is a culmination of a series of activities that all contribute in one way or another to the car we finally ride in.

The taxi

The person who grinds the valves on the engine can feel that he or she is making an essential contribution to the finished product. The car will not work without properly ground valves. The immediate beneficiary of the valve grinder's job is the engine assembler. The valve grinder's customer is the engine assembly company.

The engine assembly company sells the completed engines to the motor manufacturer which may be a separate company or a distinct part of the same organisation. The manufacturer benefits from receiving assembled engines. The motor manufacturer is therefore the engine assembly company's customer.

The motor manufacturer sells complete taxis to its customers – the distributors. The distributors sell the taxis to their customers – the purchasers of the taxis. The purchaser of the taxi is the customer of the final product, but is not the final beneficiary. Ultimately the taxi passengers will be the customers who benefit and will pay to finance the whole chain of activities involved in producing the taxi.

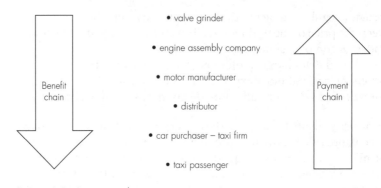

- valve grinder

- engine assembly company

- motor manufacturer

- distributor

- car purchaser – taxi firm

- taxi passenger

Benefit chain

Payment chain

Figure 6.2 Customer chains

In this example there is a clear chain of benefit passed from one customer to the next along the chain. Hence, the ultimate customers – the passengers – are the customers of the valve grinder, even though the valve grinder never encounters them and is part of a totally separate organisation. There is also a clear chain of payment which gets passed up the chain (Figure 6.2).

The chain of benefit

Just as the taxi passenger receives the benefit that results from a chain of activities culminating in a taxi journey, so does the service user in the delivery of health or social care. The example we used at the beginning of this chapter illustrated how a chain of service providers lies behind a patient's bowel operation. The pharmacy contributes the barium meal, the radiographer provides the X-ray picture, the surgeon performs the operation. There are other chains too: the works department maintains the physical condition of the ward, which is managed day to day by the ward sister/charge nurse, whose style is reflected in the standard of care delivered by the nurses. After the operation, the patient will be unable to eat normally and will need feeding intravenously. The recipe for the parenteral nutrition will be made up by the pharmacist with the advice of the surgeon and nursing staff, and will depend on the patient's metabolism and needs, information on which will come from the pathology laboratory.

So chains of service, from the point of view of service users, are not single lines, but more like a tree or river system. Although the complete network of customer chains may be complex, each strand is a simple linear sequence: the benefits flow along each strand towards the service user. The benefit chain for our example is shown in Figure 6.3.

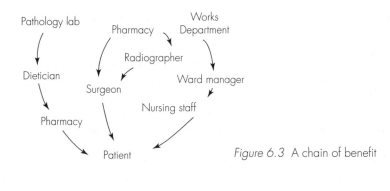

Figure 6.3 A chain of benefit

ACTIVITY 6.3

Map the chain of customers who benefit from one of your services.

Wherever you started your chain, you should have the service user as one of the beneficiaries near the end of your chain. If you work directly with service users, your chain may be quite short. Most managers, however, will have several links in the chain.

The specification chain

Returning to the taxi manufacturing example, taxi purchasers will decide which colour and model they want to buy. This will put demands on the distributor, which will have to specify what it wants from the manufacturer. These specifications will then be translated into requirements for components from their suppliers, so the engine assembly company will receive a specification for engines that will include a requirement for valves to be ground by the valve grinder. There is thus a chain of customers playing the specifying role which percolates through each element of the chain right back to the valve grinder. In taxi manufacturing, specification follows the benefit chain in the reverse direction. In health and social care, however, the chain of specifying customers is often somewhat different from the chain of benefiting customers.

ACTIVITY 6.4

Map the chain that results in the specification of services that you or your department provide.

Your chain of specifying customers is unlikely to follow your chain of benefiting customers. It will probably have additional links for third parties defining specifications on behalf of their customers. If you work in the health service, you are likely to have a GP in the chain, acting as an agent for the patient, and the primary care trust may have something to say about the quantity and quality of service. There may also be professional bodies offering advice on specifications – the British Thoracic Society, for example, provides guidelines on the management of asthma. If you work in children's services, the local Children's Trust will be part of the chain of specification, as may be voluntary organisations that take an advocacy role in relation to children at risk. National government will also have a part to play, for example through the requirements laid down in the 2004 Children Act or *Every Child Matters* in England, and the Protection of Children Act in Scotland. This plethora of specifiers may occasionally give rise to conflict if there are different priorities and interests.

By drawing these diagrams you will see that your department is at one end of the customer chains and the service user is at the other end. Broadly, these chains transmit the benefits in one direction and the specifications for what is required in the other. The payment for the services provided may arrive through another, quite different, chain of customer links.

Although we have examined the chains for each of the customer roles separately, some would suggest that, when the different roles are combined, the chains meet at the ends to form a closed loop. Those who ultimately benefit from the services (the service users) also ultimately pay for them as taxpayers. This apparent closure, however, is a simplification, as many service users are not taxpayers and many taxpayers are not service users. By separating out the different roles that customers play, the relationships between your services and each of the players can be made clearer.

The complete chain is not likely to end with you or your department. It almost certainly extends backwards to other people, departments or agencies, either internal or external to your organisation. Your department is their customer because you either specify, participate in, pay for or benefit from the goods and services that they provide for you. Hence you are a customer as well.

We are building up a picture of chains of service in which you are receiving services from your suppliers so that you can provide effective services to your customers. Like all chains, the ability of the customer chain to do its job is only as strong as its weakest link. The effectiveness of the relationships between the linked customers provides the chain's strength and improves its chances of reaching its ultimate goal without breaking.

As a manager, this means that as well as having responsibilities as a provider, you have responsibilities as a customer. If you play several customer roles in relation to a particular supplier, you will have a lot of influence in enabling the chain to operate smoothly. If you play only one or two roles, you will be less in control of what you receive (though there may be organisational benefits from specialist people or agencies performing the different roles).

SERVICE USERS' REQUIREMENTS

Having reached your service, a service user becomes involved in a process of explanation and negotiation as a result of which a specification for treatment or care is established. Let's explore some of the elements in a service user's requirements by considering the following episode.

Jim Matthews' back

Jim, who worked in the local furniture factory, had been suffering from back pain. Initially he felt confident that it was only muscle strain which would be better within a week or so, but after two weeks of severe pain he decided to see his doctor.

He made an appointment and saw Dr Smith. She asked him questions, examined him and decided he needed an X-ray before she could complete her diagnosis. In the meantime, she prescribed painkillers and they agreed that Jim should come back to see her a week after the X-ray, by which time she should have received the results. She filled in the necessary forms and advised him where he could get his X-ray taken.

Two days later, Jim went to the radiography department of his local hospital for the X-ray and he made an appointment to see Dr Smith a week later.

At the second meeting, Dr Smith informed Jim that he had compaction of one of his vertebral discs and she suggested a range of treatments. After discussing the implications of these, they agreed on a course of treatment involving painkillers, bed rest and physiotherapy. Dr Smith advised Jim to make another appointment with her if there was no improvement after a month.

We'll use this example to examine four aspects of service users' requirements – whether they are defined in terms of outcomes or means of achieving them, how tightly they are defined, how far the service user is involved in defining them, and what the service user's expectations are.

Outcomes and means

The first point to pull out of this episode is that service users have wants and needs that they express in different ways. At Jim Matthews' initial visit to his doctor he knew what he wanted. He wanted outcomes – he wanted to find out what was wrong with his back and he wanted it to be better. However, he didn't know what was necessary to achieve these outcomes. At the initial consultation, Jim's need was simply to see the doctor: it was Dr Smith who specified the means by diagnosing the problem. When Jim visited the X-ray department he knew his requirement: he needed an X-ray of his back. Later on, Dr Smith prescribed a suitable course of treatment: further means to match Jim's second required outcome.

To generalise this point, some customers may express what they want as the overall outcome required from the service. Expressing the outcome they want is equivalent to stating their objective in using the service. Some service users are happy to leave the decision about how the required outcome can be achieved to professional judgement. Other service users may express their requirements in terms of means – which treatments, protocols, procedures or processes they wish to be used.

How does this distinction between outcomes and means map on to your experience? Does the service for which you are responsible more readily satisfy those who are interested only in outcomes or those who wish to specify means? If your customers define the outcomes and not the means, there is scope for interpreting their requirements and then choosing the means by which the outcomes can be achieved. If your customers also define the means, you will have less scope for flexibility or for choosing between alternatives. The more specialist your services, the more likely it is that service users' requirements will be expressed in terms of means rather than outcomes. Particularly in chains of internal customers, the further away you are from the end-user, the more precisely defined the means are likely to be.

Tightness of definition of requirements

Jim Matthews's initial requirement of Dr Smith was a few minutes of her time and expertise. This requirement was defined only in terms of when it was going to happen and not what was going to happen. Dr Smith had little idea in advance of what resources would be required to deliver this initial service. The requirement of the X-ray department was quite the reverse. The radiographer didn't know when the service would be required until Jim had made his booking, but she knew exactly what was involved in delivering the service – it was specified on the form that Jim took with him.

ACTIVITY 6.5

For one of your customers who defines the means by which your service should be provided (whether a service user or an internal customer), use the following questions to explore how tightly the requirements are defined.

How closely does your customer define each of the following?

- How the service should be delivered (who delivers it, what procedures should be used, what equipment should be used).
- When the service is to be delivered.
- Where the service is to be delivered.

Make a note of how the tightness with which the requirements are defined will influence the way you deliver the service to your customer.

The more tightly your customers define their requirements, the more precisely you know what you have to do. Precise instructions can make life easier, but they can also put pressure on your service to deliver exactly what is required. For your customers to be able to define their requirements so tightly, they must know fairly accurately what they are. If you are concerned that their definition is too tight, it might be worth checking that they really do know their requirements so exactly. Perhaps you can negotiate a looser definition that is in both your interests.

Service user involvement

A third point in Jim's episode with his doctor is the way he participated in deciding what was required. At the first visit, he was involved in the diagnosis of his complaint. At the second visit, he was involved in agreeing a treatment: he was presented with some options and made an informed choice from what was on offer. Guided by Dr Smith, his selection was based on considering what was appropriate for his condition, what was available and what was acceptable to him. By contrast, Jim had no involvement in agreeing what was required of the radiographer. She simply had to respond to the requirement established by Dr Smith.

Stepping outside health and social care for a moment, experience shows that involving suppliers at an early stage in new developments leads to better utilisation of resources by both suppliers and their customers. Collaboration between customers in the chain in specifying requirements can make it easier to meet the requirements.

Service user expectations

Before deciding to see Dr Smith, Jim Matthews expected his bad back to be better in a couple of weeks. After seeing Dr Smith, his expectation had been modified. Dr Smith could not provide a service that would match his expectations.

We all have expectations of what is necessary for a reasonable life, including good health and social well-being. Expectations arise from comparisons with our families, friends and colleagues, from previous experience, from what we are used to, and from information about services and treatments. For example, we have a number of expectations of the health service. We may expect:

- our illnesses to be accurately diagnosed;
- that most conditions will be treated successfully;
- a friendly and courteous service;
- to be able to take advantage of the latest diagnostic and therapeutic technologies;
- to be treated with respect and dignity.

However, there are often problems with expectations, leading sometimes to disappointment:

- Expectations are not always explicit, so the supplier may not know what, in their heart of hearts, customers are expecting.
- Expectations are not always reasonable, so the supplier cannot match extremely high hopes.

This second problem is particularly difficult. Managers have to be very careful about their definitions of 'reasonable'. There is a danger of trying to shape service users' expectations to fit what you perceive is available from your service. There is also a danger of failing to acknowledge that service users may be right, even if your service is not able to meet their expectations.

It is, however, conceivable that expectations that are impossible to meet might need modifying as part of the process of specifying requirements. There may be evidence from a variety of sources – research, clinical audit and reviews conducted by the Care Quality Commission and the Audit Commission or the National Institute for Health and Clinical Excellence in England and NHS Quality Improvement, Scotland – indicating that particular treatments or interventions are more effective than others. Being alert to developments in practice is important, especially in these days when information is available both to health and social care professionals and to service users from a wide range of sources, including the internet.

ACTIVITY 6.6

	Yes	No
1 Are all your customers explicit about their expectations when they express their requirements?	❐	❐
2 Do you ask them what they expect?	❐	❐
3 Do you consciously modify their expectations as part of agreeing their requirements?	❐	❐
4 What about your suppliers? Do they give you the opportunity to express your expectations of them?	❐	❐

Matching the expectations of the customer to what can be delivered is essential if a quality service is to be provided. In the process of working towards an agreement about what customers require, you need to ensure that:

- you know whether or not the means of achieving the outcomes are included in the customer's requirements;
- it is clear how tightly the requirements are defined;
- customers are involved in setting the requirements at the earliest stage possible;
- customer expectations of the service are addressed.

GETTING FEEDBACK FROM SERVICE USERS

There are a number of ways in which you can seek to develop a picture of how service users view your service. Here are two examples.

Working with children and young people

During 2006 and 2007, the Liverpool Children and Young People's Participation Unit sought feedback from children and young people who receive services from the Child and Adolescent Mental Health Service (CAMHS). The aim was to gain their views on the services, what was good and what improvements they would recommend.

The Participation Unit worked with senior staff in six centres across the city and consultation meetings were arranged after the children and young people's treatment sessions. It was decided that face-to-face interviews would be preferable to sending out questionnaires. The study was designed to elicit both qualitative and quantitative data. All data were anonymised.

The participants were invited to take part through colourful posters and letters to parents and children and posters of the interviewers and facilitators were placed in the waiting rooms. Participants were rewarded for giving their time with a gift voucher.

The team used individual semi-structured interviews (total of 51) and focus group discussions. In the focus groups, the young people worked on group scenarios with a chosen service user taking a star part. Through working on the drama, they discussed their own experiences and feelings about the service and also suggested improvements. This methodology helped them discuss their concerns in a more abstract and anonymous way. Although parents were often present, the focus was on the views of the children and young people.

In addition, the researchers developed a rating scale with pictures, which young people could use as a means of expressing their feelings about certain issues. They could also write or draw messages on a postcard to be given to the service managers.

Findings differed between age groups (age 7–10; 11–14; 15+) and in older age groups, between young men and women. In general, there were concerns about knowing what to expect from their first appointment and not being addressed directly. Most of those interviewed were keen to have their own letter, text, email or information on a web page. Privacy was very important to the participants and they were not keen on appointments at their schools. They were all keen to contribute ideas about how the reception and waiting areas should look and regarded them as part of the whole experience.

Recommendations for the service included improving publicity, ensuring that the children and young people were negotiated with directly and had their own letter (or email or text), avoiding schools as a venue unless appropriate, working in partnership with schools, and improving the waiting room activities for the older age group, particularly young men.

Seeking feedback from children and young people, and involving them in research more widely, is a sensitive issue. However, it is important to include their voices and opinions in evaluation of services.

(Based on: Liverpool Children and Young People's Participation Unit, 2007)

Specialist palliative care social work

This study focused on what service users want from specialist palliative care social work – user-defined outcomes. This area of social work includes practitioners working in multidisciplinary teams drawn from statutory and non-statutory agencies. The social workers primarily work with people with life-limiting illnesses and people facing bereavement.

The research was supported by the Joseph Rowntree Foundation and was based on a sample of service users. A total of 111 people were interviewed: 39 were men, 72 were women and 9 per cent identified themselves as black and/or members of minority ethnic groups. Of the participants, 61 were bereaved people, 52 had life-limiting illnesses and conditions. They were based in hospices, hospital oncology units and palliative care day centres. In-depth interviews were conducted in a mix of either individual or group discussions.

The research took a 'user involvement' approach, i.e. service users were involved in the research but did not take a lead or collaborative role. The interview questions were developed with the help of service users, particularly those involved with the advisory group, and they also contributed to analysis and dissemination of the findings.

A number of themes emerged from the study. One was the service users' positive attitude towards the service and, in particular, the relationship they built with the social worker, highlighting the development of trust and a bond. A key element of this was how they regarded the relationship as a friendship.

The participants also appreciated a participative and responsive model of practice, such as determining their own agenda in partnership. There was no feeling of social workers having a judgemental attitude: they were treated with respect, social workers had time for them. They also valued the continuity of support.

As well as gaining service users' perspectives on their service, the researchers felt the study gave them insight into wider issues, such as 'what social work is and should do', and how it should reflect user-centred support.

(Based on: Beresford, Croft and Adshead, 2008)

We are not suggesting that you should initiate large-scale studies like these. But more explicit public consultation and involvement are now considered an important element within health and social care services. How much you are directly involved in getting feedback from service users will depend on your job, the service you manage and the policies and practices of your organisation. However, getting involved in the process of consultation or getting access to its outcomes can provide useful information about who your potential service users are and what they require.

The next Activity should help you to be clearer about the kind of information you need and encourages you to think about how you might obtain it. Gathering this information is not a one-off project: it is a long-term process that you need to keep in the forefront of your work as a manager.

ACTIVITY 6.7

Make notes in response to each of the questions below. For each question consider:

■ whether you know the answer
■ if not, how you could set about getting the answer.

  1 What do people want from your services?
  2 Why are people satisfied or dissatisfied with your services?
  3 What is the image and reputation of your services locally?
  4 What services would people like to see increased or improved?

Some of these questions can be answered by making use of the feedback your staff receive from service users day by day. Staff who work directly with service users often receive expressions of gratitude and thanks, sometimes with detailed comments about what worked particularly well. Managers rarely receive this feedback directly. All feedback from service users provides information about how they view the service that they have received. You can learn a great deal by developing systems to gather feedback about day-to-day service delivery that works well (or badly). You need to analyse and interpret this *ad hoc* feedback to decide what implications it has for the delivery of your services. Some feedback will confirm that things are running smoothly. Some will suggest minor improvements and adjustments. Some will indicate that there has been a serious failure.

If, in addition to making use of day-to-day feedback, you decide to use a more systematic approach to gathering information, here are some pointers for success:

■ Ensure that all those involved are clear about the purpose of involving service users.
■ Acknowledge that real involvement and partnership between health and social care organisations and the community may take time to achieve.
■ Make sure that the method you choose for involving the community is suitable for the task in hand (for example, is the objective to secure support for a change in services or is it to assemble information to guide planning?).
■ Work collaboratively with other local health and social care organisations and share information with them.
■ Recognise that well informed service users can encourage services to change.
■ Use language carefully – avoid health or social care jargon.

HANDLING COMPLAINTS

Dealing with complaints about public services has become a key aspect of 'good governance' and a means to improve service delivery; although most organisations have embraced a more consumerist model for addressing complaints, there are concerns that this can weaken values of citizenship such as fairness and social justice (Brewer 2007).

When things go wrong in health and social care settings, they can go very wrong. Mistakes can sometimes result in unnecessary pain and distress and even in the early death of a service user. However, many people who complain are not seeking revenge or even financial compensation, they often just want an explanation and an apology.

Most health and social care organisations have an established complaints procedure: many are required by legislation or government guidance to do so. Some complaints procedures require adherence to a strict timetable. The aims of a complaints procedure should be:

- to resolve complaints as quickly as possible;
- to ensure that the individuals involved and the organisation as a whole benefit from the experience;
- to learn from any mistakes made and make adjustments to the service to reduce the likelihood of them happening again.

A typical complaints procedure

Complaints procedures typically have four stages (based on the Department of Communities and Local Government website).

Stage 1: the informal stage

The first stage is an attempt to resolve the complaint informally: the complainant should explain the problem to the person they have had direct contact with (by letter, fax, email, telephone). That person's manager should be involved even at this early stage. The member of staff concerned should provide an informal response, explaining how and why they have come to their conclusions and, if they do not accept the complaint, they should explain why not, and advise what to do next. They should provide the name and contact details of their own line manager in order for the person to pursue their complaint formally.

Stage 2: the formal stage

If resolution at Stage 1 proves to be impossible, a complainant can request that the complaint be formally investigated. The significance of Stage 2 is that other people are involved in the consideration, discussion and, possibly, investigation of the complaint. The person should set out the complaint clearly, in detail and stating that they want it treated as a formal complaint. Organisations are obliged to keep records of all formal complaints, so they need to agree a detailed, written statement. For example:

- make sure that the complaint is clear;
- check that the Stage 1 procedure has been completed;
- review, with the person who dealt with your initial approach, the reasons for their response;
- consider the issues afresh;
- consult lawyers if there any doubts about the relevant statutory powers;
- decide upon their own findings in the light of these considerations and write to the complainant setting out their findings.

Particular consideration also needs to be given to people with disabilities and in cases where English is not the first language. Instead of insisting on a written letter, other options may need to be offered.

Stage 3: the complaints manager

The next stage is for the complainant to communicate to a complaints manager, who is usually independent and ensures that the issues are considered by lawyers.

Stage 4: review by the ombudsman

If the complainant is still dissatisfied, he or she would need to approach the relevant ombudsman for an independent review of the complaint and how it has been handled.

As a manager, you are most likely to be involved in the first of these stages. However, you might be required to provide evidence if a complaint against your service reaches the second or third stage. You might also be appointed as the officer responsible for investigating a second-stage complaint. At Stage 1, your responsibilities are to ensure that:

- the complaint is properly acknowledged;
- it is properly investigated;
- it is referred to a senior manager if it has wider implications;
- an appropriate response is provided to the complainant;

■ careful records are kept of the complaint and how it has been handled.

The last point is important for two reasons. First, you will need to have a proper record if the complaint reaches Stage 2 or Stage 3. Second, complaints – whether or not they are well founded – are an opportunity to learn: they can provide a valuable source of information about users' perceptions of your service and so may provide ideas for service improvements.

Ways in which complaints are resolved

Essex and Wide (1996) identify a number of ways in which complaints are resolved. In some cases, more than one of these processes may be at work simultaneously.

1 The people involved reach a new understanding of the situation. Complainants might say: 'Maybe I was being a bit unfair.' Staff might say: 'Perhaps we could have handled that differently.'
2 The people involved get over the original hurt or anger they felt at the time. Complainants or staff might say: 'It doesn't bother me any more. It's in the past.'
3 The people involved feel that they have been heard and understood. The complainants receive an apology or explanation and feel that they were justified in complaining. They might say: 'I got a full apology.'
4 The organisation offers a remedy and the focus shifts from the complaint to the solution. Complainants might say: 'I got what I wanted.' Staff might say: 'We can now see how we could deal with a situation like that differently in the future.'
5 The people involved accept the judgement of a trusted arbiter. Complainants or staff might say: 'I lost' (or 'I won') or 'I was right' (or 'I was wrong').
6 The people involved accept that they will get no further with the complaint. Complainants might say: 'I've stopped banging my head against a brick wall.' Staff might say: 'I don't agree but I suppose I'll have to get on with the job.'

To be the subject of a complaint, or to be a complainant, is often a painful experience. The situation needs to be handled with openness and sensitivity. Unnecessarily defensive behaviour on the part of the service can be frustrating for the complainant and reduce the likelihood of resolution. It is important to keep the focus of attention on the lessons to be learned both by the individuals involved and by the organisation, and to look for possible service improvements.

As a manager, you may need to take a lead in establishing the facts of a case. You will have to balance the perceptions and expectations of those making a complaint with those who may be the subject of the complaint. The members of staff involved may be under considerable stress and in need of support to deal with their feelings. You may have to suggest ways to resolve the situation for all parties in an environment where resources are limited but expectations about the level and quality of services may be increasing.

In this chapter we have focused on understanding what users require from your services. We have looked at who your customers are, how service users define their requirements, how you can get feedback from service users, and at the stages involved in handling complaints. No one likes receiving complaints, but one positive way to respond is to try to learn from them.

REFERENCES

Beresford, P., Croft, S. and Adshead, L. (2008) '"We don't see her as a social worker": A service user case study of the importance of the social worker's relationship and humanity', *British Journal of Social Work*, vol. 38, pp. 1388–407.

Brewer, B. (2007) 'Citizen or customer? Complaints handling in the public sector', *International Review of Administrative Sciences*, vol. 73, no. 4, pp. 449–556.

Clarke, J., Newman, J., Smith, N., Vidler, E. and Westmarland, L. (2007) *Creating Citizen-Consumers: Changing Publics and Changing Public Services*, Sage.

Department of Communities and Local Government <http://www.communities. gov.uk/corporate/about/freedom-of-information/complaints procedure> (accessed 20/6/2009).

Essex, S. and Wide, M. (1996) *A Matter for Investigation*, Educational Broadcasting Services Trust.

Horizon House, Bromley, Kent <http://www.zen99560.zen.co.uk/hhmenu. html> (accessed 03/3/2009).

Liverpool Children and Young People's Participation Unit (2007) *It's not just about talking: A Consultation with Children and Young People who use Liverpool Children and Adolescent Mental Health Services, 2006–2007.* <http://www.liverpool.gov.uk/Council_government_and_democracy/About _your_council/Consultation/Consultation_exercise/Closed/user_feedback_ research.asp > (accessed 03/3/2009).

CHAPTER 7

MAPPING THE SERVICE ENVIRONMENT

If you are to understand how your service 'sits' in its environment, you need a mental map that shows how the important elements of the environment relate to each other, and to you and your area of work. We begin this chapter by suggesting a way in which you can map the components of your organisation's environment and categorise them. We identify three major parts of this map – the *internal environment*, the *near environment* and the *far environment*.

The remainder of the chapter focuses on the near environment. We discuss how and why organisational boundaries can change in response to changes in relationships with the near environment. We examine the concept of *stakeholders*, and invite you to identify the main stakeholders in your area of work and their interests. We consider some approaches to managing your relationships with your stakeholders and thus influencing your near environment. We complete the chapter by considering the nature of 'needs' and 'demands' and their impact on the environment of health and social care organisations.

COMPONENTS OF THE SERVICE ENVIRONMENT

Organisations exist to provide services or to make products – to meet needs. They can be very large and complex or they can be small enterprises with only one area of work. Both the size of an organisation and its shape – for example, why certain activities are carried out within it and why others are purchased in or contracted out – are determined by environmental factors. Your organisation does not exist in isolation: it is part of a large and complex network of service users and their carers, suppliers, competitors, regulators, and so on. In addition, the economy, social trends and technological innovations have an impact on it. We can represent this complex network in terms of three environments (Figure 7.1).

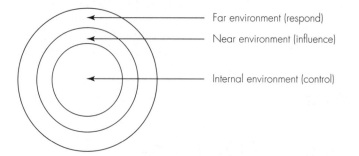

Figure 7.1 The three environments

There is a dynamic relationship between these three environments:

- The *internal environment* is composed of the staff, resources and facilities within the organisation. These components can be *controlled* – to a large extent, at least – by the organisation's managers. The internal environment is, however, influenced by the near and far environments, which the organisation is unable to control.
- The *near environment* includes service users and carers, contractors, suppliers and competitors. It also includes local politicians, other organisations that are partners in service delivery and local pressure groups. These components of the environment are all close to the organisation and they interact with it in a variety of ways. They cannot be controlled by the organisation, but they can be *influenced*.
- The components of the *far environment* are those factors that can neither be controlled nor influenced from within the organisation. They include a wide range of social, technological, economic, environmental and political factors. Every organisation has to *respond* to the impact of these external factors. Some respond more thoughtfully, quickly and successfully than others.

Each organisation and area of work has different components in these three environments. You might have staff teams or groups of volunteers in your internal environment, along with internal administrative services or resources like buildings, facilities and equipment. In your near environment you might have those who use your services, services in other organisations or agencies with which your organisation regularly works, and local people and organisations that have an impact on your organisation in some way. Components of your far environment might include new legislation that requires your service to change and developments that change the nature of the local community (for example, your locality becoming an increasingly popular holiday destination).

The boundaries of an organisation

If a new acquaintance asked you where you work, would you reply giving the name of an organisation like 'I work at Barsetshire Council' or 'I work at the Royal Hospital', or would you say something like 'I work in social care' or 'I work in the health service'? The acquaintance might then ask you to explain a little more, to give some idea of what your work involves and how it relates to other services. This sort of discussion is often about boundaries. It is similar to discussions you might have about your own job, and where the boundaries are between your responsibilities and those of others. Like jobs, organisations have invisible boundaries that define what is 'inside' the organisation; they are part of the way in which an organisation carries out its purpose. They also define what is 'outside' the organisation, but contributes in some way to its work.

Organisations differ in where they draw the boundary between their internal and external environments. There are lots of examples:

- Some residential care organisations carry out all their catering and cleaning activities themselves and others buy in these services from external suppliers.
- Some doctors' practices collaborate to run out-of-hours services whereas others use private deputising services.
- Some local authorities carry out services such as home care with in-house staff whereas others use contractors.

There may sometimes be a special relationship between a contractor and its client organisation, for example where the contractor's staff are people who formerly worked for the client organisation and now sell their specialist service back to it. Other types of special relationships are partnerships or network arrangements (such as the information services run by rail companies) or franchises (such as most fast-food outlets and many hotels).

These examples illustrate that organisations have choices about where they set their boundaries. The activities that are included within the organisational boundary and those bought in from outside may change over time. The main choice is between carrying out activities *in-house* and using contractors (*outsourcing*). If you use outsourcing, you are buying services from what is available externally – from the 'market' – looking for levels of quality and price that meet your organisation's needs. If there are many potential suppliers, you can make choices and demand exactly the service you want. But if there are few suppliers, it might be difficult to buy in the service you want at the price you want to pay.

It can be very frightening for staff who are accustomed to being valued employees of a stable organisation to hear about the possibility that their service area may be outsourced. But there are many advantages and disadvantages of outsourcing that need to be considered.

In-house services are often valued for their 'fit' with the organisation because they are managed within the same policies, structures and culture (although specialist services such as personnel and training often have their own cultural flavour). However, in-house services may have high overhead and management costs, particularly if the volume of service is not large enough to justify the infrastructure required. There may be difficulties in reducing or increasing the volume of the service quickly enough to respond to needs. Also, small in-house services may not be able to keep up to date with developments that enable new ideas and technologies to contribute to improving the quality of service delivery within an organisation in which the core work and investment are focused on other activities. Investment for development can sometimes be found by creating external partnerships – one form of outsourcing.

If organisations become very large and carry out a wide range of different activities, they may become difficult to manage and difficult to change. Skilled staff who perform well may often be the best people to continue to carry out the activities being considered for outsourcing. It may be possible to transfer them so that they can do so under different management arrangements in new organisations. This has become common practice in public services, leading to the creation of many organisations that are able to deliver specific and focused services. Creating these new organisations requires new skills, such as contract management and quality assurance.

Communication becomes increasingly important to ensure that they work well together. Integration of services is an important theme in health and social care nowadays, to ensure that service users receive an appropriate set of services to meet their particular needs. If there are different service providers, with parts of services outsourced, effective co-ordination is essential.

The advantages and disadvantages of in-house provision and outsourcing are illustrated in Table 7.1.

Table 7.1 Advantages and disadvantages of in-house provision and outsourcing

	Advantages	Disadvantages
In-house	Control Reliability Flexibility (resources can be reallocated) Accumulated experience Quality control	High overhead and management costs Costs inflexible if requirements change Limited economies of scale Lack of access to new ideas and technologies Lack of specialist skills
Outsourced	Easy to expand/reduce resources Access to specialist suppliers Reduction in in-house fixed costs Overall cost savings	Loss of in-house expertise in key areas Need for contract management skills Possible loss of quality control Possible loss of short-term flexibility

ACTIVITY 7.1

Consider an activity currently carried out inside your organisation that could possibly be outsourced. It might be a catering service or support for a technical function, or perhaps even provision of a professional or specialist service. Make a note of the advantages of the current in-house provision and compare these with the potential advantages of outsourcing.

You may conclude that – at least for the time being – the advantages of keeping the activity in-house outweigh the advantages of out-sourcing. There is a tension between keeping all services within the ethos of an organisation, and the potential financial and quality advantages of outsourcing. Many organisations prefer to retain their core services and contract out the facilities that support these. However, as the environment in which your organisation functions continues to change, there will be pressure to keep these options under review, particularly if financial resources are limited. It is impor-tant to ensure that the organisation is investing its resources in the services it is required to deliver (its core services) and to focus on how these services could be improved, rather than keeping a support activity in-house if it is performing less well than it could if it were outsourced.

Organisational boundaries are not fixed. They can change in response to political pressures or pressure on costs or the introduction of new technology. In their efforts to improve the quality of the services they provide, organisations are constantly seeking the best balance between short- and long-term objectives, between operational and strategic considerations, and between the needs of their different stakeholders. It is to the interests of stakeholders that we now turn.

STAKEHOLDERS AND THEIR INTERESTS

In the first half of the last century, political meetings throughout Europe would be interrupted by shouts of 'What about the workers?' More recently the shift to a more consumer-oriented society has changed the concern to 'What about the customers?' Employees and customers are both examples of stakeholders – people who have a 'stake' in an organisation in the sense that they have a keen interest in what the organisation does and how it does it. In the voluntary sector, stake-holders include funders, donors and volunteers. In the public sector, they include the general public in their capacities as citizens, taxpayers who fund public services, and beneficiaries of those services as service users.

All organisations have internal stakeholders: employees, managers, directors, trustees, and board and committee members. They also have stakeholders external to the organisation, but strongly linked to or affected by it: service users and other customers, suppliers, funders and possibly competitors. Other external stakeholders are more indirectly affected by the organisation: the local community, the general public, local involvement networks in health and social care – LINks (in England) or community health councils (Wales), pressure groups, local councillors and Members of Parliament. (These three categories correspond to an organisation's three environments.)

It is important for you, as a manager, to be aware of who your stakeholders are because these are the people who can influence the working of your organisation. Some stakeholders' interests are protected by law. Employment legislation and health and safety legislation provide increasing protection for employees. Contractual relationships protect the interests of partners in service provision. The legislation governing services for children regulates most aspects of care involving children.

Different stakeholders have different interests, which may conflict. For example, the interests of employees in security of employment and increased earnings may conflict with those of funding agencies which may be seeking short-term cost reductions. The interests of taxpayers may conflict with the interests of those who depend on public services. A proposal to build a new bail hostel or motorway is often opposed vigorously by local communities. The culture, structure and governance of an organisation will determine how these conflicts are resolved and, in some cases, the interests of one stakeholder group will have a dominant influence. Organisations may have to work hard to ensure that the interests of other stakeholder groups are not compromised.

Your internal stakeholders will include your colleagues, other employees of the organisation and possibly staff in other parts of the organisation who provide services linked with those in your area. Near environment stakeholders include all those who use or purchase your services, and others who come to your organisation for a particular purpose. They might also include those who take an overview of the services provided by your organisation, including external quality assessors and external organisations to which your organisation is accountable. Professional bodies may be part of your near environment because of their concern for the maintenance of professional standards. However, professional bodies could also be considered to be part of the far environment: it depends on how you view the strength of their influence. National bodies, such as government health departments and agencies are likely to be part of your far environment.

Analysing stakeholders and their interests is important for two reasons. First, it emphasises that different stakeholder groups have different interests and that managers have to balance these interests when making decisions. Second, it helps you to appreciate the relationship between your organisation and its external environment.

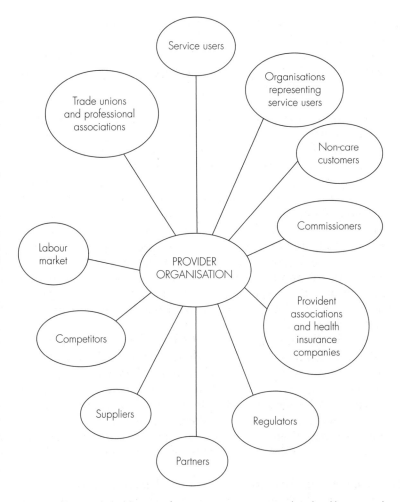

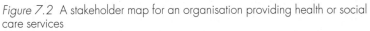

Figure 7.2 A stakeholder map for an organisation providing health or social care services

Identifying stakeholder groups in your near environment

If you work in an organisation that provides health or social care services, you will have a number of groups of stakeholders. Some of these are shown in the form of a 'stakeholder map' in Figure 7.2.

Here are a few comments about each of these groups of stakeholders:

■ *Service users* include their relatives and carers, who may receive services in an indirect way. This group could also be described as your external customers, in the sense that they come from outside your organisation and are consumers of the services you offer.

- *Organisations representing service users* include voluntary organisations such as MIND and Age Concern, as well as your local LINks.
- *Non-care customers* are those to which your organisation may sell services (other than care services) to generate income. For example, hospitals may rent space to shops or sell franchises to photographers of newly born babies.
- *Commissioners* are also customers, since they are paying for the services that you provide. They act as the agents of service users. They include health trusts, health boards in Scotland, primary care trusts, and social care organisations. As the emphasis on joint working and integration between health and social care increases, local health care commissioners and local social care commissioners will both be important to you, whether you work in health or social care. There will certainly be arrangements for joint consultation. For example, the local social services department is responsible for commissioning social care for your local population: as a manager in an organisation providing health care, your work may have an impact on that responsibility of the local authority – as well as on its housing, education or environmental health departments – and on the police.
- *Provident associations (such as BUPA) and commercial health insurance companies* are probably the main purchasers of your services if you work in a private hospital, although some patients will be paying directly from their own resources. (In the case of independent health care, which forms only a small part of health services in the United Kingdom, the user and the purchaser are one and the same.) Even if you work for a public-sector provider, you may still have services for private patients, again mainly purchased by insurers.
- *Regulators* are responsible for ensuring that service provision is of a sufficiently high quality and meets agreed standards. At a local level, some forms of regulation are part of the function of commissioners, but there is an increasing emphasis on the development of national bodies to ensure that health and care services are provided equally effectively in all geographical areas, for example the process is streamlined in England through one body for health, social care and mental health (the Care Quality Commission).
- *Partners* include any other organisations with which your organisation collaborates in delivering services. Partners may work together in order to share expertise across a wider service area, or they may have pooled their resources because they are then better able to deliver co-ordinated services in a geographical area. Partnerships are usually formed because there is a clear advantage for both partners, and they may have varying degrees of formality. When the need to work closely is very strong, organisations may even merge rather than retaining distinct characteristics as in a partnership. At the other extreme, many organisations have loose alliances within which they have mutually beneficial working arrangements.

■ *Suppliers* are the firms and organisations from which you buy goods and services – from food to high-tech equipment to domestic services to management consultancy.

■ *Competitors* are other organisations (whether in public or private ownership) providing services that commissioners may see as actual or potential alternatives to the services you provide. Service users have a degree of choice about which service provider they use, and commissioners can select service providers that most closely meet their criteria. Organisations which can demonstrate that they attract high numbers of users are likely to attract continuing funding and thus survive more easily than organisations that are not the first choice of service users.

■ The *labour market* is made up of individuals who actually or potentially possess the skills and knowledge needed in your organisation. You cannot provide services without sufficient numbers of suitably qualified staff. Your organisation has a reputation within its environment and staff recruitment may be assisted or damaged by its reputation as an employer.

■ Some *trade unions* and *professional associations* will have members within your organisation, but you may occasionally find yourself dealing with them as external organisations, perhaps in educational or disciplinary matters or over the recognition of a training post in your organisation.

If you work in a commissioning organisation rather than in an organisation that provides services, the organisations that provide services will be an important group of your stakeholders. Some of the group of stakeholders in Figure 7.2 (such as service users) will be just as important for you as for provider organisations, while others (for example, competitors) will be less significant than they are for provider organisations.

You may have been surprised at how many different groups of stakeholders can be identified, particularly if you have recognised some that you have not previously considered as having a particular interest in what you do and how you do it. If you are considering a change in a service that you offer, each stakeholder group will take a view of the proposed change from their particular perspective. You and your colleagues may see the benefits to be gained by making a change, but some of your stakeholders may feel that the disadvantages outweigh the benefits of the proposal or may want to propose a different way of achieving similar benefits.

The interests of each stakeholder group will vary according to the circumstances. If a proposed change will have immediate consequences for a particular group, it is easy to see that their interests should be taken into account. However, changes often have less obvious repercussions for other groups and it is helpful to think about any proposal from a range of different perspectives in order to consider how each group of stakeholders might perceive it. Your organisation probably has a variety of ways of keeping in touch with its stakeholders' views. However, team leaders and other first-line managers are often closer to the stakeholders who are in direct contact with their services and are in a good position to ensure that the stakeholders' views are understood within the organisation.

INFLUENCING THE NEAR ENVIRONMENT

The near environment consists of people and organisations (stakeholders) with whom, in a loose sense, your organisation has to 'trade'. Either you need things from them, or vice versa, or both.

One way of thinking about the relationships in an organisation's near environment is to consider the choices and constraints that exist because of the availability of the resources that the organisation needs in order to operate effectively. This approach was called *resource dependence* by Pfeffer and Salancik (2003). They took the view that no organisation can be completely independent – all need resources, including money, materials, personnel and information. Organisations acquire these resources by interacting in their environment with others who control the available resources. There is a constant struggle for balance as an organisation confronts difficulties and constraints imposed by these external circumstances. As all organisations experience similar difficulties in obtaining resources, those which work geographically close to each other or which deliver similar services are often interdependent. One organisation may be dependent on another to buy its services, another may be dependent on those that provide it with services or goods. These dependent relationships are more or less important, depending on how critical the resource is.

It can be useful to think about what is the scarcest resource that is critical in enabling you to provide your service effectively. In some cases it is availability of skilled professionals – for example, a serious shortage of nurses and junior doctors in some parts of the country. In other service areas there are shortages of transport, sheltered housing or hospital beds. Some resource shortages might be resolved if more money were available, but many would take a considerable time to develop, even with additional funding. Sometimes the solution may be to find an alternative source (doctors and nurses from overseas) or a substitute for it (physiotherapy aides to do some of physiotherapists' more routine work). In other cases a new process can change the demand for resources – for example, minor surgical operations are now often carried out in GPs' surgeries without the need for patients to be treated in hospitals. Developments like these change the balance of dependency: organisations then have to respond to different levels of demand, and demand for different types of services needing different types of resources. Pfeffer and Salancik suggested that there are four ways in which an organisation might balance its dependencies.

1 *Adapt to the conditions.* This could be done by reducing levels of service, restricting use of resources, slowing down the speed of response to demand or influencing the types of demand made on its services. For example, a small hospital might reduce the number of different services offered, and specialise in treating a particular condition or a particular group of people (for example, admitting only older people or only children).

2 *Alter the interdependencies.* This could be done by merging with another organisation that controls some of the needed resources. It could be done by growing and providing a wider range of services, so that the organisation is not dependent on providing only one type of service. For example, a small community-based home care service might link with a community health service to provide care for people who need support at home when they leave hospital.

3 *Negotiate the environment.* This could be done by creating partnerships with other organisations to deliver services jointly or to share resources. One way in which this is increasingly happening at the present time is integration between social services and health services, or working with the voluntary sector.

4 *Change the environment by political action.* This could be done by influencing decision makers to change the conditions in which the organisation operates. An example would be lobbying local Members of Parliament in an effort to prevent the closure of a hospital or to try to obtain subsidies or special financial allowances when the demand for a service increases unexpectedly (as often occurs for health and social care organisations in harsh winters).

All organisations have relationships with other organisations and may have to adopt one or more of these strategies to ensure that they are able to access sufficient resources to continue to deliver their services. All these relationships can be – and need to be – managed. Part of the role of management is to manage externally in this sense. Although this may not be a central part of your role as a first-line manager, you do not need to become the chief executive to be involved with this near environment. In the language of systems theory, such managerial roles are part of *adaptive systems* – those whose function is to help fit the organisation into its environment and thereby to ensure its survival.

We have introduced the idea of creating a map of the environment of your organisation as a first step towards understanding – and thus managing – its relationships with the wider world. Many managers in health and social care are involved in working jointly across traditional boundaries in order to develop service provision. An understanding of the environment of your service and your organisation is helpful in enabling you to think ahead and to be sensitive to the ways in which you and your organisation respond to the influences of the environment while respecting the interests of your many stakeholders. You are in a position to influence the ways in which relationships with your stakeholders develop.

However, managers in health and social care also have to consider the influence of 'needs' and 'demands' on their organisational environment and strive to be responsive to both need and demand.

NEEDS AND DEMANDS

The concept of need is somewhat problematic in health and social care. If you have acute appendicitis, you definitely need a surgical operation, but there are other cases where an alleged need (for example to have your tattoos removed, or for you or your partner to be provided with *in vitro* fertilisation) would be the subject of fierce contention. It is not difficult to make a conceptual distinction between need and demand: *need* is usually thought of as the ability to benefit from a service, while *demand* constitutes people claiming services. However, despite the conceptual clarity with which this distinction can be made, there are real problems in *using* them: people may demand what they don't need and vice versa and different groups of people have different perceptions of need:

- perceptions and expectations of the population;
- perceptions of professionals providing the services;
- perceptions of managers of commissioner/provider organisations based on analysis of data;
- priorities of the organisations commissioning and managing services – linked to national, regional or local priorities.

(National Institute of Clinical Excellence 2005)

Demand is not a simple concept either, because it has overtones of the consumer-led market. But in modern public services it can be seen as emphasising an appropriate focus on the service user.

Many people prefer to think in terms of health and care services responding to demand. None the less, variables such as the demographic structure of the population, the known pattern of mortality (death) and morbidity (illness), and the extent to which various services are utilised are often treated as indicators of need when forecasts of future expenditure or plans for future health and social care services are being made. Let's look briefly at each of these variables.

The *demographic structure* of a population is an important determinant of need for health and social care. This occurs in two ways. First, the age structure of a population determines whether more or less of a particular service is needed. For example, if the birth rate falls there will be less need for maternity and child health facilities (as well as for playgroups and infant schools). Second, and more importantly, people of different ages tend to have different patterns of usage of health services, with different cost consequences. In general, very young children and older people are much more expensive to provide for than other age groups. In private health insurance, these differences are reflected in the premiums that subscribers have to pay.

Mortality rates and the causes of death within a population are regarded as important information about a population's needs for health care, as well as about its health in a broader sense. The attraction of mortality as a measure of these needs is that death is both unequivocal (except in the relatively few cases of people in a persistent vegetative state) and it is the subject of statutory recording through death certificates. The causes of death recorded on certificates are, however, a matter of medical opinion (confirmed by post-mortem examination in a minority of cases) and, over longer periods, are susceptible to changes in medical knowledge and perhaps diagnostic trends.

Morbidity is the prevalence of disease in the community. The diagnoses of hospital patients are sometimes used to assess morbidity, but this only reflects illness among people who have *both* approached a doctor (usually a general practitioner) *and* been referred to hospital. To obtain data on illness across the whole population, whether under treatment or not, it is necessary either to undertake special research (something which is normally only feasible in a specific geographic location or among a particular social group) or to rely on answers to questions about health that are included from time to time in data-gathering exercises such as the Census or the General Household Survey. Since such data are self-reported, they cannot provide accurate objective information about needs for health and social care. Nevertheless, they provide useful information, for instance about the prevalence of long-standing disabilities.

Utilisation rates are measures of the extent to which the public use health and social care services. They are sometimes assumed to represent need and they certainly reflect demand. However, it is not always clear how the demand created by professionals interacts with the demand created by service users (for example, you cannot be admitted into hospital without a doctor's agreement).

Furthermore, given the increasing emphasis on a holistic approach to defining health (for example, as the World Health Organization highlights, health is 'the state of complete physical, mental and social well-being') it may also be appropriate to consider the contribution of a wider set of statistics when considering need: housing, income, education, employment, crime rates, and so on.

At this point, it is useful to consider separately how health and social care services each meet needs and demands (although bear in mind the increasing integration of elements of these services and moves towards a single assessment process).

Meeting need and demand in health services

There are many difficulties in bridging the gap between acknowledging that health services and service managers are affected by public need and demand, and knowing what can be done about it. But it is important to recognise that people's health problems are *filtered* by the services that exist. Various studies have demonstrated that the health service deals with only a small proportion of the health problems present in a population at any particular time. Most people do not contact any formal services when they have symptoms of illness. The term 'symptom iceberg' was coined to draw attention to this situation. Consider some of the following evidence:

- A survey of 1,000 adults in London found that only 49 were free of symptoms in a two-week period. Of the remaining 951, only 21 per cent had seen a doctor for their symptoms. The majority had treated themselves with medicines purchased at a pharmacy.
- A group of general practitioners asked a sample of young and middle-aged women in their practice to record symptom episodes in a health diary. When they compared the evidence of the diaries with records of attendance at the surgery, only one in every 37 symptoms had been presented to the doctors.
- Serious illnesses may go untreated. With problems as diverse as hypertension, rheumatoid arthritis, diabetes and psychiatric disorders, the number of cases in which treatment has not been sought may be as high as the number of patients receiving treatment.
- Among those over the age of 85, one-third will not have reported problems of poor hearing, giddiness and heartburn to their GPs and one-quarter will not have reported problems they experience with their feet.
- Social background appears to have a significant influence on whether a doctor is consulted. Among women, the ratio of medical consultations to rates of illness in Social Class I is 2.0 compared with 0.7 in Social Class V. In other words, women from professional backgrounds are nearly three times as likely to consult their GPs.

In meeting health care needs it is useful to think of three filters: the individual, the GP and the hospital consultant.

A number of considerations are involved in *individuals'* decisions whether to seek health care in relation to a health problem. For example:

- Are the symptoms worrying?
- How painful/uncomfortable are the symptoms?
- Are the symptoms to be expected?

- Do the symptoms disrupt daily life?
- Is it appropriate to seek care for this particular problem?
- Can the doctor do anything for the problem?
- Would it be embarrassing to take this problem to the doctor?
- What are the costs of consulting the doctor in terms of time and inconvenience?

Perhaps symptoms such as headaches or changes in energy may be considered trivial or to be expected as part of everyday life. On the other hand, a sore throat may be considered a problem for which the doctor can prescribe treatment, and a pain in the chest may be considered life-threatening. From a medical point of view, many of these perceptions may not be well founded, but they are powerful influences over behaviour in relation to illness. They can change over time as health services change. Suppose that a general practice began to provide and promote awareness about migraine clinics. Consultations for headaches might increase as people became aware of the availability of services.

General practitioners manage virtually all health problems initially and refer patients to hospital care only when primary care is insufficient. They may filter patients' problems in at least two ways.

First, there is considerable research evidence that GPs may not be aware of many of their patients' problems:

- Half of patients' disabilities may not be known to their GPs.
- Two-thirds of patients' mental disorders may not be recognised by their GPs.

This kind of evidence suggests possible shortcomings or limitations in primary care that can lead to undesirable filtering of health problems. The introduction of the Quality and Outcomes Framework (QOF) has led to some improvement in this area, for example in monitoring patients' smoking behaviour and blood pressure.

The second way in which GPs can act as a filter is in their decisions to refer. Some of the most puzzling data for the health service can be found when the rates at which GPs refer their patients to hospital are calculated. In one study, GPs with the highest referral rates were found to send patients to hospital four times more frequently than GPs with the lowest rates. The differences could not be explained in terms of patients' demands. Also, when GPs do refer their patients to hospital, their goals and expectations may be different both from those of the patients who are referred and from those of the hospital doctors. One study examined whether the primary purpose of the referral was diagnosis, treatment, investigation or reassurance: the GP, consultant and patient all agreed in only one-third of the referrals.

Once patients reach hospital, *consultants* decide whether and how to treat them, what X-rays and pathology tests to request, whether to admit them as inpatients, and when to discharge them. Just as there are substantial variations in GPs' practice, there are also substantial variations in consultants' practice. For instance, rates of tonsillectomy vary between different parts of the country by as much as four to one.

The management of public need and demand therefore involves a complex mixture of internal variables (for example, the doctors) and external variables (the public).

Meeting need and demand in social care

The process of assessing people's social care needs has changed dramatically in recent years. In general, this has entailed an emphasis on the individual and their full participation in the assessment process. It has also involved giving service users the right to buy and manage their own care: direct payments enable service users to choose, and pay for, a care service of their choice. Furthermore, the single assessment process should, in theory, streamline the process by reducing the number of forms to fill in, enable professionals to share information more effectively, and result in a less stressful experience for service users. The sharing of personal information has, however, proved to be a complex issue, both in terms of ethical concerns as well as the need to train staff in inputting and storing electronic data.

Assessments of need cover a range of issues, including people's housing circumstances, the financial resources available to them, their physical and mental incapacities, their family and social environments including the needs of informal carers, and the transport available to them. The type and cost of services supplied vary according to the needs identified, the preferences of the people concerned and the resources available to the local authority. Thus a person who requires help with washing, dressing, going to the toilet and cooking is deemed only to need help with these activities. This is rather different from describing people as 'needing' a particular service, such as residential care or day care.

The financing of social care services is very different from the financing of health services. Some social services have always been available for private purchase. Some services are available from local authorities, but are subject to charges. Local authorities are not required by law to provide or commission a service on behalf of service users at no cost to them, although they may do so. Pressure on resources has increasingly led to higher charges for services such as care in the home, coupled with raising the threshold (or eligibility) criteria – the level of need required before a service will be provided. Evidence of this can be seen in residential care homes. Forty years ago most residents would have been able to wash and dress themselves, and those with greater care needs would have been in a hospital or nursing home. Now most residents of care homes require more intensive personal care. This has led to considerable changes in the type of accommodation and care services available, both in the public and independent sectors.

Unlike most health care services, social care services are often required for life (for example by those with learning difficulties, physical disabilities, mental health problems or frailty in old age). They are also required to provide for the whole person – not just for physical care, but also for the emotional and social aspects of life. This has major implications both for the long-term cost of services and for the range of services that are required.

A challenge for social care professionals and managers is to keep in mind the needs of people who are excluded from services by eligibility criteria. As the severity of the needs of those who receive care rises, more people with mild or moderate needs are excluded from receiving social services unless they can afford to pay for them themselves. The preventive effect of providing low levels of care to help with everyday needs is gradually lost, thus increasing the number of people with higher levels of need. Similar processes apply in the provision of services for children and families.

WORKING WITH YOUR ENVIRONMENTAL MAP

You should now have a better understanding of how your service 'sits' in its environment and of how the important elements of the environment relate to each other, and to you and your area of work. You should be able to 'map' the main implications for your organisation of the *internal environment*, the *near environment* and the *far environment*. As an operational manager, your work will probably be most affected by the internal environment, but your understanding of the issues arising from the near and far environments will help you respond to the impact of the different pressures as they change over time.

You should also be able to identify the main stakeholders in your area of work and their particular interests. You have many opportunities to influence your near environment through the ways in which you manage relationships with your stakeholders.

We completed this chapter by considering the nature of 'needs' and 'demands' and their impact on the environment of health and care organisations. It is often difficult to respond positively to everyone's needs and demands when your resources are limited. Every manager of health and social care services may expect to be involved in contributing to the improvement of services as they change to address newly identified needs and demands.

REFERENCES

National Institute of Clinical Excellence (2005) *Health Needs Assessment: A Practical Guide*.

Pfeffer, J. and Salancik, G. R. (2003) *The External Control of Organisations: A Resource Dependence Perspective*, Stanford University Press.

World Health Organization <http://www.who.int> (accessed 20/6/2009).

CHAPTER 8

ENGAGING WITH SERVICE USERS

In many areas of public policy, including health and social care, the trend in recent years has been to encourage service users and the general public to participate on a more equal basis than has previously been the case in the design, delivery and evaluation of public services that are funded by taxation.

In this chapter, we begin by examining the different meanings of participation in the context of health and social care and describe the different kinds of relationship that may exist between those who pay for services, those who design them, those who deliver them and those who benefit from them. No 'one size fits all', however: different types of participation and different types of relationship may be appropriate for different services or for the same service in different local environments.

In order to decide what is appropriate in particular circumstances, a manager may have to find out what existing service users, potential future service users and/or the general public want – in other words, to collect evidence. So we next turn our attention to the nature of evidence and what kind of evidence is needed. In order to collect evidence, managers may need to conduct – or commission – an appropriate investigation. We conclude this chapter, therefore, by examining some of the investigative techniques that are available to collect evidence – surveys, interviews and focus groups.

SERVICE USER PARTICIPATION

There are numerous ways in which to model the different levels of service user participation: one approach is to differentiate between a 'consumerist' view of services in which the providers of services offer options for the service users to make choices from (they are consulted but not involved in service design) and the 'democratic' view which emphasises the active participation of service users in the process of designing the options and therefore engages with service users at a strategic level. Based on notions of citizenship and civil rights, the democratic approach should lead to transfer of power and control to service users (SCIE, 2006). Webb (2008) defines participation in terms of three related forms:

■ *action* – for example, talking, listening, attending, responding to questions, sharing information;
■ *processes* – involvement in decision-making, relationship-building, agenda setting;
■ *values* – participation is underpinned by concepts of citizens' rights, inclusion, democracy, power relationships.

Participation is usually modelled in terms of a continuum, whereby the initial stages involve simply providing information or consulting on an individual level progressing in intensity through to the final stages as a true partnership and user-led initiatives (see Figure 8.1):

■ *Information*. Gathering information about service users and carers, ensuring that relevant information reaches them, and sharing ideas and plans about services with them (for example, by means of surveys, leaflets about services and discussion groups).
■ *Consultation*. Asking people's views and advice on plans, policies and services (for example, by means of advisory groups, focus groups, user panels and public meetings).
■ *Partnership*. Working as equals to set objectives, make plans and decide funding priorities (for example, through service users being members of planning, review and evaluation committees and groups).
■ *User-led services*. Giving authority and money to service users, carers and the wider community to plan and implement services (so that services are actually run by service users and by the community of which they are part).

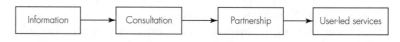

Figure 8.1 The service user participation continuum

Although many health and social care services are making considerable progress at the information/consultation end of the continuum, full partnership and delegated control of services are still relatively rare. Figure 8.2 shows examples of services for people with disabilities mapped on to the user-participation continuum.

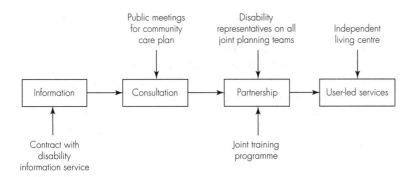

Figure 8.2 Examples of services for people with disabilities

ACTIVITY 8.1

Where do the services you are responsible for lie on the user-participation continuum at present? Following the example in Figure 8.2, map them on to the continuum.

Thinking about your services in this way may have shown that not all your services involve service users to the same extent. This may be because it is sometimes more appropriate to provide or gather information than to consult, enter into partnership or delegate control. As Carr (2004) highlights however, it is important that the *choice* for different levels exists but participation is contingent on various factors: the amount of activity participants themselves are able or wish to contribute, the stage of development of a particular project and the objectives of the project. Your strategy for involving service users and carers does not have to be an 'all or nothing' approach. Service users will appreciate it if you are honest and clear about what you are aiming to do. For example, if user-led services is not on your agenda, don't disguise the fact: it will be evident from the way you work with service users, and fudging the issue is likely to end in cynicism and a withdrawal of interest.

Mapping relationships

Another way of thinking about service user participation is to consider the relationships between those who pay for, design and deliver services, on the one hand, and the service users and carers who benefit from them on the other. We are now going to map the relationships between these 'key players' by using four circles depicting those who pay for services, those who design them, those who deliver them and those who benefit from them.

Figure 8.3 shows the relationships in what we might call the *bureaucratic* model of health and social care services. There are close relationships between those who pay for, design and deliver a service. Those who commission a service are involved in both paying for it and designing it. Staff are involved in both designing and delivering it, with managers functioning at the interface of payment, design and delivery. The service is then delivered to the service users and carers who benefit from it.

The *responsive* model is illustrated in Figure 8.4. The aim here is to develop and sustain a dialogue between, on the one hand, those who pay for, design and deliver the service and, on the other, those who benefit from it. However, although the beneficiaries' views and wishes are gathered and acted on, they are still excluded from decision making and do not have any power in planning and designing the service.

Figure 8.5 represents one version of an *empowering* service model. The 'design' circle in Figure 8.5 includes the specification of services and the way in which they are planned, and is the crucial element in this model. In contrast with Figures 8.3 and 8.4, almost all the key players,

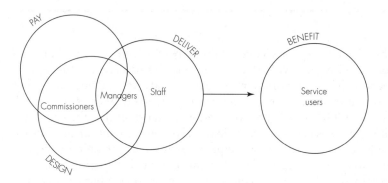

Figure 8.3 A bureaucratic service

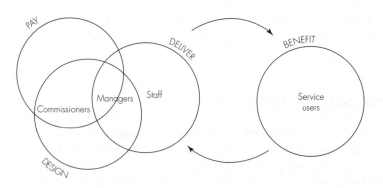

Figure 8.4 A responsive service

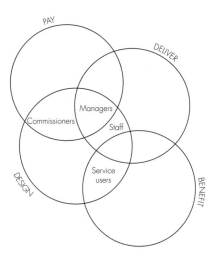

Figure 8.5
An empowering service

including service users, are now included within the design circle, whatever other circles they may also be part of. This suggests that the power relationships between service users and the other players will be worked out in the design circle: it is here that the amount of influence or power each key player has over service design will be resolved. Service users and carers can only be said to be empowered if they have direct influence in this sphere. Working with the inevitable difficulties this creates – in a situation where a clash of interests is certainly possible – is the central challenge for managers in developing modern health and social care services.

Interestingly, there has also been a shift from the bureaucratic to the responsive model in the relationships between key players *within* health and social care organisations. Ideas have changed about how different departments – and different levels within departments – should relate to one another. Similar diagrams can therefore be drawn for support services, showing the relationships between different parts of an organisation. A crucial move, in the interests of developing a service that empowers staff as well as service users, is to bring those who deliver the service and those who benefit from it inside the design circle.

ACTIVITY 8.2

1 Which of the three models described in this section most closely describes the main service for which you are responsible?
2 Using this model as a starting point, map the relationships between the key players in this service. (Don't forget to identify yourself in the diagram!)
3 How would you like to see these relationships change over the next two or three years?

One of the immediate effects of empowering service users and carers – or internal customers if you work in a support service – is that relationships and roles become more complex. Understanding and clarifying roles and relationships are important both to you and your team and to those who use your services. Changing the roles and relationships may crucially affect the nature of the outcomes that are required of your service by those commissioning it and by those using it – as well as the means of achieving them.

The rest of this chapter explores how you would plan a consultation with service users.

THE NATURE OF EVIDENCE

If you are to base your decisions on evidence or to present evidence in support of your claims, it is important to understand the nature of evidence. It would be very reassuring to be able to say that a claim is true if there is evidence to support it. But evidence may or may not be convincing in the way it is used to support a claim. Evidence is not a truth that cannot be challenged, because it can be used in different ways for different purposes. The nature of evidence and how it has been collected are important in considering how it can be used effectively.

Evidence usually takes the form of data relating to the issue under investigation. Data might include numbers, statistics, written statements, oral statements or photographs. For example, if you want to prove that you are competent in carrying out a management activity, you might present evidence including:

■ letters or emails relating to a particular occasion or event;
■ papers or reports you have prepared;
■ witness statements from people who have seen you carry out the activity successfully;
■ your own statement explaining how you did it.

However, your belief that the evidence supports the claim will not necessarily be sufficient to convince others, because data do not become information until they have been interpreted in some way.

Interpretation is often personal and subjective because it relies on knowledge and experience from which beliefs and values arise. For example, you might believe that you act in an efficient and effective way in carrying out your management activities. However, your judgement is related to the knowledge and experience that you have. A more experienced person with more knowledge would be able to make a judgement that draws on a broader range of examples. He or she might corroborate your opinion or might challenge it. Interpretation is based on judgement; judgement is about comparing things and coming to a conclusion based on the comparison.

In addition, it is important to remember that data have to be collected before they are presented as evidence, and the way in which they have been collected will shape the evidence.

ACTIVITY 8.3

Imagine that it is widely known that the reception area for your service is to be moved to a new location that has yet to be agreed. Several members of your team come to you with a suggestion that it should be transferred to a site close to the new shopping centre. They are sure that this is a wonderful opportunity because it would be much more convenient for everyone. They show you evidence that service users have been consulted and agree that it is a good idea. Would you be convinced? Make notes of anything that you would want to ask them.

You would want to know how they had collected the evidence that they are presenting to support their argument. If they are so convinced by this idea, they may not have looked for any alternative ideas or even noticed if any objections were presented to them. People tend to seek out and present only data that can be interpreted to support their case. You would also want to know whom they had consulted. For example, did they seek the views of different service users, including those with mobility difficulties? Did they consult different age groups, or representatives from support services or partner or linked services? Did they consider the financial aspects? Questions such as these – and the answers – would lead you to form an opinion about the extent to which you could have confidence in the evidence presented.

Evidence is data interpreted as information and used as proof to support an argument. If you are to be convinced by the argument, you need to be convinced that the evidence is acceptable. The tests that can be applied to help you to decide whether evidence is acceptable are:

- Is it sufficient?
- Is it authentic?
- Is it valid?
- Is it current?

Sufficient evidence

Is there enough evidence to support the claim that is made? If you are told that 100 service users were asked for their views, you would want to know how many had responded. You might also want to know whether various categories of service user were represented among those that had responded – older and younger, male and female, able and disabled, and so on.

Authentic evidence

Is the evidence what it is claimed to be? In the example of relocating the reception for a service, were all those who responded users of your service? Does it matter whether they were current or past users or whether they have never used your service but would be entitled to do so if the need arose? Who collected the data? Are you seeing the raw data – in the same form as when they were collected – or have they been analysed or interpreted in any way? If so, are they still representative of the original data or have they been interpreted to present the proposal in a better light?

Valid evidence

Does the evidence demonstrate what is claimed? How was the evidence collected from the 100 respondents? Did they understand what was being asked? Were they asked whether they would like the suggested new location or were they asked which of a number of possible locations they would prefer? Their answers may depend on how the questions were asked. How closely do they represent what service users really think? How real or truthful is the evidence? Does it prove what is claimed? Could it be interpreted in any other way? Is too much being claimed on the basis of too little evidence? Have opposing views been sought?

Current evidence

Is the evidence up to date? This is important in situations where there is rapid change. What people think about an issue may depend on whether there has been a recent event that may have influenced their attitudes or opinions.

It is not easy to produce evidence that is convincing when you are investigating an issue that concerns a number of people or groups of people with potentially different interests.

PLANNING AN INVESTIGATION

Evidence is obtained by investigation. Data are collected and analysed to provide information that can be used as evidence to support decision making or to demonstrate whether standards have been met. We will introduce some approaches and techniques that can be used to carry out an investigation, using the example of planning a consultation with service users. This will help you to think through some of the issues involved in planning an investigation in which other people are involved either in giving you information and opinions or in working with you to develop ways of improving the delivery of a service. The issues are similar if you manage a support service such as finance or estate services, and are planning to consult the colleagues who are your direct service users.

But what does it mean to *consult*? How might you go about it? What kind of evidence does consultation produce – and how useful is it?

ACTIVITY 8.4

What do you think are the strengths and weaknesses of each of the following approaches to planning and conducting an investigation?

Ask the questions you think should be asked and then interpret the answers that you receive.

Involve those you are consulting in deciding what questions should be asked and how the answers should be interpreted.

If you ask the questions you think should be asked, you will be focusing on the issue as you understand it. You may, however, miss some of the wider issues that concern service users. For example, you might want to ask what seems to be a simple question about whether service users can easily contact your organisation by phone. However, some service users may not have a phone and therefore prefer to visit an office; others may find it difficult to talk or to hear on the phone and prefer to meet face-to-face. Even if phones are answered promptly, some service users may have found those answering unhelpful. Some service users may prefer to access your services through a website or email.

If you ask a question like, 'Do you find it easy to contact this organisation by phone?', you may receive a range of different types of answer. Some people may simply say 'yes' or 'no'. That doesn't tell you what they consider 'easy' or 'difficult'. Service users are often very grateful for a service and may want to be obliging and say 'yes' rather than offer criticism. Some may say 'no' because they would prefer other means of contact rather than because there is any particular problem with using the phone.

Involving those who are being consulted in deciding what questions should be asked is often preferred because the issues may be complex and getting a range of different views and perspectives is helpful. This approach is likely to lead to a richer understanding of the range of people's feelings and opinions. From the perspective of a service provider, it is easy to make assumptions about what constitutes a 'good' service. The viewpoints of service users frequently demonstrate priorities and concerns that are different from those of providers. If you only ask people the questions that occur to you, you may only get the answers that you anticipated. If you engage people in carrying out an investigation with you, you may get some surprises and some information that is new to you.

Consultation and partnership

As we saw earlier, *consultation* means asking for people's views; *partnership* implies that those views are respected and acted upon.

Consultation implies a degree of partnership. A consultation in which the views of people are sought but then ignored would be a pointless exercise, and would not be regarded by those consulted as any kind of partnership. If service users think you have no intention of taking their views into account, they may become angry or cynical about service provision. It is important to demonstrate that their views have been heard and understood. However, this does not necessarily imply acceptance of their views. Where views are not accepted, or not acted upon immediately, you need to ensure that the reasons for the decisions you take following the consultation are explained fully and clearly.

So the first decision you need to make in planning a consultation is what you wish to consult people about. In particular, you have to think about what those consulted might expect or anticipate as a result of the consultation. Engaging in consultation has important consequences for service managers and professionals, but it also has important implications for those who are consulted, not least for their willingness to co-operate. If they are not convinced that the consultation is genuine, they are less likely to be responsive. Partnership implies a willingness to act on the information arising from a consultation which, in turn, implies that the information obtained must be in a form that can be acted on.

Planning a consultation exercise from a partnership perspective – from a perspective that regards the views of service users and carers as important – helps you to do the following:

- Think about your own and your staff's willingness and ability to listen to what service users are saying and to respond to it.
- Ensure that the responses you obtain from a consultation are in a form to which you can respond.
- Determine the scope of the consultation – limit it to gaining information on which you have the authority to act.
- Be clear, realistic and honest about the extent to which you are prepared to share power with service users.
- Ensure that the consultation process is sufficiently sensitive to pick up the underlying concerns of service users. For example, you might undertake a survey of satisfaction among residents in residential and nursing homes from which it is apparent that most people rate the staff and the care they receive very highly. However, you may fail to discover that most of the respondents would have preferred to be cared for in their own homes.

Attitudes to consultation

Part of the process of planning a consultation is, therefore, understanding the reasons for the consultation and making sure that all those involved understand them. This includes making sure that staff, who may be asked to adopt different working practices as a result of the consultation, understand the thinking behind it. In other words, you need to consider your own and other people's reasons for listening to service users.

ACTIVITY 8.5

Jot down at least three benefits of consulting people who need long-term care about service provision.

Thinking about this puts you in a better position to judge what to ask and who should be included in a consultation. The benefits arising out of consultation might include:

- getting feedback about services;
- improving services;
- improving the status of service users;
- assessing the impact of participation upon service users and the organisation;
- increasing public accountability and thus contributing to clinical governance and 'best value';
- increasing the trust of service users and the general public;
- getting a better understanding of the threats and opportunities facing services.

Different people may place a different emphasis on these various benefits. For example, some will recognise that there is an expectation that managers will act upon the information gained to improve services. However, others may see the requirement for consultation as just another government initiative to which they must respond with the minimum of effort. In some organisations the responsibility for undertaking the consultation will be passed on to a policy or quality assurance unit that is somewhat removed from operational units and professionals. Either of these responses would potentially undermine the intended benefits.

Consulting service users can be merely a token exercise in which the results are ignored or acknowledged with reluctance. Alternatively, it can lead to a better understanding of how services contribute positively and negatively to the quality of people's lives, and an improved under-standing of the priorities of service users. It can also provide valuable insights into conflicts of values and priorities that need to be better or more explicitly managed.

ACTIVITY 8.6

What value does your area of work place upon consultation with service users?

What are the implications of this for you and the service you manage?

WHAT KIND OF INFORMATION DO YOU NEED?

Referring back to the idea of a continuum of participation (Figure 8.1), we can see that there are different types of consultation. One is concerned with obtaining feedback from service users about the extent to which agreed standards have been achieved. The other is a more fundamental review of whether services are meeting their needs. These require different kinds of consultation. One is asking a *closed question* – 'Did we do X?' – to which the answers are limited to 'yes' or 'no' (or perhaps 'partially'); the other is asking an *open question* – 'What do you think about X?' – to which there may be as many responses as there are respondents.

All purposeful activity relies upon feedback and evaluation to provide information about how successful it is. This is true whether the activity is striking up a friendship or delivering a service. Implicitly or explicitly, purpose is translated into action through a plan, and the information required is two types: 'Are things going according to plan?' (feedback) and 'Is the plan producing the desired results?' (evaluation). This is represented by the quality control loop in Figure 8.6.

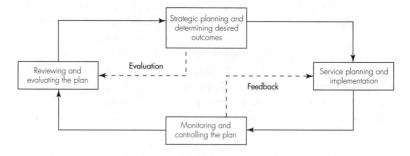

Figure 8.6 The quality control loop: two kinds of involvement and consultation

In this model there are two sub-loops. One is relevant to managers of services who need feedback on whether their service plans are being implemented effectively. The other involves a wider range of stakeholders, including service users, and is concerned with evaluating whether the plan being implemented is the right one. The first one is about the extent to which certain targets have been achieved – such as the number of patients treated or whether all service users have their own care plan. The second is about whether the treatments and care plans have delivered the desired outcomes for individuals.

Most performance management schemes involve collecting information about the achievement of targets. This is straightforward when the performance is easy to measure. For example, a standard might be that a request for assessment will be responded to within two working days: whether this standard has been achieved can be monitored by keeping a dated record of all requests and responses to them. This record provides the evidence of achievement. Examining the record – or perhaps a statistical summary of it prepared at intervals during the year – provides feedback about achievement against the standard.

ACTIVITY 8.7

How would you set about finding out whether service users feel able to complain about your service?

1 How might you monitor performance against this standard through records kept by staff?
2 From the perspective of one of your service users – or perhaps one of their carers – what would have to be in place for this standard to be met?
3 What steps might you take to monitor achievement of the standard through consultation with service users?

From an internal service perspective, compliance with this standard might be based on assurances by staff that it is being complied with. This might be supported by a procedure requiring that people be informed about their right to complain, or there might be a leaflet explaining how to complain. Perhaps staff are required to keep records confirming that they have informed people about their rights. As a manager, you may be confident that members of your team are doing all they can to meet the standard.

However, from the perspective of service users, your confidence may be regarded with some scepticism. In one survey of over a hundred users of social and community health services and their carers, fewer than 40 per cent said they knew whom to contact to make a complaint. But this is not necessarily evidence that they had not been informed.

A leaflet or a verbal explanation might have been given to them at some time in the past, perhaps when they were being assessed for services. This might have been at a time when they were faced with a crisis in their lives. Even in ordinary circumstances, giving information is only one half of the process of communication: information also has to be heard and understood (and perhaps also has to be readily available when it is needed) for communication to be effective.

In any case, the standard refers to 'ensuring that people feel able to complain', which is a rather different matter. In the survey referred to above, fewer than 50 per cent of those interviewed said that they would feel confident about complaining. The reasons they gave included fear of loss of service or reprisal, and unwillingness to get their support worker (nurse, social worker, home carer, etc.) into trouble.

Using records to show that information has been provided about how to make a complaint is therefore not sufficient to demonstrate that service users feel able to complain. Records of complaints that have been made, who made them and the circumstances in which they were made are useful. But if you want to know whether your service is meeting this standard, you need to ask service users for their views. Three of the principal methods for doing this are postal surveys, face-to-face interviews and focus groups. We'll consider each of these briefly in turn, and then conclude the section by considering some of the issues involved in asking questions which apply to all of them.

Postal surveys

The problems with postal surveys are summed up in an article about the surveys of the satisfaction of users of care services, which are conducted by the Social Services Inspectorate and Audit Commission Joint Review Team.

Professor Hasel Qureshi heads the Department of Health funded research programme into outcomes of social care at York University's Social Policy Research Unit. She points out that the joint review survey has got some important shortcomings, including an average response rate of just 42 per cent:

> As a researcher, you simply would not be able to use this data as evidence. To be seen as respectable you must have a minimum response rate of 60 per cent. It is also likely to be a biased sample – because only the views of people who are able to read and fill in a paper questionnaire are being represented.
>
> (quoted in Fickford, 2000)

Even leaving aside these methodological problems with the survey, Qureshi points out that previous tick-box surveys have also shown high satisfaction rates among adult users of community care services, and suggests that other approaches may elicit more useful information.

Satisfaction is multi-dimensional. It is important to separate out people's views of the workers who help them from their views of the agency. Most people like the workers and are satisfied with them. They see them having to rush around and wouldn't want to complain or risk getting them into trouble.

(Fickford, 2000)

The critical issues raised here are the low response rate, the difficulty people may have in responding and – a point already noted – a reluctance to complain.

ACTIVITY 8.8

What are the implications of Qureshi's comments for you, as a manager, when thinking about how to obtain feedback about your service from users and their carers?

First you need to be clear about what sort of information you want. Do you need to survey all the users of your service, or obtain a response rate of at least 60 per cent? If you want to know what proportion of your service users know how to complain, you do. But if you want to find out if a standard that should apply to everyone is being achieved, a smaller sample may be sufficient. Even if you survey only ten people, their feedback will provide some independent evidence to support a claim that you are meeting the standard – or to demonstrate that you are not achieving it.

It is perhaps more important to find out *why* people feel inhibited about complaining, rather than simply to discover the proportions of service users who do or do not feel inhibited. It is only by exploring the reasons that you may be able to think of ways to resolve the problem. If the type of information you require is qualitative rather than quantitative, a low response rate to a postal survey may not necessarily be a problem. However, the type of information that postal surveys generate is an issue. They tend to ask closed questions, to which respondents have to answer 'yes' or 'no', choose between two or more alternatives or mark a point on a scale from, say, 1 to 4. Postal surveys are a good way of generating quantifiable information. If you ask 100 people if they know how to complain and 60 say 'yes', that provides a useful snap-shot about performance. But if you ask an open question in a postal survey such as 'Do you think the complaints procedure is good enough?', a hundred different replies provide you with a challenge to find a way of organising the responses other than by simply counting them.

Face-to-face interviews

A major advantage of face-to-face interviews is that they do not rely on people's ability or motivation to fill in a form. Interviews also provide opportunities to ensure that questions are understood, to cover all the questions you want to ask and to ask follow-up questions. It is possible to establish rapport and thus to gain deeper insights into people's experience as users of your service. Questions about experiences, preferences and feelings usually need to be discussed and are therefore easier to deal with by interviewing than by postal surveys.

The major disadvantage of interviews is that they are very time-consuming. It is unlikely that you will be able to obtain the views of as many people by one-to-one interviews as by a postal survey – even one with a poor response rate. However, you can count responses to closed questions, as well as adding depth by asking open questions that invite people to describe their experiences and make judgements. Interviews can therefore provide both quantitative and qualitative information.

Focus groups

A focus group is a group of people who are invited to meet to discuss a particular issue.

ACTIVITY 8.9

Imagine inviting a number of users of your service to a meeting to discuss how you and your colleagues can best ensure that service users feel able to complain if they feel the need to do so. Make a note of some of the advantages and disadvantages of such an approach to consultation.

You may have thought about the difficulties of arranging for possibly severely ill or disabled people to attend a focus group. And how likely is it that people would feel able to discuss their personal experiences and feelings in such a setting? Some would, no doubt, but the meeting might be dominated by a few vocal people. So how representative would the views expressed be? You are unlikely to be able to record the number of people who agree or disagree with a certain proposition.

However, participating in a group discussion might encourage some people to have the confidence to make comments they might otherwise not make, especially if they discover that their experiences or feelings are shared by others. Focus groups can, therefore, generate useful feedback, and can help you to understand the strength of feeling about an issue that might not be apparent from one-to-one discussions.

For many service areas, advocacy groups, such as Age Concern, or support groups, such as a stroke club, can be a valuable source of information and feedback. They have a special interest in an area of work, and can be well informed about what they expect and what is good practice. However, their interest may be somewhat broader than yours as a service manager and their emphasis on service evaluation rather than providing feedback on current standards of practice.

How successful a meeting is in terms of getting useful feedback about your service depends on how it is structured and managed. Inviting 50 people to sit in rows in a large room is unlikely to be conducive to an open dialogue. It is easier to put people at their ease in smaller groups. A larger group can be divided into smaller discussion groups, each with a facilitator, to address a particular question or topic and then report back. As in all approaches to consultation, it is important to be clear about the purpose of the discussion, and to ask appropriate questions in appropriate ways using appropriate language.

Asking questions

A major strength of postal surveys is that they are relatively neutral and anonymous. In face-to-face discussions – whether with individuals or groups – your presence, wittingly or not, inevitably influences the consultation. Service users may not wish to give offence, and you may not want to hear negative comments. Your influence may be more limited in group settings, but it is then more difficult to control the agenda to make sure that you cover the full range of issues that you want information about. However, focus groups are more likely to generate information that you had not anticipated – what you want to know about may not be what your service users want to talk about. Face-to-face interviews can be carried out in people's homes, so that even severely disabled and ill people can be included, but in these settings it is even more difficult to avoid exerting your personal influence.

How, then, can you guard against unduly influencing people when you are consulting them? You need to consider using both open and closed questions, to be consistent in the questions you ask, to be aware that people attach different meanings to words, to ask simple direct questions, and to avoid defensiveness.

Open and closed questions

It is a good idea to have a mix of open and closed questions so that you can collate the answers to closed questions, as well as obtaining more detailed views through open questions. People often feel more comfortable if you start with a closed question and follow it up with an open one.

Consistency of approach

If you are going to be able to count the answers to a specific question (such as 'Would you feel able to complain if something went wrong?'), you have to ask the same questions of everyone. This may seem obvious but, especially if there is more than one interviewer, questions may be asked with varying degrees of emphasis or slightly different wording, and explanations about the meaning of a question might differ. All these can give rise to a lack of consistency.

The meaning of words

However you conduct a consultation, it is important to avoid professional jargon, to use everyday words as far as possible and, where difficult words are unavoidable, to explain them. For example, if you are seeking feedback about the requirement that everyone who is receiving community care services should have a care plan, it is unwise to assume that everyone knows what a care plan is.

Even more tricky is the use of everyday words that may mean different things to different people. For example, if you ask 'Did you feel involved in drawing up your care plan?', 'feel involved' is open to alternative interpretations. For some people, being informed of the nature and possible side effects of a treatment may be sufficient for them to feel involved; others may only feel involved if alternative possible courses of action are discussed with them. It may therefore be necessary to ask questions about the activities that underpin the idea of helping people to feel involved. This might include asking whether service users were given a choice between different courses of action, whether they think their views were taken into account when the care plan was drawn up, and so on. In this way, you can form a judgement against your professional understanding of what it is to involve people in planning their care and treatment.

Ask simple direct questions

In designing a questionnaire or drawing up a list of questions you are going to use in interviews or focus groups, you need to be clear what information you want. Consider, for example, the question 'Do you have a care plan?' There are at least three possible meanings for this apparently straightforward question depending on where the emphasis is placed, and each may prompt different answers according to how it is heard by the other person:

■ Do you have a *care plan*? (This might be asked as part of the process of finding out if the person knows what the term 'care plan' means.)

■ Do *you* have a care plan? (This may be asking the person whether he or she has something he or she calls a care plan, which may or may not be the document that you have in mind.)
■ Do you *have* a care plan? (This might mean 'Do you have a care plan in your possession?' or 'Do you know if there is one, maybe held by someone else?')

This illustrates the importance of being explicit about the purpose behind each question – of spelling out your information objectives. You need to divide the objectives into simple discrete questions and make sure that whoever is conducting the interview is clear about what information is being sought by each question. It is often helpful to try out your questions on a few colleagues and then on a few service users to ensure that they are understood in the way you intend them to be.

Avoiding defensiveness

If a question elicits a criticism, it is very easy to respond with an apology, a denial or an explanation. This may be appropriate, but it may not be. If the purpose of consultation is to obtain feedback, entering into a debate can distort the process. On the other hand, appearing indifferent to a problem or concern that has been expressed can be equally unhelpful. It is important to think through some 'What if . . .?' scenarios so that you can be prepared – or prepare others – to handle such situations.

ACTIVITY 8.10

Select three standards (preferably from among those that are already in place for your service). Examples might be:

■ all service users have a care plan
■ service users are involved in planning their care
■ service users feel able to complain if necessary.

Imagine that you and a colleague have set yourselves the task of interviewing 20 users of your service over the next few weeks to see if, in their experience, these standards are being met.

Design two questions – one closed and one open – that you are going to ask about each of the three standards to get this feedback.

Planning and carrying out an investigation that will be robust enough to produce reliable information are not trivial activities. They take considerable time. An investigation also demands time from other people and you have a responsibility to avoid wasting their time or raising expectations that you may be unable to fulfil. As in so many areas of management, to carry out an effective investigation you need to plan carefully, ensure that many different viewpoints have been taken into account and take time to reflect on your actions as you progress your plans.

In this chapter, we have considered the nature of evidence and the tests you can apply to decide whether evidence is acceptable – whether it is sufficient, authentic, valid and current. We have explored some of the issues involved in planning an investigation, using as an example the requirement to consult users of long-term care services and their carers. In conducting an investigation of this kind, you have three main options for collecting information – postal surveys, face-to-face interviews and focus groups – each of which has both advantages and disadvantages. All of these involve asking questions, and we concluded by examining some of the pitfalls to be avoided in designing questions.

REFERENCES

Carr, S. (2004) 'Has service user participation made a difference to social care services?' *Position Paper No. 3*, Social Care Institute for Excellence.

Fickford, F. (2000) 'Are customers always right?', *Community Care*, May, pp. 25–31.

Social Care Institute for Excellence (2006) 'The participation of adult service users, including older people, in developing social care', *Guide 17*, Social Care Institute for Excellence.

Webb, S.A. (2008) 'Modelling service user participation in social care', *Journal of Social Work*, vol. 8, no. 3, pp. 269–90.

CHAPTER 9

MANAGING OUTCOMES WITH SERVICE USERS

This chapter begins by emphasising the importance of being clear about the purposes of the services for which you are responsible, and of identifying their intended outcomes in ways that enable you to measure the extent to which you are achieving them. This may seem self-evident, but it is not always easy to achieve the intended outcomes in health and social care, where many services have multiple purposes, with outcomes that are difficult to define and measure.

We also explore the importance of providing health and social care services that are effectively integrated. Many service users require a range of services from different parts of the same organisation or from different organisations. In order to ensure that a complex array of services is provided in an integrated way to each individual service user, managers need to focus their attention on the boundaries between their services and other related services.

PURPOSE AND OUTCOMES

The purposes of health and social care services as defined today have often evolved over many years. Many services now provided by statutory organisations started with a voluntary organisation recognising a need of a particular group of people and raising money to meet that need. For example, the Women's Royal Voluntary Service played a significant part in identifying that older people living alone are often unable to prepare a hot meal for themselves. They prepared hot meals in central kitchens, which they delivered to people in their homes. People not only liked the hot meal, but also the contact with the person who delivered it. Community meals services now serve a wider variety of purposes, including, for example, enabling the earlier discharge of people from hospital.

A variety of powerful influences determines the purposes of services. National government has a major role in deciding what services will be provided and for what purposes, both through legislation (for example the various NHS Acts, *Every Child Matters* and the Mental Health Act) and through policy guidance (for example, the Quality and Outcomes Framework). Local commissioning authorities (primary care trusts, hospital trusts and social care agencies) have developed sophisticated methods of determining local needs, identifying gaps in services and determining priorities. All these players control substantial funds, which they use to commission services from statutory and independent service providers, and thus determine the purposes, quantity and quality of the services that are provided.

But even though the statutory framework for provision of a service may largely determine its purpose, there is often scope for individual managers to influence this, and they certainly have influence over the way in which it is delivered. How front-line managers interpret a service's purposes can have a significant effect on its outputs and outcomes.

It is important to distinguish between outputs and outcomes. In health and social care, *outputs* are usually procedures and processes completed – for example, numbers of patients treated or numbers of care plans prepared – and they are generally fairly easy to measure. *Outcomes* tend to happen outside the service, back in the service user's own home, and are only partly within the control of those who specify and provide services. In a health and social care context, outcomes include crucial events such as healthy births, quality of life and protection from harm. The desired outcomes of a service are not always easy to define, and are often difficult to measure. For the recipient of health or social care, the outcome should be better than what would have occurred if no service had been provided: 'This is the acid test of effectiveness, and in a world of finite resources we need to think about how to apply this acid test' (Riley and Riley, 1998).

A statement of a service's purpose should specify clearly who the service is for and the nature of the service provided, and it should be possible to relate this statement to specific and measurable outcomes. However, in health and social care it is not always easy to write an explicit statement of purpose and it is even more difficult to link the purpose to measurable outcomes.

For example, the National Service Framework for Mental Health (Department of Health, 1999) included the following statement:

> *Any individual with a common mental health problem should be able to make contact round the clock with the local services necessary to meet their needs and receive adequate care.*

It goes on to say that achievement of this standard should be assessed in terms of 'evidence that services respond to mental health needs quickly, effectively and consistently 24 hours a day, 365 days a year'.

This raises a number of different kinds of questions. First, there are questions of interpretation, for example:

- What does 'making contact round the clock' mean?
- Does it mean that every possible type of service should be available round the clock?
- What does that imply for the skill mix of the personnel required?
- Is every service expected to be accessible to everyone in its catchment area?
- What constitutes an effective response to a mental health need?

Second, there are questions about making people aware of the service. For example:

- How do people know that the service exists?
- If they know that it exists, do they have the means to access it?
- Is it perceived as credible and helpful by all the people who might use it?

Third, there are questions about outcomes, for example:

- Is such a service likely to reduce the incidence of suicide?
- If the incidence of suicide reduced following the introduction of the service, how would you know what contribution the round-the-clock service had made to that reduction?

These last two questions – about identifying outcomes and finding a way of measuring whether they have been achieved – are particularly challenging ones.

Let's look at two examples of service outcomes and how they are measured.

Outcomes for cancer treatment

The aim of the NHS Cancer Plan (2000) was to improve the prospects of survival for cancer patients. A team of researchers explored national data on cancer patient survival in England and Wales up to 2007, by comparing survival trends in England and Wales before, during and after the implementation of the plan and also taking into consideration the cancer strategy for Wales 'Designed to Tackle Cancer' (2006).

The researchers found improvement in one-year survival in England and Wales for men and women diagnosed during 1996–2006, with annual trends higher in Wales than England during 1996–2000 and 2001–3 but higher in England than in Wales during 2004–06. They concluded that there was some beneficial effect of the NHS Plan for England (Ratchet et al., 2009).

In this study, the outcomes for patients resulting from a government strategy were measured in terms of the length of time patients survived after diagnosis – a straightforward measure. However, there are many other possible measures of the outcomes of cancer treatment and care, for example, in terms of the quality of life experienced by the patients and the economic costs to the health service and the community. There is also increasing interest in the 'deprivation gap': the different survival rates between people from affluent social classes and those from deprived backgrounds.

Outcomes for children's services

The broad outcomes for children's services are based on *Every Child Matters* (Department for Children, Schools and Families (2008):

- Be healthy
- Stay safe
- Enjoy and achieve
- Make a positive contribution
- Achieve economic well-being

and are then mapped against other national frameworks, for example:

Outcome: Be healthy

Children's Plan Goal: Enhance children and young people's well-being, particularly at key transition points in their lives.

National Public Service Agreement: Deliver successful Olympic and Paralympics games with a sustainable legacy and get more children and young people taking part in high quality PE and sport.

These statements start to indicate what care services should set out to achieve for the children concerned – the outcomes – but finding appropriate ways of measuring whether they have been achieved is not easy. Some of the performance measures identified for the 'Be healthy' outcome by the Department for Children, Schools and Families are:

- Emotional health and well-being – as measured by the perceptions of children and young people.
- Prevalence of breastfeeding at 6–8 weeks from birth.
- Obesity among primary school age children in reception year.
- Percentage of 5–16 year olds participating in at least two hours per week of high-quality PE and sport at school and the percentage of 5–19 year olds participating in at least three further hours per week of sporting opportunities.
- Rate of hospital admission per 100,000 for alcohol-related harm.

Such data will need to be drawn from national and local databases and may also entail interviews, focus groups or questionnaires with service users, professionals and managers.

ACTIVITY 9.1

Choose one of the services that you have some responsibility for. Review any existing statements of its purpose(s) and outcomes that you can find. (You might, for example, look at government guidelines, national service frameworks, professional guidelines, the Quality and Outcomes Framework, or the reports of regulatory bodies for health and social care.)

1 Encapsulate, as clearly and briefly as you can, the purpose(s) of this service.
2 Specify two intended outcomes of this service.
3 Identify one performance measure for each outcome.
4 Consider how you would involve service users in measuring outcomes.

WORKING ACROSS BOUNDARIES

In this section, we explore a number of the issues involved in working together to provide integrated care for service users. Partnership working within health and social care has become second nature now and is mandatory in many areas of service planning and delivery. It was enshrined in government policy from the late 1990s onwards but locally based initiatives pre-dated this and the NHS and Community Care Act of 1991 also provided a stimulus. Working in partnership, whereby separate organisations collaborate together, has increasingly moved towards integration by the formation of new multiprofessional teams and services and the erosion of traditional boundaries between a 'health' organisation and a 'social care' organisation. As a manager in any part of the complex health and social care system, you need to be aware of the interfaces – the boundaries where the work you do needs to be integrated with the work of others.

Boundaries may be marked by geography, professional differences, different sources of funding, organisational structures, or differences in values and priorities. Service users will often not understand these boundaries. They – and you – may see them only as a hindrance. Nonetheless, it is frequently at the boundaries between services that crucial decisions are made about the care of a service user. Conflicts may arise because you do not fully understand how those on the other side of boundaries work and what their priorities and concerns are. The same may also be true of their understanding of your work. If some of the boundaries are unclear – and they often are – you may need to clarify where your responsibilities begin and end.

We are going to present a case study that highlights some of the issues related to working across boundaries. It is written from the point of view of the family of Mr Jones, who is terminally ill. We want you to try to understand their perspective on their experiences and also to look at the events described from the point of view of a manager who may be in a position to take action or to make recommendations to improve the processes involved. We have chosen a case study about a person who is terminally ill because, in one sense, there can be only one outcome – in clinical terms, at least. However, there are many other possible intermediate outcomes of the health and social care services provided to both the patient and his family in a situation like this.

Moving outside health and social care for a moment, Berry *et al.* (1985) conducted extensive in-depth interviews with a wide variety of customer groups in the service sector. In analysing their data, the researchers were able to identify a number of dimensions on which customers assessed the quality of the services they received. These are listed in the left-hand column of Table 9.1, with good and bad examples in the other two columns. As you read through Table 9.1, you may conclude that not all these dimensions of quality are relevant to the services for which you are responsible, but it is likely that you will be able to make at least some connections with your experience at work. This work has been criticised as too focused on the customer's experience of the service encounter, thereby ignoring the intrinsic qualities and attributes of the service (Walker *et al.*, 2006). However, this emphasis on the customer's perspective is even more relevant in health and social care at the current time given the shift to a more service user-led provision.

When asked about the issues that they regarded as most important to their situation, the Jones family identified the following:

- whether Mr Jones and his family felt psychologically safe;
- whether Mr Jones was physically safe;
- the accessibility and responsiveness of the health and social care services involved;
- who was empowered to make what decisions;
- the effectiveness of the communication between all those involved;
- the effectiveness of the integration of the various services involved.

You will notice that these concerns correspond quite closely to a number of Berry's dimensions of quality. Apart from the fact that some of Berry's dimensions are not included at all, there are three other differences. First, the Jones family distinguished between two aspects of what Berry calls 'security' – psychological safety and physical safety. Second, they combined two of Berry's dimensions in their concern for accessibility and responsiveness of services. Third, they focused

Table 9.1 Customer assessment of quality

Dimensions of quality	Good examples	Bad examples
Reliability	Punctual arrival of train	Failure to phone customer back as agreed
Responsiveness	Maintenance staff who service equipment at short notice	Long queues
Competence	Staff carry out task with skill and competence	Bank fails to cancel standing order, then charges fee for resulting overdraft
Access	Easy to find one's way Easy to get to	Poor signing Limited car parking
Courtesy	Polite and helpful staff	Senior staff patronising and condescending
Communication	Medical staff who explain the diagnosis and alternative forms of treatment without using jargon	Lack of information, when a train is delayed, about the cause and duration of the delay
Credibility	A solicitor you feel you can trust and depend on	A salesman who uses hard-sell tactics
Security	A feeling of personal safety and confidentiality	Unlit access at night
Understanding/ knowing the customer	Staff who make an effort to meet a customer's individual requirements	Staff who don't recognise a regular customer
Tangibles	Pleasing physical appearance of facilities	Poor or out-of-date equipment being used for the service

(Source: Berry *et al.*, (1985) *A Practical Approach to Quality*, Joiner Associates Inc. © Oriel Incorporated, formerly Joiner Associates, reprinted with permission)

on who was empowered to make decisions and on the issue of integration of services, which do not feature on Berry's list, although both might be related to Berry's dimension of 'understanding/knowing the customer'.

ACTIVITY 9.2

Read the case study below. It is divided into six phases. Pause after you read each of these and, from the perspective of the Jones family, make a brief note of how you think they may have felt at this point about the first three of the issues listed earlier: psychological safety, physical safety and accessibility/responsiveness of services.

The story of Mr and Mrs Jones

Phase 1

Mr Jones was 83 and suffering from terminal cancer. He was gradually getting weaker, and was confined to bed most of the time. He wanted to die at home, although neither he nor his wife were sure how the illness and his care needs would progress. Since the diagnosis had been confirmed three months before by a scan, his treatment plan was in the hands of his GP, who visited weekly. The GP's treatment plan was minimalist – not intervening with drugs unless absolutely necessary and choosing a time to allow the inevitable infections to take their course – a plan with which the family had no disagreement, given Mr Jones's age.

Co-ordination of practical care was in the hands of the district nurse. Auxiliary nurses were helping with washing Mr Jones, but for the rest of the time his wife (also aged 83) was his carer, looking after everything to do with finances, cooking, shopping, washing, etc. with a little help from neighbours who provided transport and other bits of practical help.

The local council's social care services department had been contacted and had supplied information, but had not carried out an assessment as yet.

No one had suggested that Mr Jones was entitled to an attendance allowance from the Department of Work and Pensions (DWP), but fortunately his daughter knew about the fast-track arrangements for people with terminal illness. Mrs Jones got the necessary form, completed it, and left it with the receptionist at the GP's surgery, who said she would get the GP to countersign it and forward it to the DWP. Having heard nothing, Mrs Jones telephoned the DWP two weeks later. They had not received the form, and further enquiries revealed that it had been filed at the surgery. Eventually, the money came through. Mr Jones was becoming too weak to stand unaided.

Phase 2

One Saturday evening Mr Jones got out of bed by himself to use the commode, and fell. The nurses had advised Mrs Jones that, if he were to fall, she should call the ambulance service for help in lifting him. So Mrs Jones called the ambulance service, expecting that they would help her to get him back into bed. Instead, they examined him, and took him off in the ambulance to the local accident and emergency department, ten miles away. Mr Jones was not able to cope – physically, intellectually or emotionally – with this situation on his own, and some time later his wife was called to the hospital. Fortunately a neighbour was able to give her a lift and stay with her at the hospital.

Phase 3

After more tests that night, Mr Jones was admitted to hospital and Mrs Jones went home. Mr Jones's bed was in a general medical ward housing mainly younger patients. A urinary infection was suspected and a drip set up to reduce his dehydration.

When relatives visited the following day (Sunday), they found that he had been left alone at the end of the ward furthest from the toilets, without a call bell, bottle or commode, and was therefore unable to cope with going to the toilet. The humiliation of wetting the bed was horrible.

Phase 4

On the Monday morning, the hospital started Mr Jones on a course of antibiotics for the suspected urinary infection (which had not yet been confirmed). The reason for prescribing an antibiotic was not given to the relatives, or to the GP who visited later that day.

By the end of Monday, Mr Jones had been fitted with an extremely uncomfortable continence aid, and was deeply distressed and unhappy. He told his wife he was lying there 'trying to die'. All the parties to his treatment – relatives, nurses, and the GP – had questioned why he was in hospital. The hospital social workers were contacted to arrange care for him on his return home.

Phase 5

Two days later, care had been arranged. The ambulance service had been contacted, and on Wednesday he was taken home. On arrival at home, the ambulance staff helped him walk up the two flights of stairs to his bedroom – a task that took more than half an hour. That evening the first carers arrived from the private care service that had been called in by the social services department. No one had been informed by the hospital that Mr Jones had a urinary infection, so the antibiotics were stopped.

Phase 6

By the following weekend, Mr Jones was very ill. He had slept for an entire day following the exhausting task of walking up two flights of stairs. He was incontinent and in severe pain from the ineffective continence aids that were being used. His daughter had to arrange a case conference with the GP and nurses to get these arrangements changed. Mr Jones's mind was wandering, and he had become incapable of co-operating in his care. For the only time in his whole illness, he was rude to his carers.

A week of extreme stress for Mr Jones, his wife and his daughter ensued, during which they had to do the following:

- adjust to twice daily visits from carers and explain the situation to every new carer who arrived;
- deal with the fact that the professionals often arrived while lunch (the main meal of the day) was being cooked or about to be served;
- explain to a number of different nurses what the circumstances and difficulties were and persuade them to do something about it;
- deal with the fact that very few of the visitors realised that Mr and Mrs Jones had poor hearing and were therefore often unable to understand what the visitors were saying, even when this was pointed out to them;
- chase around the area finding pharmacists who could supply appropriate continence aids, as well as collecting prescriptions, aids and adaptations;
- learn the working arrangements of Crossroads care attendants, twilight nurses, nightcare nurses, Macmillan nurses, hearing aid suppliers, collectors of contaminated refuse, community dentists and the private company supplying care assistants.

There had still been no assessment or review visit from the social services department. It took more than two weeks to resolve the problems triggered by the decision to remove Mr Jones to hospital. However, no long-term harm appeared to have been done and a new and more stable situation then emerged.

Our perspective on these events can never be the same as that of the Jones family, so there are no right answers. Our notes were as follows.

Phase 1

Psychological safety: good – Mr Jones at home, with Mrs Jones in charge and providing security.

Physical safety: becoming problematic because Mr Jones is now too weak to stand unaided.

Accessibility/responsiveness of services: GP seems to have been accessible and responsive, organising nursing support; social services department was accessible, but not very responsive; no help given in contacting the DWP.

Phase 2

Psychological safety: lost.

Physical safety: temporarily improved.

Accessibility/responsiveness of services: ambulance service responded quickly; no help offered to Mrs Jones to get to hospital.

Phase 3

Psychological safety: completely absent – Mr Jones in despair, having been placed in a situation where he has lost all autonomy; Mrs Jones not able to be present to co-ordinate action and family very upset.

Physical safety: satisfactory.

Accessibility/responsiveness of services: no evidence of an assessment having been made of Mr Jones's needs.

Phase 4

Psychological safety: totally destroyed.

Physical safety: treatment plan changed without apparent consultation or information given to GP or family; drugs prescribed without explanation; continence aid causing great discomfort (applied for convenience of staff?).

Accessibility/responsiveness of services: hospital very slow in deciding on discharge and in beginning to make arrangements for Mr Jones to return home.

Phase 5

Psychological safety: improving.

Physical safety: making Mr Jones walk up two flights of stairs exhausted him; still unclear whether antibiotic was needed.

Accessibility/responsiveness of services: carers arrived promptly.

Phase 6

Psychological safety: for Mr Jones, poor at the beginning of this phase, but then gradually improving; Mrs Jones now under great stress, because co-ordination of care is almost entirely in her hands.

Physical safety: poor at the beginning of this phase, but improving, especially after the painful continence aid was changed.

Accessibility/responsiveness of services: professionals slow to deal with problem of continence aid; plenty of services available, but responsibility left with carers to call them in and co-ordinate them; professionals unable to recognise and respond to Mr and Mrs Jones's poor hearing.

Now let's turn to the other three issues identified by the Jones family as problematic:

■ who was empowered to make what decisions
■ the effectiveness of the communication between all those involved
■ the effectiveness of the integration of the various services involved.

ACTIVITY 9.3

Identify for each of phases 2–6 of the case study, the key decisions made – apparently without consultation with Mr Jones or his family – that had adverse consequences for psychological and physical safety. In each case, what alternative decision might the Jones family have preferred, had they been consulted?

Once again, there are no right answers, but here are our suggestions.

Phase 2

Ambulance staff decided to take Mr Jones to the hospital's accident and emergency department. (Could they have put him back in bed?)

Phase 3

The accident and emergency department decided to admit Mr Jones to hospital. (Could they have sent him home, or could he have been admitted to a more suitable ward, with access to a call bell?)

Phase 4

The hospital decided to prescribe an antibiotic for the suspected urinary infection and to provide continence aid. (Was either necessary?)

Phase 5

Ambulance staff decided to help Mr Jones to walk upstairs. (Should he have been carried?)

Phase 6

The social services department did not arrange an assessment or review visit (perhaps this was the result of the lack of a decision). (Should they have arranged a co-ordinated care package?)

Mr Jones's story is not untypical. However competent all the individual care staff, this did not prevent a severe illness and a very stressful episode. The Jones family identified the two major – and related – inadequacies in the services provided to Mr Jones as failures in communication and a lack of integration between services. The individual professionals took actions that appeared sensible to them at the time, but which did not take into account Mr Jones's overall state of health and well-being. Each handed Mr Jones on to another person, without being aware of the consequences of their actions.

It is perhaps in managing the communication between your service and other services that relate to it – and thus contributing to the integration of services – that you, as a manager, can make the greatest contribution to the development of better outcomes for service users. The individual professionals who work in health and social care are, almost inevitably, reactive: it is your job to be proactive. Mr and Mrs Jones's story would almost certainly have been very different if a multi-agency care plan had been in place from the outset.

Measuring successful outcomes in partnership and integration

The above case study has emphasised the need for greater integration and communication between professionals and with service users. Although a need has been identified, this does not mean that partnership working and integration are easy to achieve. As Dickinson and Glasby (2008) highlight, some stakeholders have become quite sceptical about collaborative working, including the Audit Commission, and in fact some long-established partnership arrangements have even started to be dismantled. These authors, however, are relatively optimistic about the impact of the personalisation agenda on partnership and integration, i.e. it is changing the nature of partnership. They suggest that as joining up services is now more driven by the needs of individual service users than by organisations, it is resulting in a conceptual shift from an *interorganisational* focus to a *citizen–state* partnership focus. They add, however, that interaction at the interface is more imperative than ever: service users need to be able to join up and access their own services and that cannot happen without adequate inter-agency working.

Various researchers have explored the principles that can assist working in partnership, and thus help to provide more integrated and effective provision for service users.

- Specifying outcomes for partnerships is crucial. Government policy is vague on how success in partnership could be measured. In the words of Dickinson and Glasby (2008): 'if outcomes are never specified, then partnerships can never fail. But similarly, partnerships can also never succeed if it is not clear what it is they are supposed to attain.' We need to know that partnerships are producing 'better' outcomes for service users than other forms of delivery (Dowling *et al.*, 2004).
- Consider the costs and benefits of partnerships: involving more stakeholders in decision-making is generally more complex, time-consuming and financially costly (Dowling *et al.*, 2004).

■ Good leadership is required in bringing together – and sustaining – people from different professional and organisational cultures (Cook *et al.*, 2007).
■ Dealing with the 'dominance' of health in partnerships and integrated services is crucial to effective working in the new teams (Cook *et al.*, 2007).
■ Indicators of successful outcomes may include quicker responses from service providers, distribution of services relative to need, costs of services and whether there are resulting reductions in duplication and overlap between services, changes in working conditions and job satisfaction for staff, improvements for service users in their quality of life and ability to live independently (Dowling *et al.*, 2004).

ACTIVITY 9.4

For the main service for which you are responsible, identify one other service that lies on its boundary. It might be another service within the same organisation or part of a different organisation.

1 Describe briefly how you work with it.
2 Are there differences between its methods of working and yours that help or hinder you?
3 Describe briefly any areas of conflict between these two services.
4 How effective is the communication between you that directly affects patients or service users?
5 How could you work together more effectively to improve outcomes for service users? How would you know if you had been successful?

We began this chapter by considering the importance of being clear about the purposes of the services for which you are responsible and identifying and measuring their intended outcomes. We concluded by focusing on the importance of managing the boundaries between your services and others. As a manager in health or social care, it is likely that you will be increasingly required to work collaboratively with other services to seek more effective outcomes for service users. A good understanding of the part that your service plays within the whole process of care is important. This will help you to spot opportunities for service development and improvement, to take a service user perspective and to manage more effectively and in a more integrated way.

REFERENCES

Berry, L., Zeithaml, V. and Parasuraman, A. (1985) *A Practical Approach to Quality*, Joiner Associates Inc.

Cook, A., Petch, A., Glendinning, C., and Glasby, J. (2007) 'Building capacity in health and social care partnerships: key messages from a multi-stakeholder network', *Journal of Integrated Care*, vol. 15, no. 4, pp. 3–10.

Department for Children, Schools and Families (2008) *Every Child Matters Outcomes Framework* <http://publications.everychildmatters.gov.uk/eOrderingDownload/DCSF-00331-2008.pdf> (accessed 20/6/2009).

Department of Health (1999) *The National Service Framework for Mental Health*, Department of Health <http://www.dh.gov.uk/prod_consum_dh_digitalassets@dh@en/documents/digitalasset/dh_4077209.pdf> (accessed 20/6/2009).

Dickinson, H. and Glasby, J. (2008) 'Not throwing out the partnership agenda with the personalisation bathwater', *Journal of Integrated Care*, vol. 16, no. 4, pp. 3–8.

Dowling, B., Powell, M. and Glendinning, C. (2004) 'Conceptualising successful partnerships', *Health and Social Care in the Community*, vol. 12, no. 4, pp. 309–17.

Ratchet, B., Maringe, C., Nur, U., Quaresma, M., Shah, A., Woods, L. M., Ellis, L., Waters, S., Forman, D., Steward, J., Coleman, M. P. (2009) 'Population-based cancer survival trends in England and Wales up to 2007: an assessment of the NHS cancer plan for England', *The Lancet Oncology*, vol. 10, pp. 351–69.

Riley, C. and Riley, J. (1998) 'Outcome indicators: friends or enemies?', *Managing Community Care*, vol. 6, no. 6, pp. 246–53.

Walker, R. H., Johnson, L. W., Leonard, S. (2006) 'Re-thinking the conceptualization of customer value and service quality within the service–profit chain', *Managing Service Quality*, vol. 16, no. 1, pp. 23–36.

PART 3

MANAGING SERVICES

CHAPTER 10

MANAGING PROCESSES

Examining how your service is delivered in order to identify opportunities for improvement can be quite challenging. If you are to make effective improvements, you need to be clear about the areas over which you have authority and decide which staff to involve in defining, planning and implementing change. You may also want to involve service users. You need to recognise the boundary issues to be dealt with – to identify any parts of your service area that link with or overlap with other organisational or professional areas. Any change may involve crossing several boundaries between services, agencies, organisations and professions. If you work in a large and complex organisation, such as a hospital or a social services or social work department, your scope to influence elements of the pathway may be limited to your own area of work, but any changes you make will have implications for those whose services link in any way with your own area. In a small organisation – perhaps an advisory service or a small voluntary organisation – you may be able to influence the whole range of service delivery more directly. Many managers will have considerable influence over one area of work and some influence over a number of others.

Whatever your situation, you may be called on to participate in reviews of the effectiveness of service delivery, to contribute ideas for improvement, and to implement and monitor improvements or changes that have been agreed. This will require you to focus on values, purposes and results. You will need to make use of feedback from service users, use your 'people management' skills to help your team to contribute ideas and adjust to change, and use your skills in setting standards, handling information and feedback, planning and monitoring. It is also important to remember that the service is provided for service users and ensure that any improvements you consider making will benefit them. This chapter offers some signposts and tools to help you in this complex process.

The range of health and social care services provided in any geographical area have developed over time, often without any attempt to link one with another. Many years of joint planning and commissioning have improved the links between services, but gaps are regularly revealed, often when service users are failed by the systems. Many managers now find themselves not only managing an area of work within their own organisation, but also managing the relationships between their own area of work and services that supply their area or purchase from them. Integration between service areas is an increasingly important aspect of the quality of provision and many managers will have some responsibility for delivering cost-effective services to people with complex social and health care needs.

Many service users need a sequence of services, often described as a 'pathway'. Our focus in this chapter is on the pathway that service users follow through the range of services and support that they encounter in health and social care. If an older person has a fall, they may need emergency and hospital services immediately, but the reason for the fall must be investigated and, before the person can be discharged from hospital, he or she may need additional support provided in their home, tests for sight or hearing, review of medication, or other services. A well integrated care and support pathway would assess and meet service users' needs in a timely fashion and respect their views and their dignity throughout their 'journey'. A pathway might pass through a series of boundaries between organisations and professions. In a well integrated pathway, these boundaries would appear seamless to the service user or to those delivering the different services. For example, a pathway developed to integrate care of older people with complex needs crosses boundaries of different professions and agencies:

> The falls care pathway, as described in the NSF [National Service Framework] and NICE [National Institute for Health and Clinical Excellence] guidance, involves primary prevention (environment and lifestyle issues); case finding of people who have fallen or who are at risk of falling; multi-disciplinary assessment for falls risk factors; and an individualised multi-component, multi-agency intervention for falls prevention.
>
> (Department of Health, 2007)

In this chapter, we consider how well integrated pathways through health and care can be developed and managed.

DEFINING AND MAPPING PROCESSES

Defining and mapping the processes that contribute to a care pathway are the first steps in planning better integration. The NHS in Scotland has developed a toolkit that offers this advice:

Process mapping helps to identify and examine existing journeys of care from the perspective of staff, service users and informal carers. Teams can begin to see where changes or improvements can be made by identifying gaps, overlaps, strengths and weaknesses of current services and processes. This exercise alone can help to build good team working and develop shared goals and responsibilities.

A process mapping exercise should:

- identify current patterns of service delivery and available resources
- examine the journey of care for service users and informal carers
- establish the strengths and weaknesses of current service provision
- quantify demands on the services
- identify the gaps in services
- identify gaps in staff skills and competencies, and
- identify how the journey of care can be improved.

(NHS in Scotland, 2009)

The outcome of a process mapping exercise would be the process map (or maps) and any associated reports, together with action plans based on the recommendations of the process mapping.

It might be helpful at this stage to clarify a few of the terms used in talking about service delivery processes. *The New Oxford English Dictionary* suggests the following definitions of a process:

> *a continuous series of actions, events or changes . . . especially a continuous and regular action or succession of actions occurring or performed in a definite manner; a systematic series of actions or operations directed to some end.*

A process consists of a number of *activities* that are organised into an appropriate sequence and co-ordinated to achieve a specific purpose. We could describe a process as a number of activities that transform inputs (materials, skills, etc.) into outputs.

A *service* is made up of a number of processes that work together to deliver the service. The word *system* is used to describe all the services, processes, activities (and people) involved in the delivery of a particular aspect of health or social care. The contact that an individual service user has with particular processes and services as they move through the system can be described as a *pathway*.

These concepts can be examined from different perspectives. For example, a system may look very different to a service user from the way it looks to you as the manager of a particular service. Let's consider the sort of experience a service user might have. His or her first encounter with a health or social care service is likely to include a number of discussions and possibly some tests. These activities may be

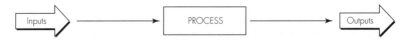

Figure 10.1 A transformation process

followed by a decision about providing some help or treatment that should lead to a successful outcome. In 'systems thinking' terms, this can be described as a *transformation process* (Figure 10.1).

Figure 10.1 shows inputs being transformed into an output by a process. However, this diagram does not give us any information about the nature of the process or processes that contribute to the transformation. The inputs may not all necessarily happen at the same time or only once. Nor may the outputs necessarily all happen at the same time. Figure 10.2 is a more helpful diagram that illustrates how a process may involve a series of inputs being made at different times, with a number of different activities contributing to the achievement of the output or outputs.

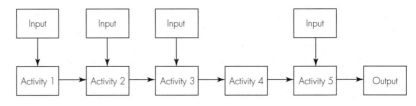

Figure 10.2 Flow of transformation processes

Process flow

The sequence of inputs, activities and outputs can be described as the *process flow*, implying that there is a smooth progression from one activity to the next until the output is achieved. This way of thinking helps to identify where improvements to processes can be made. Once the flow of a process is understood as a sequence of inputs and activities with links between them, it is possible to identify where there are bottlenecks or blockages in the flow of the process. By examining each input in relation to each activity, you can be more precise about the resources that are needed to provide each input and when they are required to carry out each activity.

The following case study illustrates how this way of thinking can be applied to improve a service area. It describes the work of a steering group that is seeking to improve the pathway (or trail) patients follow through elective surgery.

ACTIVITY 10.1

As you read the case study, focus on each activity and the inputs that contributed to it. Remember that inputs can include staff as well as materials and equipment. Make a note of the sequence of activities and the inputs that contribute to each.

The 'patient trail'

The Steering Group has generated a series of process flow diagrams for the various stages of the 'patient trail' – which begins with an outpatient department referral and consultation, and ends (it is hoped) with the cured patient's discharge. Members of the Steering Group have also been speaking with staff, at all levels, involved in theatre work.

One of the diagrams shows the segment of the trail which takes the patient through the operating theatre. Let us assume that you are the third patient on the morning list for theatre 4 on Wednesday, and that the operation concerns a hernia repair; this should take around 45 minutes 'at the table'. The list for this theatre session will have been drawn up some days ago, but will only have been finalised on Tuesday afternoon or evening. For many different reasons patients 'drop out' from and are added onto the list up to the last moment. When the second patient's operation is drawing to a close – say, with about ten minutes to go – the theatre sister fills out a 'patient request ticket'. She takes this to the holding area and either gives it to a porter or puts it on a board for the next available porter to collect. The porter then walks to the ward to collect you, and brings you down to the theatre suite with your ward nurse as escort. All patients must be escorted by a porter and a qualified nurse. When you get to the theatre holding area the ward nurse transfers you to an operating department assistant and they check your details to make sure that you are indeed expected. You are then transferred onto a special theatre trolley and wheeled into the anaesthetic preparation room outside the operating theatre. This is where you wait until the previous operation is over and the theatre has been made ready for you.

If something goes wrong with the previous operation, you could be here for some time. If the nurse on the ward has given you any pre-medication, you should be relaxed and free from anxiety. Here also you meet again your anaesthetist, who visited you on the ward yesterday or this morning to check that you were fit to anaesthetise. When the theatre and surgeon are ready, the anaesthetist will induce anaesthesia, give you a breathing tube, and wheel you into the theatre where the team will lift you onto the table.

The surgeon is now ready to start your hernia operation. A typical surgical team includes the surgeon, anaesthetist, a senior registrar, a scrub nurse (who looks after the instruments), an operating department assistant (who supports the anaesthetist) and one or more theatre nurses to assist too. When the surgeon has finished, the anaesthetist reverses your anaesthesia and removes your now redundant breathing tube. Seeing that all is going well, one of the nurses or the operating department assistant wheels you into the recovery area where the anaesthetist leaves you, if all is still well, to return to the theatre and to attend to the next patient. You are now in the temporary care of the recovery nurses, who phone your ward when you are fit to travel back with a porter and your escort nurse.

(Buchanan and Wilson, 1996)

Table 10.1 is the chart we made to show inputs to each of the activities. This chart is one way of mapping a process flow. It is not necessary to use a table as we have here – many people find that it is more immediate for them to draw a flow diagram freehand and note the inputs at each stage in a different colour.

This particular example looks only at the part of the patient's pathway immediately surrounding the actual operation. It excludes the visit to the GP, preliminary diagnosis, referral to the outpatient clinic, attendance at the clinic, pre-admission preparation, admission to the hospital, post-operative nursing, going home and care at home. Each of these processes could be mapped in a similar way.

Process mapping is widely used as a tool in planning more integrated services. An example of an approach to developing a better integrated pathway is given by Herefordshire and Worcestershire NHS Network.

Heart failure: improving the process of patient care

The process mapping event is a method of producing a description of the patient journey from presentation to the GP with symptoms suggestive of heart failure through to end of life care. The aim of the event is to bring together multi-disciplinary teams from primary, secondary, tertiary and social care of all roles and professions to create a culture of ownership, responsibility and accountability. By creating an overview of the whole pathway we aim to help staff to understand how complicated the system can be for patients and provide an opportunity for all to propose changes that will have a positive impact on patient care.

For the process mapping to be successful the Network needed to involve everyone that comes into contact with the patient along his or her journey. This could mean NHS staff directly delivering care, helping transfer them to a different department, or making sure the medical notes are available. Whatever aspect of the patient journey in which there is NHS staff involvement is an important part of the process. The Network involves people from each aspect and asks them to share their experiences.

(Herefordshire and Worcestershire NHS Network, 2009)

Table 10.1 The patient's pathway

Inputs	Activities
1 Theatre sister Request ticket	Give patient request ticket to porter or put on notice board
2 Porter and ward nurse (escort) Bed or trolley	Collect patient from ward Deliver to theatre on bed or trolley
3 Operating department assistant (ODA) and ward nurse Patient notes Trolley	Check patient details Move patient on to theatre trolley (if on bed)
4 Anaesthetist Equipment	Induce anaesthesia
5 Anaesthetist and ODA Equipment	Wheel patient into theatre Lift onto operating table
6 Surgical team (including surgeon, senior registrar, anaesthetist, scrub nurse, ODA, theatre nurses) Operating theatre	Surgeon performs operation, assisted by senior registrar
7 Anaesthetist Nurse or ODA Trolley	Reverse anaesthesia Wheel patient to recovery area
8 Recovery nurses Operation record forms	Recovery nurse waits for patient to recover enough to go back to ward Operation record form completed
9 Nurse and porter	Wheel patient back to ward

PROCESS MAPPING

The first stage in process mapping is to select the process that you intend to map and to make a checklist of the activities that are included in that process. Selecting a part of your service to examine in this way presents quite a challenge. Your service may be only a small part of the service user's pathway. It may, however, make an important contribution to his or her overall comfort and satisfaction. For example, financial assessment and billing for a service may be done separately from assessment of need and provision of the service, but these can contribute significantly to a service user's anxiety. It is important to identify the process as it is experienced and viewed by service users so that its component parts can be considered in terms of their impact on them.

The next step is to think about the output or outcome of the process. Thinking in terms of what the service user receives is helpful in identifying the outputs of any process, whether your service users are the general public or staff in other departments of your organisation. It is therefore important to consider exactly who the service users are for the process you are intending to map.

Once the outputs and service users have been identified, you are in a position to consider what your service users need, want and expect of your output. This is important in reminding you of the quality that the process must achieve.

Next, you need to identify all the people who carry out the activities that make up the process you want to map. In our operating theatre example, a considerable number of people were identified, but if you were a manager in that area and were familiar with all the activities, you would probably have been able to identify more. It is important to include the staff from support services that contribute to the process as well as those who carry out the more obvious tasks. For example, medical records staff would have been involved at various stages of the operating theatre example.

The Hereford and Worcestershire NHS Network described how they carried out their process mapping during the planning event held to improve the care pathway for heart failure. This was a practical session involving as many as possible who contributed to provision of any of the relevant services:

At the event attendees are asked to write down each step of the journey that they are involved in on a Post-it note; this can range from giving injections to administration. Network Staff then put each Post-it note onto a large sheet of paper in order to map out the patient journey. As a group the attendees then examine the full patient journey, looking for ideas, issues and challenges. By doing this the Network is able to highlight the key areas that need to be looked at. Before the event attendees were asked to think about what they do on a day-to-day basis, what steps are required in order to clerk a patient or to pass information between departments. On the day of the event the Network looked at every detail of work that each member of staff carries out.

(Herefordshire and Worcestershire NHS Network, 2009)

Once you have assembled all the information about activities included in the pathway, you are in a position to define the process in the form of a clear statement that names the process and identifies the output(s) it is intended to achieve. You are then ready to prepare a map of the process.

Here is a summary of the main features of process mapping as it is carried out at Leicester Royal Infirmary (1998):

Select a process

1 Make a list of the activities included in the process.
2 State the output or outcome of the process (the product or service that is created by the process and is handed over to the customer).
3 List the customers for your output (the person or persons who use your output: customers may be internal or external; they may use your output as an input to their work processes).
4 List your customers' requirements of your output (what your customers need, want and expect of your output).
5 List the process participants (the people who carry out the steps of the process – as opposed to those who are responsible for the process).

Define the process

Map the process

Working systematically in this way will help you to be clear about how far you want to go in looking at a pathway. There may be parts of the service user's pathway over which you have no immediate influence or control. You may decide that it is important to look at the parts of the pathway that affect service users immediately before and after they encounter your service area.

ACTIVITY 10.2

You may like to try process mapping to help to make improvements in your own area of work.

1 Select a process from your working environment that you think could be improved.
2 Make a list of all the activities that contribute to the process.
3 Identify the output of the process.
4 Identify the people who use this output.
5 Make a list of what these people want or need or expect from your output.
6 List the people who contribute to carrying out activities in this process.
7 Write a definition of the process. This should include the purpose, the inputs, the transformation and the output(s).
8 Map the process, showing the inputs and activities, as in the example of an operating theatre. Base the map on the service user's pathway through the process. Identify:

- the people involved
- any travel or transport required
- any professional or service boundaries crossed
- sources of feedback and information
- points at which decisions have to be made
- points at which delays occur
- any specialist equipment required
- other factors that are important in your process.

9 Consider the importance of this process to your organisation and who would be the major stakeholders in any proposed changes. (For example, a care management or childcare assessment process cannot be changed unilaterally by any one team, although the way it is applied in a particular team may be capable of improvement without reference to other teams.)

If there is a possibility of making some changes in your service, you will need to involve your staff, relevant partners and other stakeholders in this exercise – improving processes is easier when those affected by them have been involved in identifying the problems and designing the solutions.

Once you are confident that the process map includes all the relevant information, the next step is to analyse it to find opportunities for improvement.

Identifying weaknesses in the process

The process map is the starting point for improving the process. You are likely to have a number of sources of information that will help you identify the strengths and weaknesses in your process. For example, you will know, from supervision and appraisal sessions with your staff, which elements of the process they find most problematic. Feedback from service users may indicate where they experience difficulties with the way in which the service is run and where the process or outcomes of their contact with your service have not been satisfactory. Feedback from your management control will have made you aware of problems to be overcome, and you will know where standards – either local or national – are proving difficult to attain. Conversations with colleagues responsible for services at the boundaries of your process may be able to highlight difficulties your service causes them.

If you do not have some of this information, consider whether the information you collect and your record keeping are adequate for your management needs. It is usual to keep appraisal and supervision records confidential, but information about common concerns and training needs can be drawn from them. If you do not have feedback from your service users, you may need to conduct a survey or arrange a meeting with a group of them to find out their views. You may need to improve your records of the extent to which standards are being achieved. You may also recognise that you have insufficient opportunities to exchange views with others who contribute to the process that you have mapped.

In the operating theatre example, the Steering Group identified several problems by talking to staff and patients. Many of these involved delays of one sort or another arising from the ways in which the activities were carried out:

- the way in which the theatre list is put together (a mix of different types of procedure, the learning needs of junior surgeons, etc.) may cause difficulties in predicting operation times and in keeping to schedule;
- some of the professionals may see only their part in the process and not the 'big picture' as perceived by patients or other staff;
- the surgeon is late;
- the anaesthetist waits for the surgeon before initiating anaesthesia;
- extra demands on porters at peak times;
- the previous operation takes more or less time than anticipated.

The consequences of such delays can include cancelled operations and thus anxiety, discomfort and inconvenience for patients and their families. They can also mean that staff are unable to keep to shift times, so that they have to work longer hours than intended. There is wasted time and the potential for muddle in the links between some activities. It is not clear who is overseeing the pathway of the patient in this example or who would take action to minimise the risk and discomfort to the patient if there is a delay in any activity that contributes to the overall process.

The process map can be used to define the current situation in terms of its strengths and weaknesses, and to identify opportunities for improvement. Four useful types of analysis can be applied to identify weaknesses in the process – value-added, handover, elapsed time and process cost analyses.

Value-added analysis

An important criterion in evaluating a process is to identify whether value is added at each stage for the service user. Each part of the process can be assessed to see whether or not it represents a gain. For example, a long waiting time between referral and seeing a social worker, or between procedures in an outpatient clinic represents no gain for the service user. Time spent wandering around a hospital looking for the X-ray department also represents no gain. Activities carried out efficiently, for example taking a blood sample or supplying home care speedily when it is needed, represent added value. If any procedures are carried out inefficiently, perhaps because of faulty equipment, this will reduce the amount of value added.

Handover analysis

This involves examining how each activity is completed and the next initiated. Once again, the experience of the service user on the pathway through the whole process is the basis of the analysis. Any handover involves time and effort in passing a service user from one person or one part of the process to another. Each handover is, unfortunately, an opportunity for delay, confusion, and loss or distortion of useful information. As a service user, it can also include the frustration of telling your story to yet another member of staff!

Elapsed time analysis

This refers to the time elapsing between and during different parts of the process. You can identify the usual lengths of time involved and note the reason for each. It is useful to pay particular attention to the time taken by activities that are not essential parts of the process. For example, it takes longer for a patient to walk through hospital corridors to widely dispersed sites – X-ray, pathology, and so on – than to move from one to the other within an outpatient suite, and it takes time for a mobile service to reach a service user. Sending information online is quicker than sending it by post. Again, the experience of the service user in following the pathway through the process is the starting point for this analysis.

Process cost analysis

How much are inefficiencies in the process costing you? In seeking to improve processes, it is important to be clear about the nature of the intended benefits – are they about increasing quality or reducing costs or both? Experienced process redesigners tell us that process improvements for cost reduction alone are harder to implement because people are often less committed to making this kind of change. You also need to be aware that reducing costs in one area may only shunt them to another: if this happens to be another department or organisation, it can create friction. Some process improvements may require capital investment in new equipment or moving equipment and staff to be nearer the service user. You may not have the power to implement such changes at the moment, but you can argue the case for modest process improvements now, and present a case for the benefits and potential savings of more radical change as a later option.

Each of these analyses may have suggested potential improvements.

Identifying potential areas for improvement

If you have found that some of the activities along a care pathway offer no – or very little – added value to the service user, you could consider why they are carried out at all. Sometimes activities have been retained simply because no one has questioned whether they are still necessary. New technologies and materials can reduce the need for preparatory activities or for activities to take place in specially designed accommodation.

If staff are trained to develop a broader range of skills, it may be possible for one member of staff to carry out several activities in order to avoid handing the service user from one person to another. The location of activities is also important: how easy is it for a service user to move from one area of activities to another? If there are significant distances between activities that are frequently sequential in a pathway, it may be possible to reduce these distances. Historical reasons may have led to the locations of particular services and staff, and managers may not think of challenging this unless the implications for service users are considered.

The time taken between activities is important in contributing to the length of a process, and there are often opportunities to reduce this time by handing over from one activity to another in a different way. The handover part of a process often includes handing over information, records or notes as well as people. If time is to be saved and frustration avoided, all of the necessary information must be handed over promptly so that the next activity can take place on time and effectively.

Saving time usually results in a reduction in costs. It may seem cost-efficient to make service users wait for professionals whose time is valuable, but people who are waiting cost resources in space, furniture, support staff, heating, lighting, and the provision of refreshments and toilets. Many of these costs could be reduced if waiting areas are needed for only one or two people at a time. Also, if people are left waiting for services, their condition can deteriorate. Once a service user has been assessed as needing a service, it is likely that the service will be most cost-effective if it is supplied immediately.

If service users may need different levels of treatment as they progress along a care pathway, it might be helpful to identify this in the pathway design as a 'stepped care model'. For example, a stepped care model for a depression services pathway is described as

> *a stepped care framework that aims to match the needs of individual people with depression to the most appropriate services, depending on the characteristics of their illness and their personal and social circumstances. Each step represents increased complexity of intervention, with higher steps assuming interventions in previous steps remain relevant. People enter the clinical pathway at different steps, depending on severity and previous history. Within steps, there are choices for people about the type of treatment that suits them best. It is a needs-led process; people may move directly to the appropriate level and move between levels, to suit their needs.*
>
> (Thompson, undated)

If the processes in the care pathway cross boundaries between your area of responsibility and others, you are likely to have to negotiate your ideas for process improvements with those who manage these other activities. This may involve more senior managers than yourself or managers from another discipline or organisation. You may need to clarify who takes responsibility for the overall care of service users as they progress through the different activities along the pathway. You will also need to consider whether changes in your process may cause disruption to other activities or processes and, if so, how you could minimise such disruption and gain co-operation in making changes.

ACTIVITY 10.3

Using the information you have about the strengths and weaknesses of the process you have been examining – from appraisal or supervision, service user surveys, monitoring, and so on:

1 Apply added value, handover, elapsed time and process cost analyses to your process map.

2 List the main problems emerging from your process map and analysis.

As in the previous Activity, if you are working with colleagues on a potential process improvement you will need to carry out the analysis of the process map in collaboration with them.

You should now have identified some opportunities to improve your service for the benefit of service users. You should also have some relevant information to present to colleagues and decision makers to support your proposals. You may have identified improvements to quality that would also represent cost savings for your organisation. Once you have clear ideas about potential improvements, you need to present a clear argument for implementing them. It is often helpful to present proposals of this kind either as a written report or as an oral presentation, backed up with visual aids that support your argument. Once others are convinced that improvements can be made, the next step is to design the process improvement.

DESIGNING PROCESS IMPROVEMENTS

The design stage of process improvement may include:

- stimulating and using the creative and innovative talents of your staff, colleagues and other stakeholders, whether in making incremental or 'breakthrough' improvements;
- discovering and using new process designs, operating philosophies and enabling technologies;
- using surveys of service users and other forms of feedback to determine their perceptions of existing services and their needs and expectations of services in the future;
- designing and developing both improved and new services to meet the needs and expectations of service users.

For example, here are some of the proposals that were generated by consultations with staff in the operating theatre example:

The *senior nurse manager* in the surgical directorate has seen some recent publications on business process re-engineering. She sees a review of the theatres as a major opportunity to introduce new working practices. Re-engineering, she notes, can involve multiskilling, process teams, flatter organisation hierarchies, 'case managers', and more employee 'empowerment'.

The *business manager* in the directorate is sympathetic to this view, but feels that it is the administrative staff who assemble patient documentation, who arrange appointments and who draw up the theatre lists, who are isolated and not effectively involved in the patient trail. The hospital's computerised Theatreman system captures a lot of information about the patient flow, including operation times, outcomes and delays. This information, however, is not used systematically to monitor what is happening and to trigger improvements.

The *theatre sisters and operating department assistants* claim that the theatre lists would run to time more often if they did the scheduling themselves – once the surgeons had determined each patient's priority.

The *consultants*, however, who can claim the highest status and expertise in this context, argue that the problem lies simply with the lack of adequate numbers of ward staff and porters, and with the way these staff are used and controlled. The problem could be solved, in their view, with more nurses, more porters, more effectively managed. The data in the Theatreman computer, they feel, is inaccurate and unreliable, as information is recorded by operating department assistants and nurses under pressure, and keyed up by clerical staff who sometimes need to rely on 'informed judgement' when coding the information. They would like to see some straightforward remedial action taken immediately, to help them, to help their staff, and to help patients. A major organisational review would take time, and is not really necessary.

(Buchanan and Wilson, 1996)

What lessons can we learn from the reactions of each of these groups of people?

- Consultation with the patients in this situation is difficult because they are anaesthetised during most of the significant time. However, their views on how they experience the time they are awake – and the consequences of actions taken while they are asleep – would be informative.
- People sometimes think in terms of 'episodes' rather than in terms of 'processes' – they see problems from the perspective of their own part of the process, without perceiving the overall picture.
- Some people have higher status than others and can enforce their points of view, making it difficult for others' views to be heard.
- Major organisational review and change may be required to improve the process.
- Major change carries significant implications for costs and for disruption of services.
- Sometimes major change is not required.
- People do not necessarily agree about what the problem is.

- Problems arising from poor management of the implementation of change can lead to the usefulness of existing activities being undermined.
- There can be differences of opinion about who should be included in the 'process team'.
- New ideas take time to be accepted sufficiently to be incorporated in the creative thinking of a team.
- Some solutions can require major financial investment (for example, new information systems) which the immediate members of the process team do not have the resources or the authority to implement.
- Not everyone welcomes innovations.

ACTIVITY 10.4

Return to the process from your own work area that you examined and consider how you and the other people involved can set about designing improvements to it. Make two lists – one identifying things you need to do to redesign the process, and the other identifying things you must avoid doing as you redesign the process.

You may find it useful to refer to our lists below, which draw largely on the case study material. Your list may need to include other things specific to your working environment.

Dos and don'ts in service design and redesign

DO

Decide who the 'process team' includes and make sure they are all involved.

Check language and understanding.

Check that existing procedures are being used properly and effectively.

Think of appropriate ways to consult patients and service users that suit the situation.

Try to achieve a consensus about what the problem or problems are.

Look for technological opportunities.

Listen carefully to all points of view.

Give equal weight to all points of view.

Encourage people to think 'process' rather than 'episode' and to see their place in the overall picture.

Consider how the parts of the process fit together and communicate with each other.

Encourage creative thinking – for example, by brainstorming.

Keep your eye on the purposes and values of the service.

Make use of any outcome information.

Create opportunities for discussion and 'sparking' of ideas.

Be prepared to review the service standards to be met.

Be clear about your own powers and responsibilities.

Be prepared to think flexibly about responsibilities and skills.

Be prepared to incorporate new national standards.

Be prepared to incorporate research and good practice from elsewhere.

Consult stakeholders.

Think small before thinking big.

Check whether there are relevant National Service Frameworks.

DON'T

Force the pace.

Assume that everyone has the same understanding of the words and concepts in use.

Leave important players out of the process team.

Move to solutions before the problem is clear and has been analysed.

Forget key stakeholders.

Allow fixed patterns of thought ('this is how we do it here') to prevent creative thinking.

Underestimate the time and energy this activity may take.

The ways in which processes are carried out make a very important contribution to the quality of services and the experience of a service user as they progress along a care pathway. This chapter has taken you through the technique of process mapping and analysing process maps in order to identify opportunities for improvement in your own area of work. We concluded by considering some of the issues involved in the redesign of a process.

REFERENCES

Buchanan, D. and Wilson R. (1996) 'Next patient please: the operating theatres problem at Leicester General Hospital NHS Trust', in J. Storey (ed.) *Blackwell Cases in Human Resource and Change Management*, pp. 190–205, Blackwell.

Department of Health (2007) *Urgent Care Pathways for Older People With Complex Needs: Best Practice Guidance*, TSO.

Herefordshire and Worcestershire NHS Network. *Heart failure: Improving the Process of Patient Care*, <http://www.hwcn.nhs.uk/heart_failure_services.htm> (downloaded 20/05/2009).

Leicester Royal Infirmary (1998) *Patient Process Redesign Toolkit*, Leicester Royal Infirmary NHS Trust.

NHS in Scotland *NHS Quality Improvement in Scotland*, <http://www.nhshealthquality.org/mentalhealth/toolkit/process/standard3.html> (downloaded 20/05/2009).

Thompson, K. (undated) *Depression Care Project*, <http://www.southstaffshealthcare.nhs.uk/goodPractice/DCP/ DCPMappingSolutions_Final.pdf> (downloaded 20/05/2009).

CHAPTER 11

WORKING WITH A BUDGET

You will be aware of some of the changes that are taking place in health and social care organisations in order to make better use of finite resources in a climate of ever-increasing demand. These changes may have affected the way in which you carry out your job. For example, you may:

- have more responsibility for your decisions;
- have to consider costs more carefully before making decisions;
- be expected to contribute to the process of setting budgets;
- be responsible for controlling the budget for your service or department;
- be expected by senior managers to be more efficient;
- have to account for the money you spend.

Many of these changes arise from the way in which health and social care services are now financed – in particular the separate responsibilities of those who commission services and those who provide them. Many managers are responsible for monitoring contracts and there is a general trend in many health and social organisations towards delegating more responsibility for budgetary matters to junior managers and team leaders.

In order to do your job more effectively in this climate, you need to develop competences that will enable you to understand and to play your part in budgetary management. We begin by examining the purposes of budgeting, and also discuss a number of different approaches to setting budgets. We then turn to some of the practicalities of budgeting: the initial stages of timetabling and preparing the ground and the crucial stage of budget negotiation.

SETTING BUDGETS

The aims that organisations set themselves are like signposts that provide a sense of direction for both the organisation and its managers.

However, statements of aims rarely spell things out in any detail. They do not usually indicate precisely what has to be done, nor do they say what resources will be necessary to achieve the aims. The next stage has to be filling in the details. As a manager, part of your job is to work out – and to communicate – organisational expectations and available resources in detail. This is where budgets come in.

Budgets are plans that set out financial details about:

A *budget* is a detailed financial plan.

- ■ *income* – the resources available to an organisation and the departments within it;
- ■ *expenditure* – the uses to which these resources will be put.

Budgets contain mainly financial data. They are usually expressed in monetary terms, but some budgets use quantities. Look at the simple budget statement in Table 11.1.

It appears from Table 11.1 that senior management have estimated an income level of £500,000 and expenditure at £450,000. They expect the organisation to make a profit of £50,000 (or to carry forward this amount into the following year as reserves).

Is there any sense of direction in these estimates? Most certainly there is. Those responsible for 'selling' the organisation's services know that they are working towards a total income of £500,000 and staff know that their salaries are expected to total £350,000. Those responsible for purchasing the organisation's supplies know that they are expected to spend £50,000 and the organisation can spend £50,000 on rent. This is a clear statement of the organisation's financial plans, which provides a sense of direction for its staff.

So budgets are a practical expression of the aims of organisations. The emphasis is on the word *practical*, because the budget determines, directs and plans the actions that follow.

One important difference between budgets and aims is the time-scale. Budgets are normally drawn up for 12 months, and are regarded as being part of an organisation's short-term or, at most, medium- term planning. By contrast, aims are designed to provide a long-term framework. The period covered could be five years or perhaps even longer.

An organisation – or a department or section within an organisation – cannot be directed in enough detail if only longer-term aims are

Table 11.1 Budget statement

Income		£500,000
Expenditure:		
Salaries	£350,000	
Purchases	£50,000	
Rent	£50,000	£450,000
Profit/reserves		£50,000

available. Direction is best thought of in much shorter planning periods. Twelve months is the normal maximum length of time for which detailed planning can be undertaken. Indeed, the 12-month budget is usually divided into six-monthly, quarterly and monthly statements.

The purposes of budgeting

Budgeting has a number of important benefits – in other words, there are several purposes of budgeting.

Budgeting as a contribution to planning

We have already said that all managers must be fully aware of the aims of the organisation so that they can draw up detailed plans. The budgeting process involves managers in doing precisely that: planning their future activities in detail. Budget planning is also an essential part of contract negotiation in interagency work, involving managers at most levels in all partner organisations.

Budgeting as a contribution to communication

Budgeting, by its nature, involves senior management in briefing front-line managers and other staff about what is expected from them – in other words, in communicating. Since departments often work collaboratively, part of the budgeting process involves managers who are on similar levels communicating with one another across departments and contracted agencies about their future activities.

Budgeting as a contribution to co-ordination

Communication does not, in itself, ensure that managers work together for the overall good of the organisation. Some managers may be tempted to build a larger 'empire' and request more staff. Or they may want to develop a particular area of work because it is of personal interest to them. Some may be put under pressure to purchase goods and services they don't really need. This type of behaviour does not benefit the organisation and would divert scarce resources, damaging the organisation's ability to achieve its aims.

The budgeting process helps to influence this sort of behaviour. It forces managers to communicate with one another and co-ordinate their activities. Where departments support one another and use each other's services, the budgeting process makes sure that the right level of support is available, by identifying what resources are required and who will provide them. The intentions of managers are therefore known, and unhelpful behaviour can be identified and rectified. An overarching master budget, incorporating all the detailed activities, will be compiled to provide an overview for senior management, making effective co-ordination possible.

Budgeting as a contribution to motivation

All organisations – including health and social care organisations – are dependent on people and their goodwill. Staff need to be encouraged to carry out their tasks to the best of their ability but they also need to feel that their tasks are achievable. Most people like 'a bit of a challenge' and when budget levels are being set, a slightly optimistic view of what can be achieved may provide this. However, too challenging a budget can be demotivating if staff feel under pressure to achieve financial targets.

Budgeting as a contribution to control

The budget specifies future activities and directs staff towards achieving them. If the budget is staged on a monthly basis, it is possible to discover when plans are not being carried out satisfactorily and to take action to make sure that the targets are reached later on.

What we have just described is the controlling function of a budget. Actual performance is compared regularly with the budgeted performance. Differences can be identified and explanations sought. Action may be taken to bring activities into line with the budget. However, this may be inappropriate in some situations. For example, if the original plans were too optimistic or inaccurate, or if circumstances have changed significantly, making the plans unachievable, it may be necessary to revise the budget.

Budgeting as a contribution to assessing performance

Managers are responsible for carrying out plans. They are expected to undertake specific tasks, make the necessary decisions and manage staff. The budget helps to assess their level of success in carrying out these responsibilities, which include reporting on variations in budgeted expenditure and, if necessary, negotiating revisions to the budget. A budget does not cover the full range of managers' responsibilities, but it is useful in assessing their performance in relation to those responsibilities that involve money, although many will also have responsibilities of a non-financial nature, which cannot be ignored. Managers need feedback on the full range of activities that they undertake, in order to build up a fuller picture of how effectively they have carried out their jobs.

APPROACHES TO BUDGETING

Budgets, then, are simply plans expressed in financial terms. They help organisations to achieve their agreed aims. Budgeting is about planning for specified levels of activity with the resources available. We now turn to the examination of some different approaches to creating budgets. We'll look at the differences between 'input' and 'output' budgeting and then at 'incremental' and 'zero-based' approaches to budgeting.

Input and output budgets

Let's look at an example of a budget.

ACTIVITY 11.1

Table 11.2 is a budget statement from a day-care centre.

You will notice that, in the final column, some figures are shown in brackets: this means that they are negative (in some budgets they are shown with a minus sign, rather than with brackets).

1 What is the total annual budget expenditure?
2 What is the single largest category of expenditure?
3 Has the actual expenditure to date exceeded the budget or been less than expected, and by how much?
4 Now make a brief note on whether you think that this statement provides you with a good picture of the day centre's running costs.
5 What do you think is the main weakness of this budget statement?

The annual budgeted expenditure for the day-care centre was £241,000. The largest single category of expenditure is the salaries of nursing and care staff. Up to the date of this budget statement, actual expenditure has exceeded planned expenditure by £5,300.

We think this budget probably does provide a good picture of the running costs of the day-care centre. Its main weakness is that it does not provide any information about the level of activity that is being budgeted for.

That is because this is an *input* budget, with the costs grouped by department and function. The inputs used by each function or department – people, materials and other costs – are simply listed to form the budget. It is not possible, from this budget, to calculate the cost of providing services to any particular user of the day-care centre, so it is difficult to obtain the financial data needed to cost the day-care centre's objectives.

Table 11.2 Budget statement for a day-care centre

	Annual budget (£)	Planned budget to end of month 9 (£)	Actual expenditure to end of month 9 (£)	Budget variance at end of month 9 (£)
Pay costs:				
Nursing and care staff salaries	102,000	76,500	82,000	(5,500)
Technical staff salaries	30,000	22,500	18,000	4,500
Non-pay costs:				
Drugs and dressings	36,000	27,000	28,800	(1,800)
Physiotherapy and occupational therapy supplies	28,000	21,000	23,500	(2,500)
Cleaning	10,000	7,500	7,500	–
Building maintenance (including heat and light)	15,000	11,250	11,250	–
Administration costs	20,000	15,000	15,000	–
Total costs	241,000	180,750	186,050	(5,300)

The key point is that it is not the running costs of each department or function that we need to know in order to plan effectively. We are more interested in the *outputs* – the costs of running particular services, which may involve many functions and departments.

As a first step in determining the overall costs of operating any service, input budgeting can make a useful contribution to budget construction, but the next step takes us much deeper. We have to find out how many *workload outputs* each department or function produces and for which customers.

Information about workload outputs and customers can be used in a variety of ways:

Workload outputs are ways of expressing in monetary terms what a department or service produces or deals with.

■ to work out the average cost for each unit of service delivered;
■ to compare the services provided with other similar services, and thus find out how efficient (or inefficient) they are;
■ as a basis for pricing services or recharging costs to external or internal customers;
■ to build up financial forecasts for the future.

Output budgeting analyses the activities undertaken in workload terms to arrive at average unit costs. It is, however, necessary to exercise caution when using average unit costs to construct a budget. The signal for caution is the word 'average'. If the service you work in has a highly variable mixture of work or provides services for people with very different needs, the calculations involved in output budgeting can be rather complex.

So how should you approach budgeting? Perhaps the best advice is:

1 Analyse your costs into those that are *fixed* – those that do not depend, to a significant extent, on the number of service users – and those that are *variable* – those that vary roughly in proportion to the number of people you provide services for.
2 Use an input-based budgeting approach for those costs that are more or less fixed.
3 Base your budget calculations on estimated unit costs and projected outputs for the costs that are variable.

If you follow this guidance, the approach to budgeting for a service might look something like that shown in Table 11.3.

ACTIVITY 11.2

Can you distinguish the input-based calculations from the output-based ones in Table 11.3? Tick the appropriate boxes.

	Inputs	*Outputs*
1 Salaries	☐	☐
2 Materials costs	☐	☐
3 Cleaning, meals served	☐	☐
4 Rents and maintenance costs	☐	☐
5 Income (services provided)	☐	☐

Table 11.3 An approach to the budget plan

Items to be budgeted	Calculation
Salary costs	Either: Actual costs × Number of staff in post or: Estimated costs on mid-salary points × Funded establishment of staff
Materials or consumables used directly by the service	Average cost per unit of activity × Volume of activity
Services supplied by other departments (e.g. cleaning, meals served)	Number of units of service provided × Average unit cost
Charges for using and maintaining buildings, land and equipment	Estimated annual charges for rents, maintenance, etc.
Income	Number of units of service 'sold' to other departments or external customers × Agreed average 'prices'

We have suggested that you employ both input and output methods in assembling your budget. Salaries, rents and maintenance costs – items 1 and 4 – can most usefully be calculated by the input method. However, the costs of materials, cleaning and meals – items 2 and 3 – should be calculated, wherever possible, on the basis of outputs. Income – item 5 – should also, if possible, be calculated by the output method.

Incremental versus zero-based budgeting

Two important techniques that can be used to create budgets are incremental budgeting and zero-based budgeting. We'll describe each technique briefly, and then attempt to evaluate their usefulness.

Incremental budgeting

This approach to budgeting is heavily reliant on what has happened in the past. The costs for the previous and current year provide the starting point for the coming budget year. Incremental budgeting involves accepting fairly uncritically what happened the previous year and then updating that year's figures. Adjustments are made to cope with:

Incremental budgeting involves updating the previous year's budget.

- pay and price rises;
- the 'full year' effect of plans previously put into action;
- the effect of new projects that will come on stream in the forthcoming budget year;
- any planned 'efficiency savings'.

Zero-based budgeting

This approach to budgeting ignores the figures and assumptions of the previous year. Instead, it examines, from first principles, what is required to carry out the tasks expected of the organisation and its various components.

Zero-based budgeting involves rebudgeting from scratch each year.

First, a list of 'core' activities is drawn up. These form the essential base of the budget. Other activities are regarded as optional, and managers have to decide whether or not they will continue.

The core activities and those optional activities that have survived the first stage are then costed, and the costs are updated to take account of the effects of any new plans that will be implemented during the coming year. For example, new projects may be coming on stream that will have important financial consequences.

Which approach should you use?

The zero-based approach is better in theory, because it relates the budget directly to the tasks for which the organisation exists. But, in practice, it is difficult and time-consuming. It requires managers to be fully aware of the costs of all the tasks that have to be carried out, which can sometimes be a tall order. It also means that managers have to be completely objective when deciding which activities are essential to the delivery of the service and which are not.

Incremental budgeting is comparatively straightforward. Details of the income and expenditure in the previous year are readily available. All the manager is expected to do is to think about how the costs of the activities will change in the coming year. This is far easier than undertaking a full review. Discussion about whether current staffing is adequate and whether the heating system is efficient can be expensive in terms of time. However, no one would claim that incremental budgeting is very comprehensive.

Whichever approach you adopt, your budget will have to be submitted to senior management for final approval, and they may change the figures. Perhaps insufficient funds are available, or perhaps senior management have different priorities. Departmental managers may be involved in negotiating their budgets, but this is not the case everywhere. Some organisations impose budgets from above. It is generally considered that a 'bottom-up' approach to budgeting is more likely to encourage staff to take responsibility for managing resources. However, there is a counter-argument that, because senior management are more aware of current demands and future priorities, they should direct how the funds available should be used.

The approach taken to the allocation of funds between departments and services varies from organisation to organisation, depending to a significant extent on the management style adopted by senior staff. But inevitably, in the process of setting budgets, some departments and services will lose out while others will gain. Decisions that affect the budget can have quite profound effects on the ways in which the various parts of the organisation operate.

TIMETABLING AND PREPARING THE GROUND

The production of plans and budgets is a complex set of activities, and it needs careful organisation and timetabling. If a health or social care organisation is to secure the full commitment of its managers in building up meaningful and accurate budgets, it is vital that clear guidelines are available, showing not only where everyone fits into the budget preparation process, but also when. In order to start things moving, a timetable is essential.

Envisage yourself in a budget-planning situation. What would you want to be clear about? The range of responses that managers provide to this question is quite wide. However, the following suggestions sum up much of what people usually feel.

I want an overview of responsibility. For example, I'd like a list showing the name of each manager responsible for budget preparation. Then we could at least talk to each other.

It's important to know exactly what will be required of me: the sort of information I need to pull together and when it is required.

The process needs to be clear. For example, to whom should I pass information and in what form?

Speaking personally, I need some kind of plan or diagram – a picture if you like. A diagram showing where I stand in the scheme of things for preparing the budget would be very useful.

I need to know the stages in the process and the key deadline dates.

All these comments point towards the need for a clear timetable. Table 11.4 is an example of a master timetable for budget preparation and Table 11.5 is an example of the timetable for an individual budget holder.

Benefits undoubtedly arise from the fact that everyone involved in the budgeting process knows exactly what he or she is responsible for producing, in what format, for whom and by when. A sense of direction and clarity is essential to personal motivation and commitment. In addition, the budget preparation timetable can be used by accountants and senior management to pull the budget together by the agreed

Table 11.4 A master timetable for budget preparation

Process	Organisational level	Aug	Sept	Oct	Nov	Dec	Jan	Feb
Strategic objectives set	Commissioners/senior management	✓						
Prepare departmental and service budgets; agree recharges between departments	Departmental and service managers/ accountant			✓				
Prepare master budget; revise individual budgets	Senior management/ accountant					✓		
Issue individual budgets	Accountant							✓

Table 11.5 An individual budget preparation timetable

Service	Budget manager	Data required	Format of data and basis of collection	Date required	Required by	Budget preparation deadline
Community occupational therapy	Ms I. V. Packer	Forecast occupational therapist's travel costs for next year	Total travel costs forecast from unit personal travel records	10 Sept	Mrs O. Etoe (accountant)	16 Nov
		Forecast number of domiciliary visits for next year	Total number of visits (using sample of one quarter's figures)	5 Sept	Mrs O. Etoe (accountant)	16 Nov
		Forecast number of aids to daily living required for next year	Forecast total number of aids by type of aid (using sample of two quarters' figures)	5 Sept	Mrs O. Etoe (accountant)	16 Nov

deadline. It becomes the means by which control is exercised over the process of budget preparation throughout the organisation. Slippages can be monitored, and senior management can take corrective action when appropriate. The ultimate pay-off is a co-ordinated approach to the budget preparation process.

NEGOTIATING THE BUDGET

Having drawn up a timetable and identified the process by which the budget will be developed, you move into budget negotiation. In the political sphere, a poor diplomat can increase the chance of hostilities. Budget negotiation can be equally sensitive, and there are acceptable and unacceptable ways of going about it. Consider how you might apply the following guidance in your situation.

Be clear-sighted

You must be clear about the objectives of your organisation and be able to identify where your service fits in. Before going to any budget meeting, be clear about how your financial position fits into the overall budget and how your activities are likely to influence it.

Be brief

You should be prepared to state your service's aims and its financial objectives without too much elaboration. Be prepared to talk through a short report, which you should circulate well in advance to all those attending the meeting. Use this report to highlight your key objectives.

Be simple

Make your report as plain and simple as possible. Avoid too much detail, particularly arrays of figures. This can alienate people very quickly. You are not trying to score points, you are trying to make them.

Be well informed

You need to make yourself familiar with the overall financial climate and the policies of your organisation. For example, do you know the policies for financial control?

Be open

Try to be open-minded in your approach to finding new resources for your service. This means reviewing the situation in your service as a whole and thinking about opportunities that may be available. Before going to a budget meeting, you should have taken a cool and critical look at the main features of your service. There is no need to be afraid of thinking radically. continued

---

continued **Be factual**

You must go into negotiation knowing the facts. What are the facts on your current costs and activities?

Be prepared

You need to do your homework on the information you have gathered.

Be alert

If you are aware of opportunities that exist to save money, you may be able to use them as a bargaining point. When you identify such savings, do so on the basis that you expect some share of them to be passed back to you for the development of your service. Work out the savings as accurately as you can and calculate the time-scale over which you can make them. Don't let the finance staff – or anyone else – work out these things for you because, on the whole, they will be less well informed than you are. If you fail to take the initiative, unreasonable demands may be made on your service to deliver savings and cost improvements.

Be straightforward

If, at the end of the negotiation meeting, you feel that the resources necessary to run your service adequately will not be available for the forthcoming year, spell out the consequences in a clear and rational way. Be explicit about the quantitative and qualitative effects on your service. If the under-resourcing is likely to be critical, you could prepare and circulate a report to senior management, after the meeting is over, to record your analysis of the situation. An honest, straightforward presentation of the facts will at least form a launching pad for a later round of budget negotiations. If there is financial leeway, your stand may gain additional financial resources for your service later on in the financial year.

We cannot anticipate how you will have reflected on each of these points. 'Clear-sighted', 'brief' and 'simple' appeal to most of us when we look at what other managers present us with, but perhaps you also thought about how what you produce might appear to other people. For example, being open might involve recognising that you have not always achieved the best use of resources.

When it comes to being factual, managers mention a range of items, including amount spent to date, income due to date, the total value of orders currently placed, the number of staff in post compared with the funded staff establishment, workload to date, projected workload and a host of others.

Being prepared involves, to some extent, reading the minds of others who will be present at the budget meeting, and perhaps having some preliminary discussions with them. One manager made this point explicitly:

> *You should project forward your income and expenditure budgets for next year. In my opinion, this gives you a head start in any negotiations with accountants, because they can see that you've already constructed your own forecast based on your specialist knowledge of the service you provide.*

These suggestions are not meant to provide an exhaustive guide. However, if you do try to use them, the process of communicating your financial concerns and needs should be made easier.

ACTIVITY 11.3

Your organisation is about to enter the budget-setting season. Your departmental head has asked for your assistance in making a case for purchasing a new piece of computing equipment. The argument for doing so is that it will achieve a net saving of £5,000 per year because the department will not have to employ a part-time clerical assistant to extract the data manually from service users' records.

Jot down some key facts that you would seek to establish about this proposal. Your ideas will form the basis for a short report, which your departmental head has been asked to take to the budget meeting. Remember to think about the sorts of question that the accountant might have in mind.

Your head of department wants some facts as a basis on which to make the case. The kinds of question that need to be answered in the report include:

- Is the £5,000 per year saving an accurate figure? How has it been established, and by whom?
- How soon could you start saving this amount? Would it be dependent on staff redundancies?
- How much will the computer equipment cost and how long will it be before it has to be replaced?
- What would be the total forecast savings on the project after allowing for notional interest on the capital cost of the equipment?
- What are the running costs of the computer equipment?
- Will the equipment improve the output and quality of the service that you currently provide?

The answers to some of these questions may be complicated. For example, how soon you might start saving the money could be dependent on a member of staff being made redundant. If so, your figures would have to include redundancy costs. If not, the savings might have to wait for natural wastage. The last question involves deciding how you are going to demonstrate improved output and/or quality of service.

The report presented by your head of department might look something like the following.

Report on the estimated costs and financial benefits arising from the proposed acquisition of a computer for the Skin Department

I propose the acquisition of a computer, the costs and benefits of which are as follows.

Costs

Estimated capital cost: £2,400
Estimated life-span of computer: 3 years
Annualised cost = £2,400 ÷ 3 = £800
Plus 6% notional interest per year on £2,400 = £2,400 × 6 ÷ 100 = £144
Running costs (computer stationery, maintenance contract and power): £200 per year
Total cost per year = £800 + £144 + £200 = £1,144

Benefits

A part-time clerical assistant's post is currently vacant, and not filling this post would save £2,800 per year, so buying the computer will produce a net saving of £1,656 per year.

In addition, the efficiency of the department would be significantly enhanced, as data on service users would be accessible to all staff at any time.

Summary

This analysis demonstrates that the financial benefits of acquiring an Acne computer are unquestionable. The proposal enables a saving of almost £5,000 to be made over its three-year life-span.

Taj Surma, Department Manager

You will not have failed to notice the virtues of this report. First, it is brief and to the point. Second, the costs and benefits (both financial and non-financial) have been set out, showing net annual savings and total savings over the life of the project. Finally, it is presented clearly. The importance of this in making any financial case successfully cannot be overestimated.

TARGET-SETTING, MOTIVATION AND COMMUNICATION

You may have noted that budget reports are used as one means of communicating information to managers within your organisation about activity levels and the financial consequences of the previous month's activity. It may be that 'keeping within budget' is a performance criterion in your department or organisation, or you may work in a department or agency which does not use budgets as performance targets.

Not all organisations use budgets for target-setting or motivation, although most budget holders would be deemed not to be performing well if they did not remain within their budgets. In theory, tight budgets can be used to encourage people to think more creatively about how resources are used and this may happen in your organisation. However, tight budgets can also be demotivating, particularly if the budget holders have had no say in the budget-setting process. They may feel that the constraints imposed upon them are unreasonable, or that they are not being rewarded for what they have already achieved. In either case they are unlikely to take 'ownership' of the budget, and their commitment to it may be low.

If budget reports are used as part of performance evaluation, it is important to ensure that managers are not held responsible for costs which they do not have the authority to control. Too often managers have little real control over spending. For example:

■ The organisation may only allow one supplier to be used, so there is no scope for saving money by 'shopping around' for a better deal.
■ Salary levels and ratios of staff to patients or service users may be fixed.
■ Costs that appear in a manager's budget may be allocated from other departments (administration, cleaning, etc.) and may therefore be outside of the manager's control.

Whatever role budget reports have within your organisation, it is important to recognise that they are a form of communication. Like all communication, they need to be treated with care because they are open to differing interpretations and can have unintended consequences if their purpose is not clear to all concerned.

Budgeting and providing the financial data for setting budgets are part of the responsibilities of many managers. This is, however, a shared responsibility, as there will almost always be expert guidance readily available from accountants.

You should make the best possible use of your accountant! The two roles run together:

■ Your role as a manager is to collect and validate financial information, using your experience and knowledge of the work your service does, to provide a sound basis for financial planning.

■ The accountant's role is to respond to your need for sound and relevant advice, providing you with good quality financial information.

The key to success lies in establishing close, collaborative working relationships. Working together, managers and accountants can put together viable plans and produce sensible budgets.

CHAPTER 12

SERVICE PLANNING, ACCOUNTABILITY AND RISK

Planning publicly funded health and social care services in most countries is a function of government. Government policy has a profound influence on the proportion of national income spent on health and social care, and on the ways in which services are provided and priorities are set. This influence extends to health and social care organisations that are not directly funded by government because of the ways in which the processes of commissioning services operate. Managers who are planning service provision must therefore take account of government policy whether they are planning for:

■ a large national organisation such as the NHS;
■ a local council, as in the case of social care;
■ a primary care trust;
■ an independent service provider in the voluntary or private sectors;
■ a provider of an integrated service that no longer sits squarely in any one of these sectors.

We begin this chapter by examining the process of business planning, which enables organisations to translate government policy, the resources available to them, and the needs and aspirations of local people into plans focused on making the best use of resources to achieve their objectives. Your organisation's business plan provides the background against which you have to manage your service or department.

We then consider what accountability means to you as a manager in health or social care services. We conclude by examining the responsibilities that you have for the safety of your staff and service users, and how you can assess and manage risk in your service or department.

PLANNING HEALTH AND SOCIAL CARE SERVICES

Health and social care services in all countries in the United Kingdom are strongly influenced by changes in government policy because they are funded as public services. It may be tempting to think that changes at government level are unlikely to have much effect on your service. You may think that running a children's home or a hospital ward or assessing and providing for service users' needs is essentially the same process – with the same management challenges – whatever government is in power.

However, if there is a change in the level of resources provided by government or in national or local government policy, there may be a need to make major changes in how health and social care services are delivered. New policies can include changes of priorities in funding, different attitudes to collaboration or competition, how to measure the quality of services, and different values relating to the purposes of public services. These in turn can produce changes in emphasis, new opportunities and new organisational structures that may provide you with opportunities for improvement, change and innovation.

Consider, for example, Local Area Agreements (LAAs) in England. These are agreements between central government and local authorities and their partners on improving the quality of life for local people. The agreements provide a means to channel public resources towards local priorities, alongside national outcomes and targets. The priority areas cover children and young people, economic development and environment, healthier communities and older people, safer and stronger communities. The key elements of LAAs include:

- *an emphasis on area-based service delivery* – stronger partnership working between all local organisations on making the agreement and in consultation with local people;
- *inspection* – local authority-based inspection replaced with an area-based assessment of risks to service delivery;
- *priority outcomes* – these are linked to indicators for measuring performance and 'reward' grants achievable if some 'stretch' targets are met.

Planning guidance

Government policy directives provide the main building blocks for planning in publicly funded health and social care. For example, local authorities, in conjunction with health and other partners, must produce children's services plans that take an overview of services rather than focusing on provision by individual organisations. This approach to planning is based on the concept of integrated care pathways, thus promoting the development of services that are integrated across organisational boundaries. The requirement for services to work across traditional boundaries to provide more integrated responses to the needs of service users is seen as a national priority because failure to make appropriate links between services decreases public confidence and increases costs. Service users should also be involved in the planning process.

As a front-line manager, you are not likely to be responsible for the preparation of a plan that involves other organisations and service providers. You may, however, be asked to contribute information to such a plan, and to develop your own service to meet the objectives of integrated service plans in your locality. If you are a manager in an independent organisation, you need to keep your eye on developments that may affect your position as a service provider, and you may be asked to contribute to the planning process.

Business planning

Organisations in health and social care have to plan their own activities within the overall plans that have been developed for services in a geographic area. Each organisation develops a *business plan* to ensure that it can continue to make a valuable contribution to service provision by using the resources available effectively to meet appropriate performance standards.

Business plans are inevitably complex to develop because of the number of separate health and social care organisations that need to be involved in providing services and because organisations have to demonstrate that they offer good value, in terms of both value for money and standards of performance. Comparisons are increasingly made between services provided in different areas of the country, with the aim of bringing all services up to an equivalent standard. This approach emphasises continuous development of service provision, and managers at all levels can expect to be involved in measuring performance against standards and in planning for improved performance.

Business planning can be described in terms of three main features – it should be continuous, user-driven and outward-looking:

- ■ Business planning is unlike planning a task or a project because it has no clear end-point. There are always aims and objectives in a business plan, but they are regularly updated and replaced. Thus business planning is a *continuous* process.
- ■ Business planning is *user-driven* because every organisation, if it is to remain successful, has to meet the needs and expectations of service users and the objectives set by commissioners. Four types of stakeholder have an interest in your services – beneficiaries, participants, payers and specifiers. Failure to be sensitive to the needs of any of these can lead to failure to meet performance targets. If an organisation is unable to meet its targets, its future may be in

jeopardy, particularly if there are other local organisations that are more successful.

■ The focus of attention in business planning is partly on the organisation itself, but it must also be *outward-looking* – it must take account of external factors that could influence its future. For example, there may be imminent changes in national service frameworks or new standards may be introduced. Business planning needs to take account of comparisons with other organisations that are doing better and what any potential competitors are doing.

Since business planning is a continuous process, which implies that a business plan is constantly changing, is it worth writing it down? The answer is 'Yes'. Organisations need a written business plan because the information it contains needs to be shared both within the organisation and with stakeholders and the public. All the interested parties need to know:

■ What are we trying to do?
■ What is the best way of doing it?
■ What resources are we going to need?

Although continuous change is to be expected, some elements of a business plan will be more enduring than others. For example, organisations rarely change their overall purpose or core activities. Most organisations plan to build on what they already do successfully.

There are no absolute rules about what should be included, but a business plan will usually:

■ make clear the purpose of the organisation;
■ describe the organisation's vision of the future;
■ set out broad aims and more specific objectives that will move the organisation towards its vision of the future;
■ describe the services being offered and to whom they are offered;
■ describe any intended changes in services;
■ set short-term targets for activity levels and outcomes;
■ set targets for income and expenditure;
■ describe how the organisation intends to keep in touch with the needs and expectations of service users to ensure that its services are responsive;
■ describe quality standards and how they will be met;
■ describe the implications of the plan for staff, including how their development needs will be met.

Business plans are often written with different levels of detail for different audiences. For example, most health and social care organisations produce a business plan that covers these issues in sufficient detail to enable members of the public to be involved in consultation about them. Staff need more detail about some aspects of the business plan in order to make detailed plans for their own areas of work.

ACTIVITY 12.1

Use this list to reflect on whether you have a clear understanding of the plan for the service for which you are responsible. Put a tick against each item that you feel that you could explain to your staff and your service users.

The purpose of your service	❐
The vision of the future for your service	❐
Your service's broad aims and specific objectives	❐
The service offered and to whom it is offered	❐
Any intended changes in the service	❐
Short-term targets for activity levels and outcomes	❐
Targets for income and expenditure	❐
How you keep in touch with the needs and expectations of service users	❐
The quality standards and how they are met	❐
The implications of the plan for your staff and how their development needs will be met	❐

If your organisation has a business plan, obtain a copy and study it. This should help you understand how you can contribute both to working towards achieving its objectives and to developing future business plans. If any aspects of the plan are unclear to you, you may wish to discuss these with your manager or other colleagues. If your organisation does not have a formal business plan, discuss with your manager whether it would be helpful to develop one. In the absence of a plan, it is difficult for staff at any level to set objectives that contribute to the aims of the organisation and thus to work towards a common purpose.

In addition to the characteristics of the business planning process that we described earlier (it is continuous, user-driven and outward-looking), you may have noted that a business plan includes:

■ components that can be described as strategic (for example, vision and aims) and those that are operational (for example, targets for income and expenditure);
■ a range of different time-frames, from the long term (vision) to the short term (objectives and targets).

Your task is to identify how your service is going to contribute to improvements in the health and well-being of your local population, in the context of national and local policy. Business planning should enable managers at all levels in an organisation to contribute to the planning process and to take responsibility for organising activities that are directed towards achieving the purpose, aims and objectives of the organisation.

ACCOUNTABILITY

If you are *accountable* for something, you are the one who has to explain or is held to account if something goes wrong (or right!). It implies that you have *responsibility* – that you have to undertake duties and make decisions. Organisations give *authority* to job holders so that they can carry out their responsibilities and be accountable for the outcomes. Organisations also design structures that define who is responsible for each area of work and to whom each manager is accountable. These hierarchies are called *lines of accountability*.

Accountability and responsibility thus go together. As a manager, you may be asked to account for the areas of work for which you are responsible. Your organisation is accountable for the quality of the services it provides and the resources it uses in providing them. Accountability is more than responsibility, in that it also brings an expectation that the responsible person or body will be able to provide evidence of the way in which the responsibility has been carried out. It includes being able to demonstrate that management control has been exercised over the use of resources to maintain quality standards. The reality in most workplaces is that, while senior managers are accountable for the overall quality of the service, first-line managers carry the responsibility for ensuring that the services directly available to service users are the best possible within the resources available.

Accountability in health and social care organisations

Health and social care are public services, and must therefore be accountable to the public. They deal with vulnerable and ill people, and carry important responsibilities in relation to the mental and physical health and the protection of individuals and communities. Governments are aware of the importance of these responsibilities, and have set up structures and processes to ensure 'good governance' – that responsibility lies with people who can be held to account for the quality and fair delivery of health and social care. Strategic health authorities, primary care trusts, hospital and community trusts, voluntary sector management committees and trustees, and local authorities all have specific responsibilities for which they are accountable.

There are a range of performance assessment frameworks for health and social care services in the UK, including national targets for particular initiatives, for example in children's services, as well as assessments on how well different localities are achieving their goals. There are national institutions that focus on identifying and disseminating good practice, such as the National Institute for Health and Clinical Excellence. There are also institutions that focus on reinforcing good practice, such as the Care and Social Services Inspectorate in Wales, and the Audit Commission and the Care Quality Commission in England, which carry out reviews and inspections of the performance of health and social care organisations. Registration and inspection authorities regulate the work of all service providers, whether statutory or independent, and have the power to close down services that do not meet the required standards. Codes of conduct – for example, for members of local councils and trustees – spell out the standards of behaviour expected of people occupying these offices.

Clinical governance

The notion of governance has become important as a means of focusing on organisational accountability in health and social care. Clinical governance is the system through which NHS organisations are accountable for continuously improving the quality of their services and safeguarding high standards of care.

The four main components of clinical governance for health service trusts were spelled out in *A First Class Service* (Department of Health, 1998). They are:

■ clear lines of responsibility and accountability for the overall quality of services, including clinical care;
■ a comprehensive programme of quality improvement activities;
■ clear policies directed towards managing risks;
■ procedures for all professional groups to identify and remedy poor performance.

The Royal College of Nursing website lists the key themes of clinical governance based on the documents on standards from England, Scotland, Wales and Northern Ireland:

■ patient focus – how services are based on patient needs;
■ information focus – how information is used;
■ quality improvement – how standards are reviewed and attained;
■ staff focus – how staff are developed;
■ leadership – how improvement efforts are planned;
■ public health – how health can be improved and inequalities reduced.

There is a similar expectation that quality in social care will be regularly reviewed and improved, but the systems are different because of differences in the structure of provision. Each local authority's responsibility for social care is regulated by inspection and by being required to demonstrate 'best value' (which includes measuring public services against similar services provided by the voluntary or private sectors).

Although there is some variation in detail from country to country, similar expectations of quality, efficiency and accountability have developed across the United Kingdom. For example, the NHS in Scotland (Scottish Office, 1998) provided a list of indicators to determine whether clinical governance is working well in a trust. In the next Activity, we ask you to apply these indicators (slightly amended to make them equally relevant for health and social care) to your own area of work.

ACTIVITY 12.2

Work through the list of indicators and make a brief note for each of any evidence of good practice in your area of work.

1 Services will be provided, organised and managed in a manner that supports the delivery of high-quality care.
2 The wider environment in which care is provided will support the delivery of high-quality care. (This could include the clinical environment, the physical environment and the culture of the organisation.)
3 Effective quality assurance and improvement processes will cover all aspects of service delivery.
4 Those providing care will be appropriately trained and have the skills and competences required.
5 Continuing professional development and lifelong learning will be taking place and there will be mechanisms for further training, retraining and reassessment.
6 Poor performance that affects the quality of care will be recognised and appropriate action taken.
7 There will be mechanisms through which staff can raise concerns over any aspect of service delivery that they feel may be having a detrimental effect on the care of service users, including the performance of colleagues or the management of services, without prejudicing the principles of service user and staff confidentiality.
8 Representatives of service users and the public will be involved in quality-related activities.
9 Evidence-based practice will be in day-to-day use and (in health care) there will be an infrastructure and support for activities relating to clinical effectiveness, including appropriate information systems.
10 Techniques such as risk management will be utilised to anticipate and minimise potential problems.
11 Techniques such as clinical audit and critical incident reporting will be in use to monitor and improve existing practice.

12 Programmes of research and development will be pursued and the lessons applied.
13 Complaints will be handled in accordance with national guidance and lessons will be learned from their investigation and resolution.
14 The codes of practice on openness and on confidentiality of personal information and related statutory provisions will be applied and monitored.

Some of these indicators of good governance may involve matters over which you have little, if any, direct influence. Others, however, may have given you ideas of ways in which you could improve your area of work. For example, in relation to item 3, you might have ideas about effective mechanisms to ensure that quality is maintained and developed or about plans for improving processes. In relation to item 5, you may have some thoughts about staff development, both to ensure that your staff have the appropriate skills and competences and to support professional development and lifelong learning. These guidelines suggest taking positive approaches to recognising poor performance and taking steps to improve it, rather than creating a culture in which it is more important to find someone to blame than to remedy a problem. You will also have noted an emphasis on openness in seeking opinions and on using information to improve practice.

Managerial accountability

Most managers are accountable for the performance of their staff and for the use of other resources in contributing to service delivery. In many organisations in the health and social care sector, managers are accountable through a traditional hierarchical structure. Increasingly, however, managers' responsibilities for co-ordinating and controlling the work of others are exercised in more complex structural relationships. Consider the following example.

Lines of accountability in project teams

Figure 12.1 illustrates the structure of a large housing association's building and maintenance department, which includes a number of specialist support services. The department has to handle a variety of projects, each of which requires different skills at different times. Each project is therefore staffed according to its needs – as the needs change, so the teams must change.

In Figure 12.1, staff member 2, Dympna Scherelsky, is a specialist in building services (for example, electrical and plumbing work). She is temporarily assigned full-time to project manager A, although he is no more senior in the organisation – he just happens to have the skills needed to lead this project. Scherelsky reports to project manager A on matters concerning the project and he, in turn, reports to the senior architect. However, Scherelsky remains responsible to her specialist manager, the senior building officer, in respect of conditions of employment, discipline and the professional quality of her work.

Dympna Scherelsky's continuing reporting relationship to her technical chief is represented by the dotted line from the staff member 2 box to the box of the senior building officer. Similarly, all the other staff members and leaders in the project teams will be linked by dotted lines to their permanent bosses (but the diagram would become rather untidy if we showed them all).

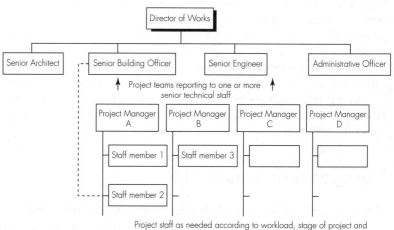

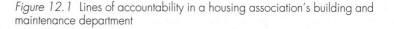

Figure 12.1 Lines of accountability in a housing association's building and maintenance department

ACTIVITY 12.3

To whom are you accountable?

How do you report to him or her?

Who is accountable to you?

Draw a chart showing the lines of accountability you have identified. Show the direct accountability to your line manager with a solid line. If you are accountable to other people for parts of your work (for example, to a human resources department or a finance department), show these accountabilities with dotted lines.

You may find your accountabilities listed in your job description. If your job description is not clear about your accountability, you could discuss this with your manager. You may be in a position where you are answerable to someone other than your line manager, perhaps for a particular project or for a particular area of work. If you are in this position, are your levels of authority clear to you?

It is important that you understand what you are accountable for – and to whom – so that you can keep the relevant manager informed of your achievements and your problems. You need appropriate authority to carry out your duties, but the extent of your authority is limited. If you find that your authority is not sufficient to deal with a particular situation, you would refer the matter up the line of accountability.

Organisations establish structures and frameworks to define, monitor and enforce accountability. Organisational charts, job descriptions, and some of the control processes (such as procedures) seek to define who is accountable at different levels and for what. In many social care organisations, the supervision process creates a structure of accountability throughout the organisation, from the director or chief executive to the care assistant. This is managed through regular supervision meetings between line managers and their staff to ensure that responsibilities, authority and reporting mechanisms are clear.

Personal and professional accountability

The concept of *personal responsibility* is crucial in the provision of health and social care services. Many staff at all levels work alone with service users. Some are responsible for toxic substances and difficult and sometimes dangerous procedures, and some have powers to deprive vulnerable citizens of their liberty. All staff carry personal responsibilities for ensuring that they do their work to the best of their abilities, without casual mistakes or deliberate abuse. They are all expected to know what they are doing, to keep themselves up to date with best practice and to maintain service quality. They need a level of confidence in their abilities to be able to operate effectively, but also an awareness of their limitations so that they seek support when necessary. It is part of a manager's role to help staff to recognise their responsibilities.

Health and social care organisations require their staff to be able to act appropriately – and sometimes creatively and imaginatively – when working alone or under pressure. The requirements of accountability to service users and the public at large tend to generate structures, frameworks, committees and inspections that can sometimes feel time-consuming and repressive. This needs to be balanced by having confidence in staff and giving them some freedom to experiment, in order to enable best practice to emerge and to develop. This is a dilemma for most organisations and is an issue you need to address in managing your own service.

Professional bodies expect their members to be accountable for their professional conduct. This includes responsibility for continuous professional development and lifelong learning. Professional bodies provide advice and support to their members on good practice. Most of them are also involved in setting standards and some have the power to remove from the register members who consistently fail to meet the required standards.

ACTIVITY 12.4

Are the staff that you manage accountable to one or more professional bodies? If so, list the main standards to which they adhere.

Are any of your colleagues, either in your own organisation or in partner organisations, members of professional bodies? If so, list the main standards to which they adhere.

If you work alongside people who have to adhere to standards set by professional bodies, it is helpful if you understand what is required of them. Difficulties in working across professional boundaries are often caused by misunderstandings about what each profession sees as particularly important.

ASSESSING AND MANAGING RISK

All staff have responsibilities for health and safety. They need to know what to do if a dangerous or harmful situation occurs. They should be aware of how to protect themselves, service users and visitors, and to be confident that they can take appropriate actions. This confidence is usually developed by rehearsing situations, for example, by holding fire drills and evacuations to ensure that buildings can be cleared quickly. They are also, as we have said, responsible for keeping up to date with best practice in their area of work.

Managing risk has become increasingly important in health and social care at all levels. First-line managers are routinely asked to contribute to risk registers.

Managers, however, have a broader responsibility to ensure that neither staff nor service users are subjected to danger and harm while they are, in any way, the responsibility of the organisation. They need to be aware of potential risks that exist because of the kind of work staff are doing, or the circumstances in which they do it, as well as of risks arising from the physical or emotional state of service users. They are responsible for taking appropriate action to protect staff and service users from harm.

What do we mean by the terms 'risk', 'risk assessment' and 'risk management'? The *New Oxford English Dictionary* defines risk as:

> *to hazard, to endanger; to expose to the chance of injury or loss.*

Aleszewski and Manthorpe (1991) define risk rather differently, as:

> *The possibility that a given course of action will not achieve its desired outcome but instead some undesirable situation will develop.*

Both definitions are useful in the context of health and social care. Parsloe (1999) goes further:

> *Risk is closely linked to dangerousness, resulting in harm. The issue here is not about defining dangerousness, which it seems to be agreed means harm to self or others, but with the extent of harm which should constitute a risk in various situations and with different kinds of people.*

All health and social care services face risks. *Risk assessment* is about recognising and predicting the potential for a dangerous situation to occur. *Risk management* is about taking reasonable steps to avoid risk, to reduce the likelihood of risk occurring, or sometimes to accept the consequences of risk.

Different kinds of risk

Different kinds of risk require different responses. Managers need to balance the likelihood of a risk occurring with the resources that are put into preventing it. For example, if it is likely that your staff will sometimes face abuse or violence from service users, you will need to invest resources in protecting them. However, if it is extremely unlikely that your staff will face such situations, you may not need to take any action other than, perhaps, to keep the situation under review.

Your responsibilities as a manager include:

■ knowing the risks involved in your area of work
■ knowing the procedures that staff are expected to follow
■ ensuring that all necessary safety equipment is available
■ taking action on any faults or potential hazards.

Let's look briefly at two categories of risk – risks from the environment and risks arising from people's actions.

Environmental risks

There are a number of potential risks in any working environment. These include the safety of the physical fabric of buildings, vehicles and equipment. Regular safety checks need to be carried out to ensure that accommodation and equipment are safe to use.

Environmental risks also include equipment and materials used in the workplace that are inherently dangerous, such as drugs, needles, high voltage electricity, radioactive sources, clinical waste and other substances that are hazardous to health, including chemicals that are volatile or may deteriorate. All health and social care organisations have procedures to protect staff and service users from the dangers of such environmental risks and it is part of your job as a manager to ensure that they are followed.

ACTIVITY 12.5

1 Who takes responsibility in your organisation for preventing environmental risks?
2 What are your main responsibilities for the maintenance of a safe and healthy working environment?
3 Is there any action that you need to take to ensure that you and your staff are aware of potential risks, or any additional precautions that are necessary to avoid harm to staff or service users?

If you are unsure of the policies and procedures that exist in your organisation, or suspect that they are inadequate, this is certainly something to follow up. Having explicit policies and procedures – and making sure that staff know what they are – are the first step towards safe practice and are the responsibility of every employer.

People risks

Risks associated with people tend to fit into three categories.

RISKS INHERENT IN THE WORK AND WORKING PRACTICES OF THE ORGANISATION

These include the risks to people's backs and shoulders from frequently lifting people or heavy objects, and risks incurred from working excessively long hours. The dangers here arise from not applying safe lifting techniques (not using suitable equipment such as hoists), and from accidents or mistakes caused by poor attention and fatigue. There are also potential risks in offices, for example, for those using visual display units, or from trailing leads or uneven flooring.

RISKS FROM EVENTS THAT MIGHT HAPPEN

These risks are difficult to predict. Anything might happen, but some things are more likely to happen than others. For example, stones might be thrown at ambulance drivers, staff working at night might have their cars stolen, or there might be attacks on or accidents to staff while they are carrying out their duties. It is difficult to predict occurrences like these, but precautions can be taken to reduce risks. For example, when staff are making visits away from their organisational base, information about where they are going and when they are expected to return should be left with a responsible person. It may be appropriate to keep a supply of mobile phones, torches and emergency alarms for staff to borrow. It may be possible to arrange shifts so that staff are not working alone at times of high risk.

RISKS ARISING FROM SOME IMPAIRMENT TO A PERSON'S FUNCTIONING

Much of the work of health and social care organisations involves working with people who are in pain, distressed, or under stress of one kind or another – people who may be under the influence of drugs or alcohol, people whose functioning is impaired by mental illness, or people who are unable to deal with their emotions. Sometimes risks may arise because a normally calm person is under great stress; sometimes the risks may be a continuing part of the way a person is. Much of the work of social care in particular, but also of some health services, is concerned with protecting vulnerable people from abuse.

An important step that a manager can take is to ensure that there are systems to protect people from human fallibility. Memory and habit are not enough when there are risks to safety. In areas of work where safety procedures must be followed, posters on the wall can remind people. You can also set up systems to remind you to carry out safety inspections and to have equipment checked.

One of your functions as a manager is to foster attitudes in your workplace that raise awareness of safety. Once a culture of vigilance is established, everyone is at less risk because everyone is aware of potential danger to themselves and to others.

ACTIVITY 12.6

Think back over an incident in your personal, professional or managerial career where harm occurred. How did this situation arise? Make a note of the action you took – or could take – to minimise the likelihood of it occurring again.

We came up with the following list of contributory factors that could lead to a fairly ordinary situation becoming a hazardous one:

- *ignorance* – not knowing that the hazard is or could be there, not knowing what type of hazard it might be;
- *incapacity* – poor judgement or loss of the ability to act, perhaps associated with tiredness, stress or error;
- *believing that nothing can be done* – hazards can occur because no attempt has been made to identify risks or take action to reduce them;
- *lack of vigilance* – staff failing to observe potential hazards;
- *lack of support* – there was no one there to help when help was needed – this can sometimes arise from a feeling of invincibility that proves to be unfounded.

We have focused on environmental risks and risks arising from people's actions. However, there are other kinds of risk.

There are also risks associated with the reputation of your organisation. As a manager, you represent your organisation to the public and you might be asked your opinion. The risk here is that, as a manager, what you offer as your personal opinion may be misunderstood to be an 'official' statement. If you are invited by a newspaper or local radio to comment about an incident in which your organisation appears to be involved, it is usually wise to seek advice from a senior manager before offering comment.

There are also financial risks in failing to anticipate essential expenditure and thus exceeding budgeted targets. In services that are responsive to demand, it is not easy to forecast expenditure accurately. However, many areas of expenditure can be anticipated by thinking ahead. For example, equipment deteriorates and needs replacing and you should be aware of approximately how long equipment will last, so that plans can be made in good time to obtain replacements. Similarly, good record keeping will enable you to plan to replace stocks of materials that are used in your area of work, avoiding the risk of running out of essential supplies.

Frameworks for the management of risk are vital to prevent unnecessary danger and harm. No matter how careful, logical and rational you are, you cannot anticipate everything that might represent a danger. However, you can take reasonable precautions and encourage vigilance. In particular, you can make sure that people are well trained and properly supervised.

The risk register

As a manager in health and social care, you are likely to have some involvement with your organisation's risk registers. You may have an organisation-wide register or several incorporating the main services.

Local authorities, for example, are required to produce community risk registers covering threats to local communities from environmental change or terrorism. Registers are also needed for addressing risk in health and social care services. What is a risk register? The Risk Register Working Group (2002) define it as:

> A log of risks of all kinds that threaten an organisation's success in achieving its declared aims and objectives. It is a dynamic living document, which is populated through the organisation's risk assessment and evaluation process. This enables risk to be quantified and ranked. It provides a structure for collating information about risks that helps both in the analysis of risks and in decisions about whether or how those risks should be treated.

The register is likely to include the following:

- *Description of the risk* e.g. 'increase in number and cost of children's placements' or 'delivery of personalisation agenda';
- *Risk rank* – a scoring from very low to very high, e.g. 1–10 based on scoring the impact and likelihood of the risk;
- *Actions required* e.g. 'use of robust project management', 'improved working with partners', 'robust monitoring';
- *Owner* – the lead person responsible for controlling and monitoring the risk.

ACTIVITY 12.7

Locate the risk register for your service and/or organisation. Ensure you fully understand each of the risks and consider how well your team is doing in addressing them.

We began this chapter by considering the context in which health and social care services are planned, and looking at what is involved in business planning. We have examined the structures that support and reinforce public accountability for health and social care services, as well as the concept of personal responsibility. We have also examined the processes of risk assessment and risk management: protecting staff and service users from harm has become an increasingly important component of the work of health and social care services and the completion of risk registers is a crucial management tool for achieving this.

REFERENCES

Aleszewski, A. and Manthorpe, J. (1991) 'Literature review: Measuring and managing risk in social welfare', *British Journal of Social Work*, vol. 21, pp. 277–90.

Department of the Environment, Transport and the Regions (1998) *Modern Local Government: In Touch with the People*, The Stationery Office.

Department of Health (1998) *A First Class Service: Quality in the NHS*, The Stationery Office.

Parsloe, P. (ed.) (1999) *Risk Assessment in Social Care and Social Work*, Jessica Kingsley Publishers.

Royal College of Nursing <http://www.rcn.org.uk/development/practice/clinical_ governance> (accessed 20/6/2009).

Scottish Office (1998) *Clinical Governance*, Scottish Office Department of Health.

The Risk Register Working Group (2002) *Making It Happen: A Guide for Risk Managers on How to Populate a Risk Register*, The Controls Assurance Support Unit, University of Keele.

PART 4

MANAGING IMPROVEMENT

CHAPTER 13

QUALITY IN SERVICES

Though 'quality' is an elusive concept, you will be well aware of the pressure there is on managers in health and social care to improve it. Knowing who your service users are, understanding what they would like from you and using your resources appropriately to meet their requirements are essential ingredients in providing quality services.

It is important to consider what 'quality' means. We begin by looking at various definitions of quality to help you identify what quality means for your area of health and social care services. This is the first step towards recognising where you are delivering good quality and diagnosing any quality problems you may have.

A great deal of attention has been given to quality in recent years. But why is quality important? In particular, why is it important in health and social care? We examine why quality is important both to those who use your services and to your staff. Quality has many dimensions and it is important to identify all those that affect your services and your service users' perceptions of them.

WHAT DOES 'QUALITY' MEAN?

So what does this elusive word 'quality' mean? If you buy jewellery from a Bond Street jeweller in London, you might think that this gives some guarantee of quality – but what about the jeweller who sells work in your local craft market? He or she might use gold and precious stones too – so can this be work of a high quality? And how about the differences between taking a Mediterranean cruise on a five-star luxury cruise liner and cruising around Poole Harbour on Joe's pleasure boat? Can we expect quality from Joe?

There are always at least two points of view – the customer or service user's view and the provider's. Therefore, one key to defining quality in health and social care is to look at differences in points of view between those who use services and those who provide them. Any definition of a quality service must incorporate the perceptions of both service users and service providers.

Quality means different things to different people. For example, your parents might offer you a top quality jacket, perhaps made of the best traditional materials. However, you know that you would never wear it because it is not a style that you would choose or one that you would want to be seen wearing. It does not fit in with the image you are trying to create. Is that a quality item of clothing? The answer is 'yes' for them but 'no' for you.

In health and social care, people see quality (or lack of quality) both in the way in which they are treated while they are using a service and in the outcomes they derive from it. If a mother with young children is moved into more appropriate housing, she will have an opinion about how she was consulted and supported during the process, as well as an opinion about the new housing and how this has changed her living conditions.

Defining quality

Quality was recognised as an important issue in developing successful services and businesses in the early 1980s and the influence of writers at that time is still important. The list below contains several definitions of quality, some of which are still widely used.

Quality is:

- fitness for purpose (Juran, 1986);
- conformance to requirements (Crosby, 1984);
- the totality of features and characteristics of a product or service that bear on its ability to satisfy stated or implied needs (International Standards Organisation, 1986);
- the degree of conformance of all the relevant features and characteristics of the product (or service) to all aspects of a customer's need, limited by the price and delivery he or she will accept (Groocock, 1986).

These definitions have many similarities. They all indicate that quality is about meeting the customer's requirements – whether they are stated or implied. If quality is about meeting customers' or service users' requirements, it is important to discover what these requirements are. If you provide services with extras that service users don't want, you will not be adding quality. So how do those who provide the services they think are needed match their ideas with those of service users who often know what they want and need? If you provide what you think are high-quality services because they are provided by well qualified and caring professionals who know what is best, will the service users agree with the professionals and think that they are receiving a high-quality service? Not necessarily! Let us consider which of the definitions we offered earlier are most useful for health and care services.

Fitness for purpose

This is a useful definition when considering what sort of support to deliver or which drugs or equipment to use. If an item fits the purpose for which it is intended, it is a quality product. On the other hand, if an item embodies the latest features or technology but is not suitable for the task in hand, it is, in this context, of poor quality. For example, if an older person needs help with shopping and cleaning, that is the support that he or she requires of a quality service. Providing a place in a residential home would not meet his or her needs, however much better the accommodation and services might seem to the provider.

Conformance to requirements

Crosby's definition means that the requirements must be specified. Such a specification is frequently described as a 'standard' and the specification should give a clear indication of what must be done if the standard is to be met. It should be easy to assess whether a standard has or has not been achieved. Standards are increasingly used in this way in health and social care services, and organisations are often required to conform to standards that are set nationally.

The totality of features and characteristics of a product or service that bear on its ability to satisfy stated or implied needs

Many requirements of those who use health and social care services are implied rather than stated. We can fairly easily predict that service users simply want to improve their health or well-being as quickly and as painlessly as possible. But they might not always know exactly what services will meet their needs. They might even expect or want services that are inappropriate or potentially harmful. To meet this definition fully, you need to tease out from service users what their implied expectations are. This can be difficult and time-consuming, but the effort is often worthwhile in improving co-operation and mutual understanding.

The degree of conformance of all the relevant features and characteristics of the product or service to all aspects of a customer's need, limited by the price and delivery he or she will accept

You might have preferred Groocock's definition because this is the only one that considers the relationship between meeting customers' requirements and cost. Cost is usually a constraint in the provision of health and social care services. A quality service cannot usually meet

John Oakland (1989) often asked students whether his watch is a quality watch. It has, he says, been insulted all over the world. Typical responses are 'No, it's cheap', 'No, the face is scratched', 'How reliable is it?' and 'I wouldn't wear it'. Rarely is he told that the quality of the watch depends on what the wearer requires from it. Oakland claims he does not need a piece of jewellery to give an impression of wealth. What he requires is a timepiece that also gives him the date in digital form. In his view, he has a quality watch.

all service users' wishes at any cost. Some residents in care homes or patients in hospital may, for example, want their own room with a private telephone and a television. However, managers would probably take the view that the value that customers put on this extra service would not justify the cost. One solution might be to make these extra facilities available but make a charge for them.

Continual improvement of quality has become a central concern of organisations since these early definitions of quality were proposed. Quality continues to be defined in different ways, but it is widely accepted that both the general public and service users expect high-quality health and care services that are at least comparable to the quality of other types of service (for example, in the leisure industry, hotels and catering, or travel). Five characteristics of quality management for the future were identified by Groetsch and Davis (2006) as:

■ a total commitment to continually increasing value for customers, investors, and employees;
■ a firm understanding that *market driven* means that quality is defined by customers, not the company;
■ a commitment to *leading* people with a bias for continuous improvement and communication;
■ a recognition that sustained growth requires the simultaneous achievement of four objectives continually and for ever: customer satisfaction, cost leadership, effective human resources and integration with the supplier base;
■ a commitment to fundamental improvement through knowledge, skills, problem solving, and teamwork.

These characteristics go beyond the early definitions of quality as meeting requirements by adding the commitment to continuous improvement – that it is no longer sufficient to be 'good enough' but that now organisations need to be continuously improving in order to keep up with the rising expectations of the public. All public service organisations face high levels of scrutiny and are expected to use resources to provide good value and high quality. Leaders are expected to set directions that demonstrate continuous improvement and no employee in health or care services will be unaware of the expectation that their skills and knowledge will be kept up to date and will be used to contribute to problem solving and teamwork.

Sustained growth in the capacity and capability of health and care services is essential if the increased demands on them are to be met. The Secretary of State for Health, Alan Johnson, said on the occasion of the 60th anniversary of the NHS:

The service continues to be available to everyone, free at the point of need. One million people are seen or treated every 36 hours, and nine out of ten people see their family doctor in any given year. In 2008 the NHS will carry out a million more operations than it did just 10 years ago. . . . The NHS already delivers high quality care to patients in many respects. The NHS Next Stage Review makes a compelling case that it can deliver high quality care for patients in all respects. It is only because of the investment and reform of the past decade that this is now possible.

(Department of Health, 2008)

Numbers of people wanting to use health and care services are forecast to continue to increase alongside rising expectations of a high quality professional service. Levels of funding will always be limited and the only way that health and care services will be able to continue to meet expectations will be by continuous quality improvement.

The quality chain

You may have a number of service users with very different requirements. Your management role may not involve delivering services directly to service users, but may be in a service that supports a number of activities, for example, a finance or information or personnel service. The concept of a 'chain' of quality is useful in considering the implications of these complex relationships. Quality is an issue in every aspect of a service so, when there are a number of different stages, and links between these stages, there is often the potential for things to go wrong. The *quality chain* uses the idea that the quality of each element and each link is crucial in determining the quality of the whole chain.

People within organisations are often customers of each other's services. For example, you are a customer of your finance department when you receive financial services but, when you provide information to the finance department, it is your customer. Often services are delivered by a sequence of different people – the receptionist may receive and record the arrival of service users, someone else may interview them to clarify their requirements, someone else may carry out tests and someone else may give them information about what will happen next. This process is often referred to as a *quality chain*. Each person or service in the organisation is both a customer (or service user) of the preceding person or service and a supplier (or service provider) to the following person or service (Figure 13.1).

The quality delivered to the ultimate service user will be a result of services meeting his or her requirements all along the chain. For a quality service to be delivered, requirements have to be met both inside the organisation – between internal providers and their customers – and across the organisation's boundary – between internal and external service providers. Increasingly, people from different health and social care organisations and agencies are contributing to a quality chain to deliver more integrated services.

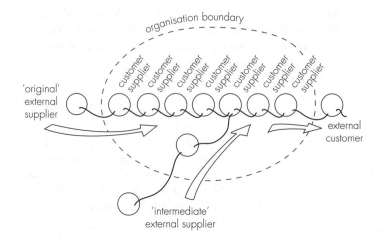

Figure 13.1 The quality chain

The quality chain may be broken at any point by a person or a piece of equipment not meeting the requirements of the customer, internal or external. In most cases this failure eventually finds its way to the service user, reducing the quality of service provided. In addition, such failure both adds unnecessary costs to the whole activity and has a negative effect on staff morale. In some situations, poor quality in one aspect of a service can damage quality across a whole service area. Consider, for example, the impact of poor infection control in a nursing home:

> *Many infectious diseases have the capacity to spread within care establishments, where large numbers of people, many of whom may be susceptible to infection, share eating and living accommodation. Infection is a major cause of illness among care home residents and may result in avoidable admissions to hospital. . . . Healthcare-associated infections may be serious, and in some cases life-threatening. Many of these infections can worsen underlying medical conditions and adversely affect recovery. Some healthcare-associated infections are resistant to antibiotics and the high media profile that they sometimes receive can be alarming to residents, their relatives and care-givers.*
> (Department of Health, 2006)

Standards and guidelines to improve infection control have been developed, but one person's carelessness can set off a chain reaction that would spread not only the infection but associated anxiety among residents, relatives and staff and the need for investigations within the home, often involving other agencies and commissioners. Have you experienced the frustration of not being able to do your job as effectively as you would wish because of a failure earlier in the quality chain?

So quality is about meeting the needs of all customers, internal and external. Even if your position in the chain in a long way from the final customer, you should think both about your immediate internal customer and about the effect of what you do on the final customer – the service user:

> Quality is needed at every link, otherwise the chain will be broken, and the failure will usually find its way sooner or later to the interface between the organisation and the patient. It is those who work at that interface who experience the problems of records or X-rays not being available, or transport not arriving, or the lack of clean laundry or shabby furniture which adversely affects the service given to the patients, but the failure has occurred some time previously at some other point in the chain.
>
> (Morris, 1989)

PERSPECTIVES ON QUALITY

To builders constructing an extension to a house, quality might mean principally the standard of workmanship they can put into it and the speed with which they can finish it. The time taken to complete the job would also be important to the householder, but on top of that would be the amount of disruption caused. To the householder, the courtesy of the builders would be a major factor, as would how far the house-holder felt properly consulted on decisions like where to put the window and what materials to use. The perspectives of providers and customers are different.

An example comes from a study of hotel conference services. The hotel staff judged the quality of the coffee breaks they provided for delegates in terms of the flavour of the brew, while the delegates mentioned factors like the speed of delivery, the timing of the coffee break, the space available for conversation and the proximity to toilet facilities.

In an organisation that gives proper attention to quality, staff will have working definitions of quality similar to those of their service users. If staff have definitions that are very different from those of their service users, or do not properly understand service users' require-ments, service users are likely to be dissatisfied.

Consider the different perspectives that might be held by users of services, providers of services, commissioners of services and the general public. Some of their concerns about quality are shown in Table 13.1.

Service users will be concerned about the outcomes of their treatment and care, about the way they are treated by staff, and about the nature and comfort of their environment. All these will differ for different groups of service users with different expectations and cultural backgrounds.

For providers, there should not necessarily be a conflict between professional excellence and the requirements of service users. Each profession has a responsibility to ensure that part of what is valued by senior members of the profession is a commitment to meeting all the requirements of the service user. However, providers are not neces-sarily a homogeneous group and different professional groups may

Table 13.1 Different perspectives on quality

Interested parties	Concerns about quality
Service users	Access to services Quality of experience Waiting time Caring and supportive environment
Providers	Professional excellence Concern for patients and service users Efficiency
Commissioners	Number of service users who receive services, related to demand Number of complaints Cost per episode or treatment Concern for service users Information about quality
General public	Fairness Value for money

have different points of view. For example, a physician may wish to treat a patient with a new drug because he or she believes that it will offer the quickest solution or be the one with least side effects, and therefore be the 'best' for the patient. However, if this treatment takes longer than conventional treatments, it may prevent the contracted target number being reached by the provider organisation.

Commissioners are likely to share service users' concerns about access to services and the effectiveness of treatment. They will be particularly interested, for example, in the number of patients treated and the cost per treatment. They will also require a considerable amount of information about quality standards in provider organisations.

Although many members of the public have used health or social care services, they may also have broader concerns, in particular about fairness, access and value for money.

ACTIVITY 13.1

1 Which groups of people influence quality in your area of activity?
2 In what ways do these groups differ in their perceptions of what constitutes a quality service?
3 How could these differences be reconciled?

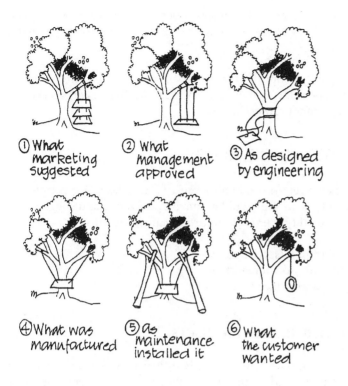

① What marketing suggested

② What management approved

③ As designed by engineering

④ What was manufactured

⑤ As maintenance installed it

⑥ What the customer wanted

Figure 13.2 Quality means different things to different people

Though your room for manoeuvre may be limited, part of your job as a manager is to reconcile different perceptions of quality. Ways of thinking that might help towards reconciliation include:

■ 'putting the service user first' as a way of setting priorities and cutting through competing requirements;
■ remembering that health and social care organisations are designed to cope with populations, but it is individuals who are service users;
■ facilitating good communication between the different parties by being open about any differences;
■ not exaggerating the differences – even the pressure to cut costs can be mitigated if providers and commissioners agree that quality is important.

Meeting all the requirements of service users, stated or implied, while keeping costs to a minimum, is often far from easy. It is well worth investing the effort in reconciling requirements because:

■ it will give you a better idea of what you are aiming at;
■ you will be better able to monitor and demonstrate the performance of your service;

■ if all your staff are on the same wavelength, your team's energy can be directed towards providing the service, rather than resolving differences.

Managers play an important role in ensuring that service users' expectations and perspectives about quality in service delivery are respected, even if they cannot always be met.

WHY IS QUALITY IMPORTANT?

In one sense, attention to quality must be worthwhile if people are concerned about it. We would go further, however, and suggest that attention to quality is important for three main reasons:

■ it is important to service users
■ it is important to your staff
■ it helps you to reduce costs.

Importance to service users

Service users not only benefit directly if their requirements are better met, but also indirectly if they feel confident that, next time they visit you, they will also be treated well.

Service users and their relatives are often worried, anxious, stressed, frightened and vulnerable. Such feelings are exacerbated by long waits, insufficient information, insensitivity to their needs and poor facilities. All that can be done to lessen these feelings and improve the quality of their experiences will be well received. When you are well, you can cope with a long wait in the supermarket, showers not working in the sports centre and a patronising bank manager – all aspects of poor quality in other service organisations. When you are in need of treatment or care, however, you are not so resilient to or tolerant of bad service and your appreciation for the good service you have received is all the greater.

Importance to staff

The majority of staff who work in health and social care have a real desire and commitment to care for people in need, often sacrificing opportunities for more money or more convenient working hours. If a service is not organised properly, staff are likely to find it more difficult to provide the level of care that they wish to and become frustrated and demotivated.

A well designed quality improvement programme, empowering staff to decide what can be done and then supporting them in their efforts to improve quality, is one way out of this spiral. The benefits to you and your staff are likely to include:

■ increased job satisfaction;
■ less frustration;
■ greater self-worth as your department's reputation grows in the community;
■ better feedback from service users.

Importance for reducing costs

It is not difficult to persuade people that improving quality will be better for both service users and staff. But it is often less easy to persuade them that improving quality can also save money.

Consider a company making microwave ovens which has, on average, 5 per cent of its products defective in some way. If it does not improve the quality of its basic processes, it will have to employ teams of checkers to pick out the ovens that are defective. It will then need to rework the defective products, incurring still more costs. Ovens may be returned by dissatisfied customers, incurring both transport and repair or replacement costs. Perhaps most importantly, the company will acquire a poor reputation and fewer people will buy its ovens. All this is a recipe for going out of business!

The cost of reducing the frequency of such problems will be small by comparison. Moreover, if quality had been built in when the plant was first designed, the extra cost of providing better quality would have been lower still and the company would have had a competitive edge both on quality and on cost.

The costs of poor quality in service industries may be more difficult to estimate, but they are nevertheless evident, as shown in the following quotations.

Service companies waste anywhere from 30–35% of their operating costs by not doing things right.

(Hutton, 1988)

In 1988 it was estimated that up to 25% of [National Westminster Bank's] operating costs were absorbed in the difference between the costs actually incurred in accomplishing a task, and the costs that would be incurred if a 'right first time' approach were to be successfully adopted.

The iceberg effect of failure costs demonstrates that above the water line are the obvious costs of failure – rework, rechecking, query handling, complaint handling, and waived fees. Below the line, and representing a far greater problem, are lost repeat business, lost customers, staff overtime, machine downtime, and bad employee morale.

(Department of Trade and Industry, 1990)

In health and social care too, studies have estimated the costs of not doing things right:

> Good quality may not always save money, but poor quality always costs and usually wastes money.
>
> (Carruthers and Holland, 1991)

At that time, such costs at Doncaster Royal Infirmary were estimated at 28 per cent of the revenue budget. At Cheltenham General Hospital, the costs of not doing things right amounted to £4 million – over 20 per cent of total costs. These costs could never be brought down to zero, but the scope for large savings and increases in the quality of care was considerable.

DO YOU HAVE A QUALITY PROBLEM?

In each of the situations in Table 13.2, there are implications for service users, for staff and for costs arising from poor quality.

It may be that these examples do not map precisely on to your service, but it should not be too difficult to see that flaws in service always carry implications further along the quality chain, particularly in terms of the time needed to sort out problems after the event. Quality, then, is not just about making things better for service users and other customers: it is also about cutting out unnecessary costs.

ACTIVITY 13.2

Estimate:

1 What percentage of time is spent by you and your staff in sorting out problems? (Consider all problems, including those caused by people outside your department.)
2 What percentage of these problems are new ones?
3 How many major quality problems can you identify in your own area of activity?

This Activity should suggest to you that there is the potential for reducing costs by better attention to quality in your department. Typical responses by managers outside health and social care are up to 98 per cent for item 1 and 4 to 5 per cent for item 2. How did you compare? Is there a fundamental message here? If there is, it will help to pinpoint the major quality problems affecting your area of activity. From your encounter with the notion of quality chains, you will probably already be able to identify which of these problems are:

Table 13.2 Quality problems

Description	Implications for service users	Implications for staff	Cost implications
Health records missing or out of date	Frustration at having to repeat history Wrong treatment offered	Histories need taking again Internal inquiries	Extra time spent searching or taking histories Extra consultations Expensive/complex remedial treatments
Insufficient car-parking facilities	Patients late for appointments	Staff late for appointments Low morale	Staff (or patients) kept waiting Capital equipment not used to fullest capacity Repeated appointments
Discharge delayed because drugs to take home are not available	Longer stay	Unnecessary work for all staff	Higher accommodation costs Slower throughput
Porters not available to move patients to operating theatre	Delays in operations Sicker patients Patients in for longer	Delays in operations Inter-staff tensions	Expensive staff and plant underused More costly treatments for patients' worsened conditions Higher accommodation costs
Patients kept waiting over an hour for prebooked appointments	Stress and frustration Car parks full	Ambulances held up Staff on the defensive	Extra staff time on explaining and mollifying Need for larger waiting rooms and car parks

- your own responsibility
- upstream of your responsibilities
- downstream of your responsibilities.

Having established where there are problems that you are aware of, it is also important to check that you have considered all aspects of quality in your area of work. So we now turn to the different 'dimensions' of quality.

DIMENSIONS OF QUALITY

Quality has many components. It is not sufficient to satisfy some requirements but not others. The aim should be to meet *all* the requirements of customers, stated or implied. Robert Maxwell of the King Edward's Hospital Fund for London proposed six dimensions of

Table 13.3 Dimensions of quality in care services

Dimensions	For example . . .
Access to services	Are services convenient geographically? Are waiting times for services, the physical design of buildings, the availability of transport and car parking acceptable?
Equity	Are services provided to all potential service users, whatever their cultural, racial or social backgrounds?
Relevance to need	Do services reflect the needs of the population served? Are there any gaps in meeting needs?
Social acceptability	Is the way services are provided acceptable to the people they are intended to serve?
Efficiency	Are services delivered as efficiently as possible within the resources available? Are services cost-effective and appropriately staffed?
Effectiveness	Do services achieve the intended benefits and outcomes in terms of the health and social care of the people served?

(Source: adapted from Maxwell (1984) 'Quality assessment in health' *British Medical Journal*, 13: 31–4, with permission from the BMJ Publishing Group)

quality in health care that have been used widely by the NHS. Table 13.3 presents these in a slightly adapted form so that they are equally applicable to quality in social care.

These dimensions have proved very useful for evaluating services. They also offer managers a checklist for setting standards for a service.

However, for day-to-day management, it might also be useful to have a set of factors that relate more closely to the requirements of individuals. For example, although each service user would like to be treated 'efficiently', he or she might have a number of more personal concerns. The Department of Health (1989) listed seven dimensions of quality that need to be satisfied for an individual patient. Slightly adapted so that they are relevant for managers in any health or social care setting, they are:

- appropriateness of treatment and care;
- achievement of optimum clinical or social care outcomes;
- all clinical procedures and professional actions minimising complications and other preventable events;
- an attitude that treats service users with dignity and as individuals;
- an environment conducive to the safety, reassurance and comfort of service users;
- speed of response to service users' needs and minimum inconvenience to them (and their relatives and friends);
- involvement of service users in their own care.

The next Activity invites you to consider how these two sets of dimensions of quality map on to your services and your customers.

ACTIVITY 13.3

Make a note of the dimensions of quality from Maxwell's list or the Department of Health's list that are most relevant to your main customers. Add any additional dimensions that are not on either list.

From this Activity you should be able to judge which classification is most useful to you, or whether you need to devise a special set of dimensions of quality for the services for which you are responsible.

The relationship between perceptions and expectations

Finally, three further pointers on quality in services may be useful to you in establishing exactly what quality means for your area. These derive from research by Berry *et al.* (1985), who carried out in-depth interviews of customers for a wide range of services.

- *Customers' perceptions of service quality result from a comparison of their expectations with their actual experience of the service.* The quality of a service is not just determined by the customer's reaction to it. It also depends on the customer's expectations. For example, an airline offering inter-city travel in the United States was experiencing problems with a flight scheduled to leave at 8 a.m. and arrive at 8.40 a.m.: it frequently arrived late. However, when they changed the schedule to say that it would arrive at 9 a.m., the plane was never late and passengers' perceptions of quality were much improved!
- *Quality perceptions are derived from the service process as well as from the service outcome.* Customers remember the process as well as the outcome. This is, of course, well recognised by staff in health and social care. One example is that of maternity services. Coming home with a healthy baby, while of prime importance, is certainly not the only matter of concern for the baby's parents. What kind of a time they had and how they were treated will be remembered for the rest of their lives.
- *Service quality is of two types, normal and exceptional.* First, there is the level of quality at which the normal service is delivered. Second, there is the level of the quality at which exceptions and problems are handled. If, for example, you were to compare the quality of service provided in different department stores, your analysis would not be complete without finding out how each store handled customers wishing to return goods.

Customers judge quality by comparing their perceptions of what they receive to their expectations of what they should receive. This point is important to understanding and controlling service quality because both expectations and perceptions are experiential states of mind rather than necessarily being real. A customer who waits, knowing it will be 30 minutes before he or she is served, may be happier than one who waits only half as long but does not know how long the wait will be.

(Haywood-Farmer, 1988)

Once you are confident that you understand the importance of working towards improving and maintaining high quality in your area of work, you need to develop some skills in analysing the causes of quality problems.

ANALYSING THE CAUSES OF QUALITY PROBLEMS

In order to solve any quality problem, you need to identify and work on its causes, rather than just its symptoms. A useful technique for analysing the causes of any quality problem is to use a *cause and effect* or *fishbone* diagram. This is a way of helping you sort out and make sense of relationships between the various possible causes that may lie behind a problem. Most problems do not have a single cause, and a fishbone diagram helps you to group causes into common themes or categories, so that you can decide what needs to be done to deal effectively with each. Drawing a fishbone diagram allows you – and others – to focus on the issues involved, and to see how they might relate to each other.

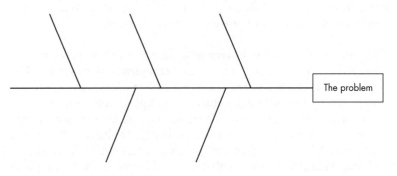

Figure 13.3 Basic fishbone diagram

Constructing a fishbone diagram

Here are the main stages involved in constructing a fishbone diagram:

1 Write the quality problem on the right-hand side of a large piece of paper or a whiteboard and draw a structure with a few branches that looks like the bones of a fish (Figure 13.3).
2 Use your own notes or discuss with your team all the possible causes of the quality problem you are experiencing.
3 Write the first possible cause on one of the branches – it doesn't matter which one.
4 Then take another of the possible causes you have identified, and decide whether it is similar or related to the first one. If it is, put it alongside the first one on the same branch. If it is different or unrelated, put it on another branch.

5 Work through all the possible causes you have identified, clustering related problems on appropriate branches. You may find you need to add extra branches, or that more possible causes occur to you while you are building up the diagram. Add them in when you need to.

6 The final stage is to look at the branches, decide what categories of cause they represent, and add labels to each branch to describe the categories.

Let's see how this approach might be applied to the following problem.

Initial complaint

The manager of an agency providing residential care for older people has received a letter from the son of one of the residents. The son complains that important information about his mother's circumstances and treatment are being sent to an old address, even though he insists that he has notified the agency of his new address. On investigation, the manager finds that the son's new address was mentioned in a letter dealing with a number of other matters, and was never entered on to the agency's computer database, which still contains the old address.

Consequences

When the manager raised this complaint at the next weekly meeting of senior staff, the discussion confirmed what she already suspected – that similar errors occurred frequently. While staff agreed that this was a quality problem, some argued that it was inevitable in the circumstances in which they were working. It was not uncommon for relatives to fail to provide information such as changes of address, no matter how often they were asked. Staff were quick to assure the manager that they always put things right as soon as a problem came to light. Indeed, they seemed to take considerable pride in their ability to fix things that had gone wrong.

After the meeting, the manager sat down to write a letter of apology. As she wrote, she began to think about the time and effort that was being wasted on 'putting things right' and wondered what she might do to get to the root causes of the problem in order to 'get things right first time'.

To help her, the manager drew the fishbone diagram shown in Figure 13.4.

In order to keep it relatively simple, we have not included in the diagram all the possible causes that the manager thought of. There are, however, enough to demonstrate the way in which the diagram is built up. You can see that the manager grouped the possible causes under

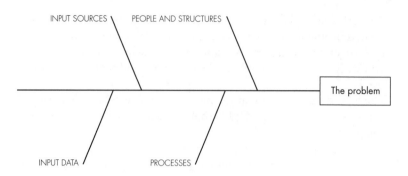

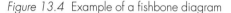

Figure 13.4 Example of a fishbone diagram

four headings – input data, input sources, processes, and people and structures. Her next step was to consider what action she could take to improve the situation.

ACTIVITY 13.4

Put yourself in the manager's position, and think about the four groups of causes in the quality problem in turn. Which causes might she regard as 'givens' – ones that cannot realistically be changed? Which causes might she concentrate on, and what actions might she take?

Here are the manager's notes to compare with yours.

> ### Input data
>
> Information like this is always likely to come in a variety of forms, and will often be mixed with other information provided for other purposes. We have to accept this as a 'given'.
>
> ### Input sources
>
> To assume that it's normal to put things right after a complaint fails to empower the residents' relatives, and often means that we have to put a lot of effort into solving problems after the event, rather than dealing with something before it becomes a problem. We can and should work with our input sources (in this case, relatives) to build good relationships, so that the information they provide is as useful to us as possible.
>
> *Action*: At the next weekly meeting, ask staff for ideas about how we might help relatives to give us the best possible information.

Processes

The database is updated twice a week by a member of the clerical staff. If changes are not notified to her in time, there will be a delay. They may even get overlooked altogether. Either way, this leads to the kind of problem we identified today. At the moment, the clerk deals only with the data that reach her. She can't be expected to go out and hunt for it. Or can she? Perhaps we can make it easier for staff to recognise information that needs to go into the database and pass it on.

Action: Devise a process for making sure that all data are sifted against a set of agreed criteria, and that relevant information then follows a simple channel into the database. We should also make the database available to all who need to use it.

I seem to have to deal with all these kinds of problems personally at the moment. If others got involved, they'd get more feedback on how well – or badly – our systems work, and they might then be encouraged to be more careful. And they've probably got some good ideas for improving things.

Action: Share and discuss difficulties regularly with staff. I've got to go about this the right way though, or they'll think I'm passing the buck.

People and structures

Our staff work hard and are often very busy. Relying on putting things right after they've gone wrong takes up the time and energy of people who should be getting on with their core jobs. If we can make changes to the system so that fewer of these problems occur, that should take some of the pressure off staff.

Action: The other action steps should have a payoff here. We could set ourselves a target for a reduction in the number of complaints about errors in our records. We need a performance indicator to tell us whether we are making progress.

But it's not reducing the number of complaints that really matters: it's getting it right in the first place. What is worrying is the 'put it right afterwards' culture. We need to shift towards a culture of 'getting it right in the first place'.

Action: I need to create a climate in which information is seen as useful to everyone. This is going to take some time. Where do I start?

You may not have agreed with everything the manager said or planned to do. You may have experience that led you to suggest different actions. Also – and this is not at all unusual – the manager seems to be reasonably clear about what she wants to do in some areas, but only at the beginning of her thinking in others. Nevertheless, mapping the causes that contribute to a problem in the form of a fishbone diagram is a useful way of focusing on the major causes of a quality problem and thus establishing a plan of action to improve the situation.

Categorising causes

When fishbone diagrams are used to analyse the causes of quality problems, the branches (or 'bones') are often not labelled at the start of the exercise. This encourages an open-ended approach and guards against making assumptions about the relationships between causes too early in the process. You often gain new insights by adding extra branches if the kinds of cause you are coming up with do not seem to relate to others you have already identified. You can always change your mind and reallocate them as your thinking develops.

However, it is often useful to label some of the branches before you start, to ensure that you focus on what you know from experience to be key areas. For instance, a typical approach when dealing with quality problems in service delivery would be to use branches labelled:

- people
- equipment/facilities
- materials
- methods
- environment.

You might find these categories appropriate to use in investigating many of the problems you encounter as a manager.

ACTIVITY 13.5

Consider a quality problem that you identify as your top priority to tackle.

1 Gather together everything you think might be useful to you in working on this problem. This might include any evidence you have about the nature of the problem (such as results, examples, opinions), as well as the analysis that led you to identify this problem as a priority.
2 Draw a fishbone diagram to help you identify the root causes of this quality problem, using the five categories of people, equipment/ facilities, materials, methods and environment. You may wish to involve other people at this stage, either in suggesting possible causes or in challenging your ideas and testing your understanding of them. Involving people in thinking through a problem is a powerful way of getting them interested in solving it.
3 Work through the possible causes you have identified and select those you think are most likely to be making a major contribution

to the problem. You will need to think carefully through the reasons for choosing some and not others. What evidence do you have?

4 Categorise those you have selected as:

- *causes you cannot do anything about* (these are the 'givens' – whatever solutions you eventually adopt will have to take account of them);
- *causes you believe you can tackle through your own actions* and through the actions of the staff you are responsible for managing;
- *causes where you will have to rely on other people to make changes* to bring about improvements (including senior managers, colleagues in other departments, information technology specialists, other professional colleagues, or your partners in joint working arrangements).

5 You should now be in a position to make an action plan to bring about the changes you have identified as being necessary. Decide the order in which you want to tackle issues. Some will be straightforward and the potential solutions will be fairly clear. Others will need thinking about rather more and may take longer to implement.

In moving forward from analysis into action, you have a number of factors on your side:

- Because you can justify your identification of a priority area for action, other people are more likely to be interested in helping to bring about change.
- You have identified the root causes of your quality problem in a systematic and thorough way. This makes it easier to share understanding and agree necessary actions.
- Where change is not possible, you will be able to explain the approach you have taken to working around the problem.

This chapter has concentrated on definitions of 'quality' and why quality is so important for service users, staff and budgets. A key element in most definitions of 'quality' is the relationship between providers' and service users' requirements and expectations. This relationship is no simple matter in health and social care services, in which expectations and requirements among the many parties in the system may be very different from each other. None the less, we have analysed some of the key dimensions of quality that health and social care services should meet, and offered you opportunities to match them against your own workplace experiences. You should now be able to begin to identify whether there are quality problems in your service and what they are. We concluded by introducing the fishbone diagram, which can be used as a method of analysing the causes of quality problems.

In the next chapter, we consider how to set quality standards and ensure that they are achieved.

REFERENCES

Berry, L., Zeithaml, V. and Parasuraman, A. (1985) *A Practical Approach to Quality*, Joiner Associates Inc.

Carruthers, I. and Holland, P. (1991) 'Quality assurance: choice for the individual', *International Journal of Health Care Quality Assurance*, vol. 4, no. 2, pp. 9–17.

Crosby, P. B. (1984) *Quality Without Tears*, McGraw-Hill.

Department of Health (1989) *Working for Patients* (CM555), HMSO.

Department of Health (2006) *Infection Control Guidance for Nursing Homes*, The Stationery Office.

Department of Health (2008) *High Quality Care for All: NHS Next Stage Review Final Report*, The Stationery Office.

Department of Trade and Industry (1990) *The Case for Costing Quality*, HMSO.

Groetsch, D.I. and Davis, S.B. (2006) 'Total quality approach to quality management', in *Quality Management: Introduction to Total Quality Management for Production, Processing, and Services,* 5th edn, Pearson Education, Inc.

Groocock, J. M. (1986) *The Chain of Quality*, John Wiley & Sons.

Haywood-Farmer, J. (1988) 'A conceptual model of service quality', *International Journal of Operations and Production Management*, vol. 8, no. 6, pp. 19–29.

Hutton, M. (1988) *Total Quality Management: The Crosby Approach*, Crosby Associates UK.

International Standards Organisation (1986) *Quality Vocabulary: Part 1, International Terms*, ISO.

Juran, J. M. (1986) 'The quality trilogy', *Quality Progress*, vol. 19, no. 8, pp. 19–24.

Maxwell, R. (1984) 'Quality assessment in health', *British Medical Journal*, vol. 13, pp. 31–4.

Morris, B. (1989) 'Total quality management', *International Journal of Health Care Quality Assurance*, vol. 2, no. 3, pp. 4–6.

Oakland, J. (1989) *Total Quality Management*, Heinemann.

CHAPTER 14

WORKING WITH STANDARDS

Quality is not achieved simply by trying a bit harder. You can be confident that you are achieving – and continuing to achieve – high-quality results only by setting up a system that will enable you to monitor them. This involves identifying what quality means for your area of work and then setting standards related to the outcomes required. Without clear and achievable quality standards, staff cannot have sufficient clarity about what is required, and have no way of knowing whether they have achieved what is required of them.

Standards provide a clear statement about the quality of service that health and social care organisations must provide and that the public can expect. This is made clear in the following statement by the National Planning Team for NHS Scotland:

> Standards . . . can guide and support the processes of clinical and service change. Equally, their existence in the public domain means that decision makers cannot ignore them. They will lead to a more informed debate about service configuration and about performance. This is of particular importance in a publicly-funded and managed healthcare system such as NHS Scotland both in terms of decision-making and accountability.
>
> (NHS Scotland, 2005)

The process of setting standards, monitoring to measure results against them and taking action if they are not fully achieved is similar to setting personal objectives, monitoring whether they are being achieved and taking appropriate action if they are not. As with objectives, standards need to be clear and unambiguous if you are to monitor quality effectively. However, there is an additional issue: once a quality standard is achieved, there is usually an expectation that this will be used as the basis for improvement. Quality is not something that can be achieved and then maintained at the same level for ever. Most quality standards need to improve steadily, even if slowly, to match the rising expectations of service users. In this session we discuss the role of standards, how they can be set, and how they relate to the outcomes required of a service.

Because it is important that a standard should be measurable, there is a temptation to emphasise aspects of a service that can readily be measured. But much work in health and social care is difficult to measure in ways that seem meaningful. For example, it is easy to measure how many people have been visited in their homes, but it is much less easy to measure whether a visit resulted in an appropriate outcome. There may be a tendency to direct activities towards achieving standards that are easy to measure and to neglect areas of work for which standards do not yet exist. Similarly, when standards are set as targets and measured nationally, there may be an over-emphasis on particular areas of work. Clare Chapman, when she was appointed as NHS Director-General of Workforce, commented that the culture of targets changed performance in the service 'from average to good', but that deep staff engagement and excellent leadership would move services to another level, 'from good to excellent'. (Jane Pickard interviewing Clare Chapman, 2009.) Managers in health and social care are expected to understand how to work with standards and within frameworks of standards and need to be able to use them in effective and meaningful ways with staff in their areas of work.

WHAT IS A STANDARD?

When you set a standard for an activity you are:

- explicitly stating a view of your customers' requirements;
- communicating to staff that these requirements are important;
- establishing that this is the target to be achieved at the present time.

A useful way of visualising the role of standards in quality management is shown in Figure 14.1. The standard is the chock that prevents the quality of service ball from rolling back down the hill. The position that has been achieved is the standard at the moment and is the position to be maintained. For example, you may have a standard that service users will be seen within 30 minutes of their appointment time. The chock is currently at 30 minutes, but to achieve real excellence it needs to be moved nearer the top of the hill, by resetting the standard to a shorter waiting time. There is, however, likely to be a cost implication of deciding to raise a standard. Resourcing levels and ways of working often have to change in order to achieve higher standards.

Once you have achieved the current standard, you will usually be expected to push the ball further up the hill and to place the chock at a higher level. This process continues until you reach the top of the hill and customers' requirements are fully met. But even when you reach the top of the hill you will find another hill – there will always be further scope for improvement. Customers' requirements are likely to change,

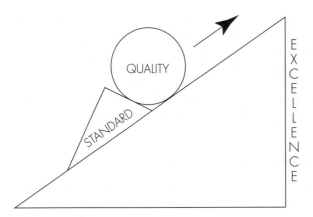

Figure 14.1 Quality 'ball on the hill'
(Source: Koch, 1991)

and research and evidence-based practice will affect the standards you set. The process is never-ending and is one of continual improvement.

ACTIVITY 14.1

A standard has been defined as an agreed level of performance negotiated within available resources.

Is this comprehensive enough? Or are there other requirements for an effective standard? Make a note of the qualities you think an effective standard should have.

Compare your notes with the following suggestions. Standards should be:

Measurable and capable of being monitored

If they are not, you will not know to what extent they are being met. Measurement does not have to be numerical, but it does involve assessing something that can be seen to have been achieved or not. You need to consider how easily a standard can be monitored – the last thing health and social care services need is more paperwork!

Realistic and attainable with available resources

It is no good having standards that cannot be achieved with the resources available to you. This would only lower motivation and morale. If the standard you can achieve at the moment is not what your customers require, you may need to make improvements in stages. You could develop a standard that goes some way to meeting customers' needs, while informing commissioners and service users that this is just an interim standard that you are making efforts to improve. The example quoted earlier is a case in point. No one would pretend that a wait of 30 minutes is ideal, but it was set because it could be achieved and it may be possible to improve on it later.

Real and important indicators of quality

There is always a temptation to set standards that are easy to monitor but are not necessarily central to service users' experiences. Numbers of people seen is an example – neither high nor low counts necessarily express the quality of the experience.

Expressed clearly and unambiguously

There should not be confusion about whether or not standards have been achieved.

Consistent with service aims and values

Your department and organisation must be able to demonstrate that they have a strategy to achieve their stated aims.

Set in conjunction with the people who will be asked to achieve them

If they are not, staff may be alienated by the standards rather than motivated by them. A key question in setting standards is who should participate in their development. If your team are to be committed to achieving a higher standard, it is often helpful to involve them in setting the standard and in planning how the new level can be achieved.

Frameworks of standards

It is important to be explicit about how standard setting fits in with your department's overall policy on quality management. You need to think about all the stages in a service user's experience and examine the quality problems that occur at each stage. Otherwise you may find that you are developing excellent standards in one area but ignoring other areas that are equally important to service users.

Setting standards in health and social care is not solely your preroga-tive and that of your staff. National standards have been established through National Service Frameworks, performance assessment frameworks and (in England) by the recommendations of the National Institute for Health and Clinical Excellence. Comparisons between the performance of different organisations against national standards are important both to ensure that they are providing value for money, and in relation to inspections by, for example, the Care Standards Commission. In setting standards you need to pay attention to the national policy context, research into the effectiveness of alternative treatments and care interventions, the results of inspections, and the policies and strategies of your own organisation.

Standards in many areas of professional work have traditionally been set and monitored by professional bodies and have often not been expressed in such measurable terms as we are proposing. Some health and social care professionals are not convinced that standards are appropriate to define their work. They argue that it is impossible to specify what a professional should do in all situations, that it is necessary to exercise professional judgement and that the aim of professional training and qualification is to prepare professionals to make appropriate judgements.

Others argue that standards based on professional consensus about good practice are useful, even if there will occasionally be circumstances that require different actions. Standards do not replace professional judgement, but set targets that can be understood by everyone involved – including both professionals and others who contribute to achieving the standards, and service users who are expecting a service of the quality indicated by the standards. The test of the usefulness of a standard is whether it is helpful in monitoring and improving the quality of service provided.

When standards are set by government agencies or commissioners, and are linked to inspection or funding, the role of managers is to organise their area of service delivery to ensure that the standards are achieved. This is often not easy because most health and social care services are essentially responsive – they are offered to those who need them when they need them. To some extent, the volume of demand can be predicted, but there are times when demand outstrips the ability of services to respond, as in flu epidemics or in very cold weather when those who can normally live safely in their own homes may need extra care. If standards are set in the expectation that demand will be steady, it is often not possible to achieve them fully when the level of demand increases suddenly. In such circumstances standards might be seen as indicators of a problem, as 'tools' to help managers to keep track of the extent to which the service is under pressure rather than as 'rules' that must be followed to avoid some sort of punishment.

Another problem is that there may be a tendency to direct work solely towards the achievement of a standard, rather than to focus on delivery of a service that meets the needs of the service user. In some cases, the emphasis on achieving standards can even lead to a temptation to subvert standards, for example, by not putting people on waiting lists so that the lists appear shorter.

Standards are not set to overrule or ignore good professional work and judgement but to acknowledge that performance in any area of care and service can vary both with individual members of staff over time, and between them.

(Koch, 1991)

However, especially when standards are agreed with the involvement of those who will work to achieve them, they can be very helpful in improving the quality of services. National standards provide a framework of expectations as the basis for developing services that offer equally high quality to service users wherever they live. The use of standards in health and social care is increasing and the ways in which standards are used can be expected to develop and change.

DEVELOPING A STANDARD

In some areas of health and social care there are not yet standards for teams to work towards and managers may be asked to contribute to the development of appropriate standards. For example, a manager in a commissioning organisation may be asked to set standards to enable a more integrated multi-agency service to be provided to replace and improve existing services. Another example would be the need to set standards for use of new procedures or equipment. The aim should be to develop realistic standards that will encourage people towards their achievement. The approach you take will depend on your understanding of the abilities, commitment and motivation of the people in your team.

ACTIVITY 14.2

Choose one aspect of the service(s) for which you are responsible that is in need of improvement and for which no standard is set currently. Who should participate in setting the standard? List all those you would include.

Service users are sure to come near the top of your list. It will doubtless include the professional, administrative and technical staff involved in your area of activity, as well as other managers and commissioners. You might also include members of staff who have had experience of developing standards in other areas. To what extent each of these groups is involved is an issue for you to decide, but it is important that none of them feels excluded from the process.

ACTIVITY 14.3

Imagine that you are managing a department responsible for providing physiotherapy services. The department's job includes:

- defining criteria for service provision
- receiving and recording referrals
- making appointments
- recording patients' attendances
- assessing patients' needs for therapy
- planning the treatment for each patient
- making sure that equipment appropriate to patients' needs is available
- delivering therapy treatments
- supervising therapy treatments
- recording the outcome of each therapy session in a patient's notes.

What information would be available to you if you were setting standards for performance in this area of work? What methods could you use to gain more information?

There will be some relevant standards that have been set nationally, for example, standards for waiting times. There will also be standards that have been developed by those commissioning the physiotherapy services or by the hospital to which this department belongs, either in this area of work or in similar areas. Previous managers or staff in this area of work may have already done some work that provides a starting point for setting standards.

A number of approaches are available if you need more information:

- You could carry out a time study for frequently repeated routine tasks such as assessing service users and recording attendances, in order to establish target times that staff are confident can be achieved. However, it is also important that the standards identify the different components of what should be achieved within the target time, for example, assessing a patient within a particular period of time, completing the form used for recording the assessment accurately and passing the information to the appropriate person.
- You may find it useful to carry out sample surveys of the most frequently performed functions. For example, you might check the availability of equipment and whether it is functioning properly. Some equipment may be shared with wards and not kept in the physiotherapy department, making the task of ensuring its availability for clinic sessions more difficult.
- You might look at past performance to establish, for example, how many service users have been seen each week in the past three months. This might be useful as a basis for establishing how many service users can be treated each week, but it may not reveal how many service users need to return for further treatment and thus have to be counted two or more times. The standard should reflect aspects of good practice that are meaningful to staff in your area.

■ In using any of these methods, you will have to involve the staff concerned if they are to feel committed to the standards of performance that are eventually defined.

Whatever standards are being set, for whatever purpose, two key considerations always apply:

■ *It is no use setting a standard unless there is a way of measuring performance.* It can be argued that, merely by setting a standard, performance can be improved even if there is no way of measuring it. However, people will realise fairly quickly that there is no monitoring, and other standards, which can be monitored, may be thrown into disrepute.
■ *The best standard is one that enables the person doing the job to see fairly easily when performance is satisfactory.* It is helpful for staff to be able to use standards to monitor their own performance. Consider, for example, drivers collecting people from their homes to bring them to a day centre. There is scope here for setting a standard that allows drivers to be flexible while still meeting a time target. They might need a target that allows them to adjust their schedule to accommodate any local difficulties that develop with individuals as they are collected.

It is important to set standards that are achievable and that help the process of service delivery rather than presenting obstacles. If standards do not enable staff to be flexible in responding to the needs of individual service users, both staff and service users will find the standard a hindrance rather than a benefit. If a standard takes a lot of work to monitor and seems to address a trivial aspect of service delivery, staff will find it tedious and irrelevant. It is also important to recognise that standards are set to address performance under fairly stable conditions and there may be times when it is impossible to achieve them.

ACTIVITY 14.4

Choose one of the processes of your department or section that does not already have a standard. This may be a procedure recently changed or introduced, perhaps involving use of new equipment or involving multiprofessional or interagency work. Devise one appropriate standard against which to measure the successful outcome of part of this process.

Now test this standard against the following criteria and tick each one that it meets:

	Yes	No
Is it measurable?	❐	❐
Is it attainable?	❐	❐

	Yes	No
Does it address quality (not just numbers)?	❒	❒
Is it clear and unambiguous?	❒	❒
Is it consistent with service aims and values?	❒	❒

If your standard does not meet all of these criteria, try to amend it so that it does.

Consider which colleagues will need to be involved in developing and agreeing this standard before it can contribute effectively to the quality of your team's work.

It is often useful to subdivide a standard into a number of component parts when an activity is complex. Smaller components can make monitoring the achievement of the standard easier. In the following example a standard developed for social workers (Smyth *et al.*, 1999) is subdivided into five elements.

Standard: The social worker works in partnership with individuals and, where necessary, carers to assess needs and to agree and plan a response to meet needs.

Element 1: The social worker seeks consent to carry out an assessment of need with service users and involves carers and others where appropriate.

Element 2: The social worker, in partnership with service users and where necessary and appropriate carers, carries out an assessment of need, taking risk factors into consideration.

Element 3: The social worker and service users agree priorities and ways of working together to meet identified needs and risks.

Element 4: The social worker and service users identify and confirm support and resources to implement the action plan.

Element 5: The social worker co-ordinates and records the agreed action plan.

Each element is then subdivided into performance criteria that clearly and specifically describe the work to be undertaken. For example, here are the performance criteria for Element 1:

■ The role and responsibilities of the social worker and the purpose of assessment are explained to service users.
■ The consent of service users is obtained to consult with others to carry out an assessment and to take any immediate action necessary within an agreed time-scale.

■ Any immediate action necessary is carried out and any services are agreed as temporary until endorsed by a full assessment.

■ Reasons for and use of assessment information given by others are clearly explained.

■ Service users are empowered to exercise their rights to give feedback on the quality of services and to make complaints.

■ Service users are advised of advocacy services available within the area.

This approach provides a great deal of detail about how the standard should be achieved. Many of the national occupational standards are written in a similar way.

Another technique is to proceed in steps. This is useful when a new standard is introduced into an area of work and it is expected that staff will speed up as they become used to the new way of working. Consider, for example, a standard to complete care plans for all patients who have been in hospital for more than 24 hours. If it is not practicable to achieve this immediately, interim targets might be set as in Table 14.1.

This gives staff time to change their practices and perhaps identifies the need for additional resources to be provided to achieve the target fully.

Table 14.1 Proceeding in steps

Months to	Percentage completed
December	70
March	85
June	95
September	100

Basing standards on dimensions of quality

In order to ensure that standards are real and important measures of quality, it is often helpful to base them on dimensions of quality. One way of doing this is to use the dimensions for quality in health and care services proposed by Maxwell (1984) – access, equity, relevance to need, social acceptability, efficiency and effectiveness. To set the standard, you need to consider quality issues relating to ensuring that the service is accessible to everyone, meets specific needs in a way that is socially acceptable and is delivered in a way that is both efficient and effective.

Another framework for dimensions of quality is the NHS Performance Assessment Framework, in which the dimensions are health improvement, fair access, effective delivery of appropriate health care, efficiency, patient/carer experience and health outcomes of NHS care. Table 14.2 shows how this framework has been used to set standards for the provision of a cervical cytology screening programme.

STRUCTURE, PROCESS, OUTCOME

Some standards are easy to measure – such as the waiting time we discussed earlier, or that an ambulance should respond to an emergency within 14 minutes in an urban area and 19 minutes in a rural area. It is relatively easy to identify such standards and to monitor whether they have been achieved. But what about setting standards for services that might be delivered over a longer period or that are more complex? Services for which it is harder to set numerical standards might include the care of older people or of people with learning difficulties. These areas require more sophisticated standards that reflect some of the complexities of the service, rather than simple counts of outcomes.

Issues like these led Avedis Donabedian (1980) to distinguish three critical components for written and measurable standards of care:

- *Structure*. The physical and organisational framework within which care is given. This includes the staff, facilities and equipment available, the environment within which the care is delivered and the documentation of procedures and policies.
- *Process*. The actual procedures and practices implemented by staff in the design, delivery and evaluation of care.
- *Outcome*. The effect of that care on the service user plus the costs of providing that care.

An example of the use of these headings is given in the following description of an adult mental health service.

Structure, process and outcome in mental health

Structure refers to aspects of the physical environment (e.g. quality of decor and furnishings, accessibility of unit to clients) and to certain characteristics of the social environment (e.g. staffing ratios, skill mix). These are all relatively static factors or fixtures which generally do not change much during an episode of client contact.

Process is concerned with events during a treatment episode. Typical process factors include the nature and speed of response to referrals, allocation of cases, decisions about treatment or therapy, therapist time per client, and case-note recording.

Outcome refers to the results of the team's intervention. It can be considered in terms of the extent to which the client has been helped or her/his

Table 14.2 Quality standards for the provision of a cervical cytology screening programme

Areas	Aspects of performance	Standard	Criteria
Health improvement	Overall health of populations, reflecting social and environmental factors and individual behaviour as well as care provided by NHS and other agencies	Health authority should only offer screening to women for whom it has been agreed that it is appropriate	Women between 20 and 65 should be offered screening every three years unless there are sound medical reasons not to do so Women who have had full hysterectomies or are already undergoing treatment should be excluded If last smear positive, women over 65 should be offered screening until they have had three negative smears
Fair access	Fairness of provision of services in relation to need on various dimensions: ■ geographical ■ socio-economic ■ demographic (age, ethnicity,, sex) ■ care groups (e.g. people with learning difficulties)	Health authority should ensure that all women have access to cervical cytology screening programme (if appropriate) at least once every three years and that this access should be made as easy as possible	There should be a register of all women in the health authority's area All appropriate women should be invited to attend for screening at least every three years Screening should be offered by all GPs and health centres Women should be able to make their own appointments Letters sent to women should be informative
		All appropriate women should be offered screening regardless of their race, creed, social class and geographic location	Access to screening services should be available in all locations in district Screening should be offered to all women residents Reminder letters should be sent to all women in district Health visitors should follow up all women who either fail to attend an appointment or fail to make one
Effective delivery of appropriate health care	Extent to which services are: ■ clinically effective (interventions or care packages are evidence-based) ■ appropriate to need	Health authority should minimise number of women who die of cervical cancer	Mortality rate from cervical cancer should be lower in population of women accepting screening than in population not accepting screening *continued . . .*

Table 14.2 continued

Areas	Aspects of performance	Standard	Criteria
	■ timely ■ in line with agreed standards ■ provided according to best practice ■ delivered by appropriately trained and educated staff		All appropriate women should be screened every three years Health authority should attain nationally and/or locally agreed targets for percentage coverage of women eligible for screening
Efficiency	Extent to which NHS provides efficient services, including: ■ cost per unit of care/outcome ■ productivity of capital estate ■ labour productivity	Service should ensure that smears are taken, processed and reported on without undue delay and at lowest cost possible, while ensuring that service remains effective and acceptable	All recall letters should be sent within three years of date last smear was taken All smears taken should be sent to appropriate laboratory within three working days All results should be reported to woman (if appropriate), place smear was taken (e.g. GP's surgery or clinic) and central register controlling programme
Patient/carer experience	Patient/carer perceptions of delivery of services, including: ■ responsiveness to individual needs and preferences ■ skill, care and continuity of service provision ■ patient involvement, relevant information and choice ■ waiting and accessibility ■ physical environment ■ courtesy of administrative arrangements	Screening service should be acceptable at all stages to women resident in district	Letter sent inviting women to attend should be sensitively expressed Rooms where smears taken should ensure women are given privacy Letters sent informing women of results should be sensitively expressed and women with positive results should be informed in person rather than by letter
Health outcomes of NHS care	NHS success in using its resources to: ■ reduce levels of risk factors ■ reduce levels of disease, impairment and complications of treatment ■ improve quality of life for patients and carers ■ reduce premature deaths		

(Source: adapted from Department of Health, 1998)

problem resolved, and is a direct measure of the clinical effectiveness of treatment or therapy. Other outcomes might relate to the degree of client satisfaction with the service or the extent to which the need for other specialised or costly services (e.g. acute psychiatric admissions) has been reduced.

(Burbach and Quarry, 1991)

All three areas of structure, process and outcome are important to any health or social care service, though possibly with differing emphases, depending on the nature of the service. For example, in the case of services for people with learning disabilities, some researchers say that the process area may be the most important. In relation to health care in general, Koch (1991) says that, 'Outcome is more difficult to define than structure and process standards and is arguably the most important of the three.'

For an example of how the headings of structure, process and outcome can be used in practice, have a look at Table 14.3, which is a standard for an occupational therapy service.

ACTIVITY 14.5

Consider how you might apply Donabedian's classification to your work area, using the headings 'structure', 'process' and 'outcome'. Choose an aspect of your service for which there is no existing standard. Many people find that it is helpful to think first about what outcome is to be achieved, then to consider what processes would achieve that outcome and finally to consider what structures are required to carry out the processes.

Once you are confident that you can draft a standard, you will be in a good position to review and revise standards for your area of work. Perhaps standard setting should be an agenda item for a meeting with your staff. Developing standards may seem like a daunting task. But many examples of good practice exist – whether in the form of standards from other parts of your organisation, from other organisations or from professional bodies. Adapting these may provide a helpful starting point.

Table 14.3 Standards for the occupational therapy service of Fife Health Board

Standard statement The occupational therapist will ensure that any child who attends Robert Hennyson School and lives at home will have an annual home visit to enhance a continuity of approach between school staff and parents and up-to-date knowledge and provision of specialist equipment.

Structure	Process	Outcome
Occupational therapist will have access to the child's record of needs	Occupational therapist will discuss child's needs and abilities with parents in areas of seating, bathing, toileting, feeding, positioning, and others as indicated by earlier assessment	Every child living at home and attending Robert Hennyson School will be visited in home by occupational therapist at least once a year
Occupational therapist will have access to other members of school staff to discuss child's current needs and functioning	Occupational therapist will offer advice and guidance to parents in above areas, and reinforce their role in using particular techniques or equipment	Parents will understand practice and principles of occupational therapy and equipment used with child, and reinforce approach used in school in home setting
Occupational therapist will discuss child with physiotherapy and community occupational therapy staff to assess need for joint home visit	Occupational therapist will discuss with family the range of statutory and non-statutory services available to them	Parents with children attending Robert Hennyson School will have access to specialist occupational therapy advice regarding home environment
Occupational therapist will ensure that time outside normal school hours is made available to carry out home visits	Occupational therapist will assess suitability of house for child and family and, where present environment is unsuitable, make recommendations as to adaptations required, or support rehousing application	Therapist will be able to meet parents outside school setting to ensure greater understanding of home situation, and parents will have opportunity to discuss child's functioning at home in that setting

continued . . . .

Table 14.3 continued

Structure	Process	Outcome
Occupational therapist will contact parents to arrange mutually convenient time to carry out visit	Occupational therapist will review with parents any equipment in the home, its use by them and its appropriateness in meeting current needs of parents and child	Written evidence will be available as to appropriateness of home environment and recommendations for any action to improve this
Occupational therapist will have transport suitable for visit	Occupational therapist will record home visits in keeping with Fife Health Board's occupational therapy policy and forward this to team members	Team members working with child will receive annual update on child's functioning in home environment, with particular emphasis on activities of daily living and use of special equipment
Occupational therapist will have records of his/her previous contacts with child in keeping with local occupational therapy policy	Occupational therapist will record home visit in monthly returns Occupational therapist will contact social work department's occupational therapist regarding any additional requirements for equipment	Occupational therapy register will identify frequency of home visits with child

(Source: based on Kitson, 1986)

FRAMEWORKS OF STANDARDS

If you are drafting standards for any health and care service that is regulated by the Department of Health, you should first make yourself aware of the guidance and requirements of existing frameworks of standards relevant to your area of work. Any new standards that are adopted by your organisation must therefore reflect the way in which standards are structured in the framework. For example, frameworks of standards are now usually expressed in terms of outcomes without explicit reference to the process by which they will be achieved, although consideration of process is always an essential part of planning.

Clinical governance was introduced to help organisations to take a strategic overview of quality and improvement of standards. The White Paper: *A First Class Service: Quality in the New NHS* described clinical governance as aiming 'to integrate recognised high standards of care, transparent responsibility and accountability for those standards, and a constant dynamic of improvement' (Department of Health 1998).

Chandra Vanu Som (2004) suggested a reinterpretation of clinical governance that would capture more of the complexity and implications for continuous quality improvement:

> *Clinical governance is defined as a governance system for healthcare organisations that promotes an integrated approach towards management of inputs, structures and process to improve the outcome of healthcare service delivery where health staff work in an environment of greater accountability for clinical quality.*

Inclusion of the word 'system' implies identifying procedures that can be monitored and controlled. Management of inputs, structure and process should link use of resources with intended outcomes and provide clarity about how standards will be achieved. This definition also acknowledges that staff who deliver services are expected to share accountability for clinical quality.

In 2004 a framework of quality standards was established that reflected increasingly joint working in health and social care. The standards in this framework were structured to enable all organisations in health and social care to interpret and achieve the standards at local levels. The standards set out in this document are organised within seven 'domains', which are designed to cover the full spectrum of health care as defined in the Health and Social Care (Community Health and Standards) Act 2003. The domains encompass all facets of health care, including prevention, and are described in terms of outcomes. The seven domains are:

- safety
- clinical and cost effectiveness

- governance
- patient focus
- accessible and responsive care
- care environment and amenities
- public health.

(Department of Health, 2004)

In each of these domains the individual standards fall into two categories:

- *core standards*: which bring together and rationalise existing requirements for the health service, setting out the minimum levels of service patients and service users have a right to expect; and
- *developmental standards*: which signal the direction of travel and provide a framework for NHS bodies to plan the delivery of services that continue to improve in line with increasing patient expectations.

(Department of Health, 2004)

These standards were intended to be measurable as an assessment tool with core standards set as the basic minimum requirement and developmental standards as improvements that an organisation should plan to achieve. An example of these standards for the 'safety' domain is given in Table 14.4, but these are updated frequently as standards are raised.

McSherry and Pearce (2007) have commented on the impact that clinical governance has had as the vehicle for delivering clinical quality through reforms in health and care services:

With an increase in the number of patients admitted with multiple needs, healthcare organisations have had to change their pattern of care delivery in order to accommodate this growing need, leading to the development of acute medical and surgical assessment units, pre-operative assessment units, multiple needs and rehabilitation units, and acute mental health assessment units. Latterly we have witnessed an increase in the development of services dedicated to maintain individuals in the community . . .

This style of service provision is about optimising the use of acute and community beds by encouraging collaborative working between primary and secondary care in the management and maintenance of the patient in the most appropriate setting. An example of this would be in the shared management of patients who have diabetes, where the care is shared between the GP and the consultant endocrinologist with the backing of the diabetic team (diabetes nurse specialist, dietician, podiatrist, ophthalmologist and pharmacist).

Table 14.4 Core and developmental standards for the 'safety' domain

Domain outcome

Patient safety is enhanced by the use of health care processes, working practices and systemic activities that prevent or reduce the risk of harm to patients.

Core standard

C1 Health care organisations protect patients through systems that:

a) identify and learn from all patient safety incidents and other reportable incidents, and make improvements in practice based on local and national experience and information derived from the analysis of incidents; and

b) ensure that patient safety notices, alerts and other communications concerning patient safety which require action are acted upon within required time-scales.

C2 Health care organisations protect children by following national child protection guidance within their own activities and in their dealings with other organisations.

C3 Health care organisations protect patients by following NICE Interventional Procedures guidance.

C4 Health care organisations keep patients, staff and visitors safe by having systems to ensure that:

a) the risk of health care acquired infection to patients is reduced, with particular emphasis on high standards of hygiene and cleanliness, achieving year-on-year reductions in MRSA (methycillin-resistant staphylococcus aureus);

b) all risks associated with the acquisition and use of medical devices are minimised;

c) all reusable medical devices are properly decontaminated prior to use and that the risks associated with decontamination facilities and processes are well managed;

d) medicines are handled safely and securely; and

e) the prevention, segregation, handling, transport and disposal of waste is properly managed so as to minimise the risks to the health and safety of staff, patients, the public and the safety of the environment.

Developmental standard

D1 Health care organisations continuously and systematically review and improve all aspects of their activities that directly affect patient safety and apply best practice in assessing and managing risks to patients, staff and others, particularly when patients move from the care of one organisation to another.

(Source: Department of Health, 2004)

MONITORING STANDARDS

Monitoring means 'continuous or regularly repeated observations of important parts of the service structure, process, output or outcome'.

(Morgan and Everett, 1991)

Developing service standards is a time-consuming process, but it can focus attention on problem areas and suggest improvements that can be quickly implemented. However, the main benefits come from sustained monitoring of performance against standards to establish the extent to which they are being met. If the service is not meeting its standards, there is work to be done to find out why and to rectify the problems. If performance is better than expected, it is still important to investigate the reasons for this in order to discover ways of continuing to improve. Hugh Koch summarised this process neatly as shown in Figure 14.2.

In designing a monitoring procedure there are many decisions to be made:

■ what to monitor
■ why you want to monitor it
■ how often you should monitor it
■ the level of detail required
■ who will collect the information and how
■ how reliable the information will be
■ if the information could be fed into a computer for analysis
■ who should receive the information
■ how the information will be used.

Monitoring can take many forms, for example, counting how many people are on a waiting list or in a waiting room, measuring service users' satisfaction with carefully designed questionnaires, or noting how long it takes a patient to recover after an operation. Deciding what to monitor and how to do it is a key task. Sensitivity may be needed to avoid monitoring being intrusive to staff or service users. Involving staff in making choices will be important in gaining their commitment to recording accurate measurements.

The methods chosen for monitoring depend to some extent on how the standards have been drawn up. Though many different factors might be measured and compared, there are essentially two main approaches:

■ Count the percentage of occasions when the standard is achieved (for example, the percentage of service users who were seen within 30 minutes of their appointment time).

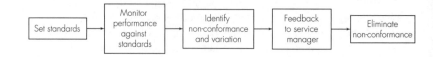

Figure 14.2 Monitoring standards
(Source: Koch, 1991)

■ Record whether the standard has been achieved, partially achieved or not achieved in the period being considered. This is especially useful where standards are set using the structure–process–outcome model. Table 14.5 shows a form from an occupational therapy service, on which a record of results can be made as well as notes of further actions to be taken.

ACTIVITY 14.6

Look back at your notes for the previous Activity. How could you monitor these standards for structure, process and outcomes?

Your answer might have included planning who should keep records of what and how frequently. You might have considered whether records should be paper-based or computer-based and how the information should be stored and used.

Monitoring is essentially about ensuring that information on whether standards are being achieved is collected regularly and in sufficient detail. In order to improve and develop service provision, the

Table 14.5 Monitoring form for an occupational therapy service

Statements of quality assurance	Achieved	Partially achieved	Not achieved	Further action to be taken
Provision of an area of privacy for treatment				
Provision of a quiet and acceptable area for patient treatment				
Provision of adequate up-to-date equipment for patient treatment				
Regular maintenance programme that keeps equipment in safe working order				
Correct staffing levels for: – inpatient treatment – outpatient treatment – day patient treatment – community patient treatment				
Fully-staffed service in line with current establishment				

(Source: Koch, 1991)

Table 14.6 Example of monitoring arrangements for patient safety

Ref	Clinical quality performance indicator	Threshold	Method of measurement	Consequence per breach
3.3	**Falls** The provider will continue to implement best practice to reduce the number of patients falling whilst in hospital and to reduce the severity of harm caused to patients as a result of a fall in hospital.	Establish robust set of baseline measures for 2009–10.	Number of patients falling in hospital by ward by severity of harm (as per National Patient Safety Association definition). Number of patients falling more than once by ward.	Subject to Clause 33 (Joint Clinical Investigation followed by Remedial Clinical Action Plan and Exception Report – escalated as appropriate).
3.4	**Hospital acquired pressure ulcers** The provider will implement best practice to continue to work to reduce the number and severity of hospital acquired pressure ulcers. Ref: NICE: Clinical Guideline 29; Pressure ulcer management (2005).	Establish robust set of baseline measures for 2009–10.	Number of hospital-acquired pressure sores, by grade, by ward (including nil returns). Quarterly audit of 10 sets of notes or 20% of patients with hospital acquired pressure ulcers against standards set out in NICE Guidance.	Subject to Clause 33 (Joint Clinical Investigation followed by Remedial Clinical Action Plan and Exception Report – escalated as appropriate).

(Source: Milton Keynes Primary Care Trust, 2008)

results of monitoring must lead to action. Table 14.6 gives an example of how standards for patient safety provision are monitored by a primary care trust.

Audit

Audit is another form of monitoring that can be a vital part of maintaining and improving the quality of a service. The term 'audit' comes from financial accountancy but is widely used in health care and includes clinical, medical and nursing audits. A definition of audit in health was given by Shaw (1991):

Audit should allow the objective peer review of patterns of care, sensitive to the expectations of patients and other clinical disciplines and based on scientific evidence of good medical practice.

Because the term has associations with investigation and appraisal, an audit needs to be carried out in a supportive atmosphere to allow open and honest discussion of the results. Though audit can contribute much to the management of quality, it tends to be a closely focused activity, examining one particular aspect of a service rather than the service as a whole.

A more recent definition of audit in health was given in a review of how boards of NHS trusts and foundation trusts get their assurance:

[A]udit should periodically review the compliance function, including operational adherence to the compliance framework and applicable legislation, and review the operation of principal financial controls within complete processes.
(Audit Commission, 2009)

In this definition, audit has its traditional role in organisations of assuring financial compliance. The criticism was made that audit should be used to ensure that all the financial operations are carried out as required, not to replace any of the normal quality assurance processes. The review went on to give a definition of clinical audit:

Clinical audit is effectively the review of clinical performance, the measurement of performance against agreed standards, and the refining of clinical practice as a result.

Again, the emphasis is on checking that standards have been achieved and reporting results, in order to provide the evidence for improvement.

The basic philosophy of quality management is getting the process and the outcomes right first time. In complex services, where many different types of staff and many different areas of work contribute to the delivery of a service, it is particularly difficult to ensure that all the stages in the process and the links between them are of an equally high quality. A well managed quality chain goes some way towards ensuring high-quality outcomes, but the outcomes for any individual service user will be viewed from a personal perspective.

Setting standards and monitoring performance against them provide a process through which quality can be managed. It is important that the standards be realistic and meaningful and that they represent aspects of the service that are worth measuring. It is helpful if the staff who are to contribute to achieving the standards are involved in setting them at a level that they agree is attainable. Once you have standards in place, performance can be measured against them. This provides the basis for taking managerial action if the standards are not being consistently achieved, and for improving the standards in due course.

REFERENCES

Audit Commission (2009) *Taking it on Trust*, <http://www.audit-commission. gov.uk> (accessed 20/6/2009).

Burbach, F. R. and Quarry, A. (1991) 'Quality and outcome in a community mental health team', *International Journal of Health Care Quality Assurance*, vol. 4, no. 2, pp. 18–26.

Department of Health (1998) *A First Class Service: Quality in the New NHS*, Department of Health.

Department of Health (2004) *Standards for Better Health*, The Stationery Office.

Donabedian, A. (1980) *Definition of Quality and Approaches to its Assessment*, Health Administration Press.

Kitson, A. (1986) 'Rest assured', *Nursing Times*, 27 August, pp. 28–31.

Koch, H. (1991) *Total Quality Management*, Longmans.

Maxwell, R. (1984) 'Quality assessment in health', *British Medical Journal*, vol. 13, pp. 31–4.

McSherry, R. and Pearce, P. (2007) *Clinical Governance: A Guide to Implementation for Healthcare Professionals* (2nd edn), Blackwell Publishing Ltd.

Milton Keynes Primary Care Trust (2008) *Terms and Conditions for the Provision of Community Health Care Services*, Milton Keynes.

Morgan, J. and Everett, T. (1991) 'Introducing quality management in the NHS', *International Journal of Health Care Quality Assurance*, vol. 3, no. 5, pp. 23.

NHS for Scotland (2005) *Drivers for Change in the Health Service in Scotland*, downloaded 12/05/2009 from <http://www.clinical governance.scot.nhs. uk> (accessed 20/6/2009).

Pickard, J. (2009) 'A healthy constitution', *People Management*, 29 January, p. 20.

Shaw, C. (1991) 'Specifications for hospital medical audit', *Health Services Management*, June, pp. 124–5.

Smyth, C., Simmons, I. and Cunningham, G. (1999) *Quality Assurance in Social Work: A Standards and Audit Approach for Agencies and Practitioners*, National Institute for Social Work.

Vanu Som, C. (2004) 'Clinical governance: A fresh look at its definition', *Clinical Governance*, vol. 9, no. 2, pp. 87–90.

CHAPTER 15

MANAGEMENT CONTROL

This chapter begins by considering some of the benefits of effective management control. It then introduces the 'control loop' – the idea that control is a cyclical process of setting standards, measuring performance, comparing performance with the standards and taking corrective action if necessary. We then look at some of the issues in measuring and comparing, and at the different ways in which control can be exercised. We conclude by focusing on how corrective action can be taken to ensure that standards and objectives are achieved.

The chapter does not set out to give you rules to work by. Its aim is to give you some ideas that you are invited to think about in the context of your own job. By the end of the chapter, you should have developed some ideas of your own as to how control fits into your managerial tasks. You should also have developed some ideas about how you can help your staff in the control they have to exercise, and what control your manager or supervisor is (or should be!) exercising over your activities and those of your department or section.

WHY CONTROL?

If you accept that part of a manager's role is to control the flow of work, you may feel that there is no need to ask this question. However, there are more benefits from control than you might at first recognise. Some of the most significant are:

- Without effective control, much of the effort that has gone into planning will be wasted, since you will not know whether your objectives have been achieved.
- Effective control helps you to obtain the best results from the available money, people, equipment and time.
- With effective control, a work group – a team, a department or a whole organisation – can be steered consistently towards its objectives.

- The standard-setting and monitoring elements of control enable systematic action to be taken to keep on target, thus reducing argument and conflict.
- Effective control can give your team a feeling of confidence, cohesiveness and purpose.
- Effective control, through measuring and comparing, provides a basis for forecasting, estimating and planning.
- Effective control of people's work helps you to assess them for promotion, transfer or training.
- With an effective control system, staff can assess their own performance and adjust their approach, leading to greater commitment and more job satisfaction.

ACTIVITY 15.1

Describe briefly a situation from your experience in which each of the statements below applied.

1 Effective control saved the day. (Was there a strong 'controller' in the lead?)
2 Absence of control resulted in damage to the organisation's interests. (What would you have done, had you been responsible?)
3 Absence of control did not cause problems. (Then ask yourself whether there was truly an absence of control.)

'Control' is an emotive word that sparks a hostile and resistant response from many people. Some find the notion of managers attempting to exercise control over staff offensive. Some writers have insisted that only inanimate items like resources, expenditure and events can be 'controlled' and that people must be 'managed'. The distinction between management and control is a fine one and you must make up your own mind about the difference.

Another reason why hostile responses might arise is that the word 'control' can be used with a variety of different meanings, some of which have overtones of coercion and exploitation. The managerial sense of the word, as used in this book, is much more akin to the control that a driver exerts over a car, keeping things on the planned course to make sure of a safe arrival at the intended destination. One of the contributions that systems thinking has made to management thinking is by providing a model of the control process. This is known as the *control loop*.

THE CONTROL LOOP

Let's take the driving analogy a little further. A minibus driver picking up people from their homes to take them to a day centre takes care that each passenger is seated comfortably and safely in the minibus. While the passengers are chatting and looking out of the windows, the driver is controlling the journey. To do this, the driver:

- continuously monitors the instruments that provide information about the minibus (its speed, its fuel consumption and reserves, the temperature of the engine, and so on) and continuously monitors the progress that the minibus is making from the final pick-up to the day centre;
- compares this information with the usual progress along the normal route, to check that everything is going according to plan (for example, that the minibus is still on track to arrive at the planned time and has adequate reserves of fuel left to reach its planned destination);
- takes corrective action if things are not going according to plan (this might include very minor interventions, such as stopping to allow another vehicle to pull out, more significant changes, such as taking a different route to avoid roadworks, or even implementing a contingency plan and diverting to a new destination if circumstances require it).

These three steps – *monitoring* what is happening, *comparing* what is happening with the plan, and *taking corrective action* where necessary – are the essence of management control.

The same three steps can be seen in health and social care. For example, if an older man who lives alone has an accident that reduces his ability to take care of himself, he may need temporary help from care services. A care plan will be prepared, the situation will be monitored as he recovers, and the level of care will be reduced and eventually discontinued when he is fully recovered.

Another example is the management of a patient in intensive care. A range of instruments provides information about the patient's condition. The medical staff monitor these instruments continuously and compare the patient's condition with what should be happening. If the data from the instruments are not following the course that they should, the staff might have to take corrective action – perhaps by administering a drug to bring the blood pressure or pulse rate within acceptable limits, or perhaps by some more drastic intervention. These processes of monitoring, comparing and taking corrective action if necessary will continue until the patient is out of danger. When, in due course, the patient leaves intensive care, the same processes of control continue, though perhaps less obtrusively. The patient is no longer wired to the monitoring instruments because it is no longer necessary to have continuous information, but the staff carry on monitoring the patient's progress by gathering information in other ways (ward rounds, observation, examinations, scans, and so on) and they compare this information with what they would expect for that particular patient. If the patient's progress is not going according to plan, they might need to take further corrective action but, if the patient is on course for recovery, they need do no more than continue to monitor his or her progress.

These three steps underlie all forms of managerial control, though in 'normal' management, such as running a section or department, the steps may be less obvious and clear-cut. Nevertheless they are there, and can be represented by the control loop shown in Figure 15.1.

The control loop implies that you must start with a plan that specifies goals (where you are going) and objectives (detailed statements of measurable standards to be attained). Your next task is to *measure* what is actually happening. You then *compare* this with what is supposed to be happening – the level and direction of performance specified in the plan. If all is well, you need only to continue monitoring. If things are not going according to plan, you need to take *corrective action* to bring the performance back on course.

ACTIVITY 15.2

List four reasons why the separate steps indicated in the control loop might appear less obvious and clear-cut in 'normal' managerial work than they do in driving a vehicle or managing the care of a patient or service user.

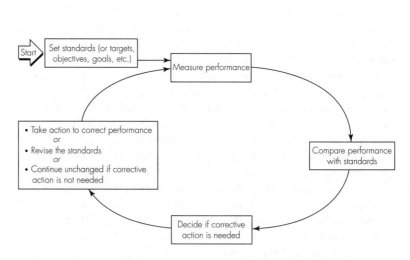

Figure 15.1 The control loop

There are many reasons why 'normal' management control is more complex than the control loop suggests. Very few managers have a plan that is as detailed and specific as the plan a driver has for a journey. Even where the destination or goal is fairly clearly defined, the standards to be attained and maintained cannot always be specified exactly. And even if some standards can be specified fairly precisely, it is rarely possible to measure what is actually happening in the workplace with anything like the same accuracy – or as quickly – as is possible in a vehicle or in many medical procedures. For example, there is often a significant delay between an event happening and the availability of data about it. Nor are the data always reliable. Moreover, a driver is controlling only one car, whereas most managers are controlling several different activities at the same time, each of which may be at a different stage of development. And a driver does not usually have to break off in the middle of the journey and turn his or her attention to something completely different such as the absence of a member of staff, a disciplinary problem or a casual interruption.

Nevertheless, the separate steps in the process of managerial control – setting standards, measuring, comparing and taking action to correct performance – are important. Many managers find the concept of the control loop extremely useful. It is a way of helping to make sense of the apparent muddle of managerial work. It helps managers to recognise the essential role of planning and objective setting. It also emphasises the fundamental importance of gathering accurate and timely information about what is going on, so that appropriate corrective action can be taken before emergency action is needed.

A systems view of control

Another equally helpful way of viewing management control is closely related to the control loop but extends some of the ideas in it. It is based on systems thinking. At the heart of systems thinking is a *process* with *inputs* and *outputs* (Figure 15.2).

You can think of most working activities in this way. It is the task of the manager to control an activity to ensure that the inputs and the process result in the desired outputs.

It could be argued that the outputs (or outcomes) are the most important. The process is ineffective and the inputs are wasted if the outputs are not right. So the manager's first task is to ensure that the outputs are right. But it is impossible to know whether the outputs

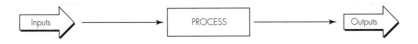

Figure 15.2 The systems process

are right unless they have been specified in detail beforehand. The manager's first job is therefore to specify the standards that the outputs must meet. These standards might be specified in terms of quantity, quality, cost, time, or other measurable characteristics. (You will recognise that this is another way of saying that the objectives must be specified in advance. You will also recognise that, up to now, this is exactly the same first step as in the control loop.)

However, systems thinking adds a new idea – that an activity cannot be controlled unless there is a *feedback* loop carrying a flow of accurate and timely information about the outputs that are actually being achieved (Figure 15.3).

The manager's second task, based on the systems way of thinking about control, is to ensure that arrangements are made for obtaining accurate and timely information about the outputs. The control loop glosses over this all-important step. It implies that managers will be able to measure performance themselves or will have ready access to a flow of information. Adequate information is not always easy to obtain.

The third task is to ensure that the information flowing along the feedback loop is used to determine whether it is necessary to take action. This is the same process as that described in the control loop. Information about what has been achieved (Figure 15.4) is compared (by the *comparator*) with the standards. If significant discrepancies are detected, an *actuator* calls for corrective action.

The control loop does not make it entirely clear how or where corrective action can be taken. The systems loop, however, shows that managers have three separate areas in which they can apply corrective action.

ACTIVITY 15.3

Look carefully at the systems loop in Figure 15.4 and identify the three separate areas in which managers can, if they think it necessary, take corrective action.

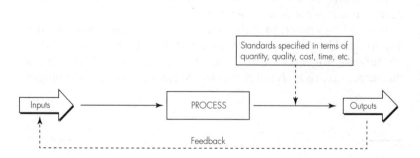

Figure 15.3 A feedback loop

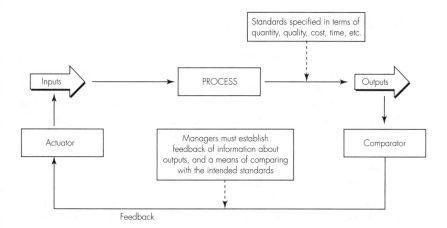

Figure 15.4 The systems loop

The most obvious area for taking corrective action is in the *inputs*. The inputs will vary greatly with the kind of work that is being carried out. They may include people, skills, equipment, accommodation, raw materials, time, finance and information. If there is a difference between the planned standards and the standards actually being achieved, managers must decide whether changes in any of these inputs might ensure that objectives could be met. For example, an additional team member might be necessary to ensure that the work is achieved within the desired time-scale.

Alternatively, managers might consider changing the *process*. This is the way in which the work is carried out. Many factors determine how work is done, for example, custom, precedent, rules and regulations, professional training and statutory requirements. Some of these can be influenced by the manager, while others might be more difficult to change in the short term. Nevertheless, corrective action might require the process to be modified.

Finally, as we saw earlier when considering the control loop, corrective action might, in some cases, require that the original plan be modified and the standards might need to be revised.

MEASURING AND COMPARING

Standards provide a basis for measurement and comparison. As we said in the last chapter, if you set standards but do not measure performance to compare it with the standards, you lose most of the benefits of defining the standards. It is the processes of measuring, comparing with expectations and then taking action to bring performance more closely in line with expectations that enable quality to be managed.

Measuring the measurable

At whatever level measurement and comparison take place, you can only measure the measurable, yet this rather obvious point does need to be considered quite carefully. It does not mean that you should avoid setting standards if there is no existing method of monitoring them but that, where there is a worthwhile standard, it is worth making an effort to find a means of measuring whether you are achieving it. However, you must be sure that your measure is a true indication of performance against your standard.

For example, put yourself in the position of the domestic services manager of a hospital. You want to measure and monitor your department's performance on cleaning work and compare it with that of the private-sector contractor that cleans a neighbouring hospital. You discover that your teams take twice as long to undertake the cleaning as do the private-sector people. You set an objective that, within one year, you will match the private-sector contractor. Six months later you have achieved your target and are very pleased.

Then someone points out that, instead of carrying out all the cleaning tasks as they did previously, your teams now do only the major ones: wiping floors and cleaning wards, corridors, sluice areas and toilets. They haven't polished the floors for six weeks, they no longer wipe down shelves and skirting boards in the wards, and they pay scant attention to clearing rubbish discarded during outpatient clinics. You believe that the private-sector cleaners have not been doing these tasks either, but you cannot be sure. You then realise that it might have been better to measure, compare and control the types of job rather than the working hours.

The choice of what to measure may have an impact beyond the range of the activities you are controlling, as Robbins and Coulter (2002) point out:

> What we measure is probably more critical to the control process than how we measure. Why? The selection of the wrong criteria can result in serious dysfunctional consequences. Besides, what we measure determines, to a great extent, what people in the organization will attempt to excel at.

People quickly become aware of the aspects of their performance that are regularly measured and will often focus on achieving the targets that are set. This can result in work that appears not to be measured being neglected or treated as though it is of less importance.

Keeping the focus on purpose

Setting measures in multi-agency work may need particular care because of the different priorities in each area of work. If some processes are contracted to other agencies, the intended quality of work has to be described in terms of standards that enable the outcomes to be measured. In health and social care the context in which these processes have to be carried out is often very complicated, with many different factors that have to be considered. Jones and Murray (2008) suggest that the task of identifying appropriate measures can be approached collaboratively to ensure that different perspectives are taken into account:

> In order to make sense of a complex social reality, we need to simplify it by identifying those factors that are of most importance to us in a particular context ... In the process of simplification and prioritisation we inevitably make choices that exclude other possibilities. This is why each decision regarding adopted choices must be justified. This is best achieved within a collaborative setting where different perspectives can be aired and a balanced judgement arrived at.

Jones and Murray advise managers to use the range of techniques available for managing projects and change in organisations to develop understanding in a systematic way. This will help to develop an evidence base which can be used to guide and justify decision making.

There will, however, be instances when it is not easy to identify a reasonable and straightforward approach to measuring performance, even when the ultimate objective is desirable and definable. In these cases, one of the following approaches may be adopted.

Objectives in sequence

You might identify a number of sequential steps necessary to achieve the objective. For example, if you have a long-term objective to ensure that all the staff working in your office have appropriate training plans, you might set an initial objective of carrying out appraisals within a short time-scale. You could set training plans for each person once their development needs have been identified.

Objectives in parallel

You might subdivide the overall objective into a number of separate objectives so that each staff group can have its own objective and control progress towards it for themselves. You would then need to ensure co-ordination between the groups so that you are satisfied that your approach results in them all working towards your overall objective.

No clear objective to start with

You might tell the people concerned that you don't yet know exactly what steps will have to be taken and so have no obvious objectives that can be used to measure progress. Make your overall intention clear and start working in that direction. While the work proceeds, look for controls that can be used (inviting staff to suggest ways of monitoring can be useful).

ACTIVITY 15.4

In each of the following situations, identify how you would set objectives and standards and monitor progress. You should consider, for example:

- how much information you might have at the beginning
- the extent to which conditions might change
- the accuracy of your information
- the flexibility with which the tasks can be carried out
- how much feedback you would need.

1 You are the co-ordinator of a community project to upgrade a large old house to a half-way home for five people with learning disabilities, using a team of about 30 relatively unskilled volunteers. (Can you follow the progress of the project if you supervise all 30 volunteers yourself? Can you forecast the project's progress? How will you maintain morale? Do you know what materials will be needed?)

2 You are the hospital works officer – without authority over other managers – advising five separate departments on the plan for moving two miles down the road into a new building. (You might have problems with staff reluctant to move, managers reluctant to listen, security of records, continuity of work, etc.)

3 You are using three temporary clerks for one week in the medical records office to assist your three experienced staff to 'pull' clinic notes for busy outpatient sessions.

We thought that, if you were the co-ordinator in case 1, the volunteer workers might not take too kindly to being controlled, so you would have to approach this carefully. You are unlikely to be able to use rigid direction and close control – if you do, the chances are that the volunteers will go home. It might be best to set objectives for completing major sections of the work (for example, plumbing, electrical, timber fixings) and to use section leaders to control the work of their own teams. Do you know of examples at work where a sensitive team of people needs to be managed (controlled) in a similar way?

If you were the hospital works officer in case 2, we felt that it would be important to consider how you could influence your colleagues and set objectives that would help all of them to move with the least disruption. If you could persuade everyone to agree overall objectives and time-scales, you might influence them to stick to the plan by having regular progress reports and by holding meetings at which you consider together how to deal with any issues that are delaying progress.

In case 3, you might decide to delegate control to your three experienced staff. They could agree together what objectives and time-scales they need to achieve in order to be prepared for each outpatient clinic. Perhaps each could manage one of the temporary staff to ensure that they meet their objectives.

Management by exception

Management by exception is one way of getting more return for less effort. It involves setting up controls in such a way that you concern yourself only with those results that are significantly different from the plans you have made. Results that are within acceptable limits – that give no cause for concern – are ignored. Only those results that fall outside acceptable limits are reported so that action can be taken if necessary.

This may seem obvious. If it is so obvious, why do so many control and information systems provide enormous volumes of data, leaving the manager to wade through them and find out whether anything requires attention? To a considerable extent, management by exception relies on having staff who are competent and on whose judgements you can rely when they tell you that everything is going according to plan. It also relies on the data presented to you being up to date and sufficiently accurate. There are, therefore, potential dangers in using management by exception and in defining, for example, what level of performance is outside acceptable limits.

Some examples of exception reports are:

The paper for next week's meeting will not be ready by five o'clock today as requested.

The chest X-rays of 1,492 patients are complete; there are four that we are not entirely happy about.

Salary awards of 3 per cent are to be made generally. Could we talk about two members of staff who should perhaps be treated as special cases?

We are 10 per cent below target on reducing the waiting list for specialty X, but all other waiting lists are within the limits agreed.

'Dear Sir, I am writing because I have been waiting for a hip replacement for far too long.'

Although the schedule of appointments generally kept to time, 10 per cent of service users waited more than 30 minutes.

ACTIVITY 15.5

Think of an instance in your work where exchanges of information would be simplified if the principle of management by exception were applied. This might be an area of work on which regular reports are made that often seem to be a waste of time because they rarely contain information that requires action to be taken. If management by exception was applied, would it:

	Yes	No
■ make your job less interesting?	❐	❐
■ clarify the picture?	❐	❐
■ allow more effective action to be taken?	❐	❐
■ save time and effort?	❐	❐
■ allow you to get to the point more quickly and with greater accuracy?	❐	❐

Identify one aspect of your management work in which you would like to adopt the principle of management by exception.

TAKING CONTROL AS A MANAGER

There are a number of ways in which a manager can take control of an area of work. In some organisations there are systems and procedures that set out what should be done.

Procedures and systems

You may have come across a 'manual of procedures' at work. *Procedures* are the way in which your organisation requires certain activities to be carried out; they are often specified in great detail. For example, an organisation may have procedures for:

■ completing the late arrivals book
■ making a weekly record of absentees

- paying expenses to people who attend for job interviews; here you may find a number of different procedures, for example:
  - where the sum is £30 or less
  - where the sum is more than £30 but less than £100
  - where the sum is more than £100
  - where the interviewee is currently employed by the organisation at another location
  - where the interviewee is not currently employed by the organisation.

A procedure defines the correct method (the standard) for doing something. If anything goes wrong, the activities performed can be checked against the standard and any differences can be recognised.

Systems are collections of procedures. It is to the system that we ascribe a purpose or an objective; the procedures are the means of operating the system. Let's look at an example.

> You are running the storeroom in a general practice and realise that you need a stock control system. You specify the objective of the system – to balance the quantities in the store with the forecast demand for goods based on historical data. The inputs to the system are data on stock used and new stock purchased. The system processes the information by adding, deleting and adjusting the information about each item. These are then output in the form of stock lists, low stock warnings and, perhaps, purchase orders.

In this example, the procedures might be:

- booking in goods received
- issuing goods to GPs' surgeries and clinics
- calculating the value of goods to the practice as a whole
- calculating the value of goods to individual surgeries and clinics
- counting each stock item
- gaining approval to purchase new stock
- approving incoming invoices.

Each of these procedures is a control device. Each defines what is to be done and the procedures thus set the standards for the system. Performance against these standards can be monitored and, if the procedures have not been adhered to (that is, the standards have not been met), either the future performance or the existing standards might be adjusted.

ACTIVITY 15.6

Are activities in your area of work done in an appropriately systematic way without going overboard on regulation? For example, are there systems and procedures for dealing with problems that arise regularly?

You might have identified areas of work in which it would be helpful to have a more systematic approach. In particular, if there are activities that are carried out frequently but inconsistently, it might be helpful to develop a written procedure that everyone could use. This is particularly helpful when staff are new to an area of work, because it helps them to perform effectively without immediate supervision. If you felt that there was room for improvement, you might discuss your ideas with your manager.

People factors

Up to now we have considered management control as the process by which managers ensure that everything stays on course or that necessary corrective action is taken. This would be a relatively easy task if the process to be controlled were entirely mechanical, but it is made infinitely more complex by the need to take account of people.

Control as a management process consists largely of encouraging people to do certain things and not to do others. How you encourage them is a measure of your managerial skills in motivating people. There are a number of factors to bear in mind:

- Individuals work in organisations to satisfy their own needs and their needs vary greatly.
- Individuals are influenced by rewards, satisfactions and punishments – in most cases more strongly by the attractiveness of rewards and satisfactions than by the fear of punishments.
- The effectiveness of rewards or punishments diminishes rapidly as the time between performance and feedback increases and the link between them becomes less obvious.
- Standards that people see as being too easy or too difficult to attain have little effect on their performance.
- Targets must be seen as desirable and achievable, and should not bear unreasonably heavily on some people and more lightly on others.
- Participation by the individual in setting a standard will increase his or her determination to achieve it.

It is most important when setting standards to obtain people's agreement to targets (either directly or through their representatives). This is often difficult and time-consuming, but it is such a key factor in managing that it must be done with determination, understanding and sensitivity.

As Balogun and Hope Hailey (2008) point out, the plans set by managers have to be interpreted and implemented by many other people before outcomes are achieved:

> *Managers can drop interventions in at the top of the organization, but the resulting outcome, in terms of the changes to behaviours or attitudes it produces, can be surprising and disappointing. Change is about managing individual expectations and inter-pretations, not just structures and systems. As a result, senior management control over outcomes, even in top–down change, is tenuous because of the way change recipients edit senior manager plans through their implementation actions. Therefore the outcomes achieved are not always as intended.*

Only close attention to managerial control can ensure that processes align with plans as intended.

Timing of control

Control can take place at three different times:

- *before* the activity – feedforward control
- *during* the activity – concurrent control
- *after* the activity – feedback control.

Feedforward control

Feedforward control is used to try to anticipate problems or deviations from plans before they occur. Setting budgets is an example, in that it involves establishing levels of expenditure across time, which are then monitored by means of regular budget statements that show actual expenditure against the plan.

'Dummy runs' are also a form of feedforward control. For example, if a new computerised data-processing system is being implemented to replace a manual system, there might be a dummy run when both systems run so that the manual system is still available if the new system fails or is inadequate in some way. This allows potentially expensive and time-consuming faults to be ironed out before the new system is fully operational.

Another example of feedforward control is setting up pilot projects. A pilot project provides the opportunity to apply an idea on a small scale and assess its impact before changing the direction of the entire organisation and then perhaps coming to the conclusion that the idea is unworkable in practice. A pilot project is often used to try out a change on a small scale when major changes would be opposed. It provides an opportunity for the supporters to demonstrate their case and the opponents to be persuaded.

Concurrent control

This is sometimes referred to as 'steering' control because any corrective action that is necessary can be taken almost immediately. An example of concurrent control is in the production of sterile packs in a hospital's central sterile supplies department. The operator of the sterilising unit has a visual control over the standard to be achieved because there is a strip on each pack that changes colour to indicate that the contents of the pack are sterile and fit for despatch to an operating theatre or clinic. The advantage of concurrent control lies in the speed at which the feedback is available.

Feedback control

All control systems provide some form of feedback, but often a considerable time after an activity has been completed. There may then be no opportunity for the outcome of the activity to be changed or modified. However, the feedback provides managers with an opportunity to influence the outcome of similar future activities. An example is an organisation's monthly or four-weekly cycle of budget reports. The financial results in certain areas of activity during the period just ended may have deviated from those planned and little can be done to correct them. But an investigation of the cause of the deviations will allow corrective action to be taken in an attempt to ensure that future periods are not affected.

Surveys of service users are another example of feedback control. They can provide valuable feedback on the quality of care, and can be used in making decisions when you review services.

Types of control

Control can be exercised in different ways:

- an informal approach versus a formal approach
- a qualitative approach versus a quantitative approach.

Informal versus formal control

In exercising control, it is important to make an appropriate choice between an informal and a formal approach. A formal approach might involve a sequence of steps that include defining a standard, monitoring performance and taking management action. An informal approach may not be discerned as control, but merely the application of common sense and experience. That does not make the informal approach any less powerful; used in the right way with the right people, it can be very effective. Consider the two statements below. The first is formal and systematic, the second informal. Both could result in effective control.

General manager to commissioning officer:

The budget for commissioning the new orthopaedic ward is shown on this computer tabulation as £100,000. We've got £10,000 for beds, £10,000 for linen, £20,000 for lockers and sundry furniture, £7,000 for soft furnishings (window curtains, bed curtains and tracking), £10,000 for utility room equipment and the balance for orthopaedic equipment. As the orders are placed according to the agreed time-scale, the costs will be allocated against the project. I will receive an updated report from the Finance Department. Please keep an accurate record of items delivered to the new ward and report to me in writing no later than five days prior to our regular Steering Group meeting.

Commissioning officer to assistant:

I'd like you to keep an eye on the delivery of furniture and equipment for the new ward. Please give me a ring each Monday afternoon and let me know how things are going.

If you choose to use an informal method, you must know the abilities of the person you are dealing with and pitch your approach accordingly.

Qualitative versus quantitative control

This distinction concerns the nature of the information and its monitoring. In the qualitative approach, the targets are defined as statements of quality rather than in numerical terms. For example:

Unless the assistant cook can improve the co-ordination of residents' meals, I'll have to transfer him to vegetable preparation duties.

All maintenance staff required to work away from their base will be provided with changing facilities in keeping with their status.

The paint colours for the office extension should be matched as nearly as possible to the existing scheme.

The quantitative approach puts the targets in terms of numbers. For example:

Unless the assistant cook can ensure that the cooked food is ready for loading on to the lunch trolleys for despatch by 12 noon, I'll have to transfer him to vegetable preparation duties.

Facilities for maintenance staff working away from their base will be as follows:

Changing room facilities	1 square metre per person
Lockers	1 per person
Showers	1 per 3 people
Toilets	1 per 10 people.

The paint colours for wall surfaces in the office extension should be matched to British Standard 1575.

Which type of control should be used?

Our aim in defining the various types of control is to make you aware of the differences. We have not proposed any clear guidelines as to where each type of control should be used. We have, however, suggested some types of problem and some types of people to which each approach may be appropriate.

In exercising any form of control, a large element of judgement is required on the part of the manager. Regardless of the form of control imposed on you from above, you must decide whether the same or a different control technique will be more effective in managing your area of work. This is a difficult but crucial aspect of exercising control. Important considerations are 'How will this action be construed by the people who are to be controlled?' and 'Will it be effective and achieve my objectives?'

ACTIVITY 15.7

Consider the relevance of some of the points made in this section to your own work.

1 Identify from your experience a situation in which each of the following has occurred:
   ■ A target has been set without agreement, and has caused resentment and discouraged effort.

- A target has been set after consultation, and has motivated people towards achievements.
- A target has been set, and fear of failure has driven people to achieve it.

2 Identify a situation in which you have used each of the following or it has been used on you:
- feedforward control
- concurrent control
- feedback control.

3 Identify one example of each of the following types of control that you have used or that has been used on you. (You may be able to identify an example that fits more than one category.)
- informal
- formal
- qualitative
- quantitative.

4 Do any of these examples show a different approach used on the controller (i.e. down the line of command as far as the controller) from that used by the controller for the same task?

TAKING CORRECTIVE ACTION

In this section we consider some of the ways in which corrective action can be taken – the last element of the control loop.

Resetting standards

We have seen how the control loop allows you either to adjust the activities that are aimed at achieving the standard or to adjust the standard itself. There are several circumstances in which resetting the standard may be justified:

- when it is clear that external factors have made the standard unrealistic;
- when the standard is recognised to be no longer meaningful;
- when the people trying to achieve the standard do not have the skills or abilities to succeed;
- when the leadership has been inadequate and the standard cannot therefore be achieved in the time available.

It will not always be clear which of these reasons is the most significant in any particular case. Nevertheless, it is important to consider why the standard needs to be reset so that you can select and plan an appropriate course of action.

When you feel that the standard should be reset, you need to consider whether you will cause more problems by changing it than by holding firm. For example, by changing the standard would you:

■ undermine acceptance of both the old and the new standards?
■ encourage people to ignore any future standards you set?
■ remove an incentive to get as close to the standard as possible, even if it cannot quite be achieved?
■ make those who have really exerted themselves feel it was a waste of effort?
■ unduly affect other aspects of your department's work or that of other people?
■ be setting a new standard that is no more realistic than the previous one?

You could, no doubt, add to this list. The important point is that you need to think through the effect of changing a standard of performance. When trying to decide whether to modify a standard, start by asking yourself, 'Would it be unreasonable to keep things as they are, even though a change is desirable?'

We have already said several times that there is little value in setting standards unless you monitor against them. Similarly, there is little value in setting standards unless you are willing to take action to ensure that the standards are met. Your choices might include incentives, motivators, persuasion, cajoling, bribing, training and coaching but, ultimately, you must be prepared to enforce discipline.

Where methods of working are laid down, objectives set or standards defined, there will be instances where:

■ people work deliberately against them
■ the standards are known but ignored
■ the targets have not been understood adequately.

In the first two of these situations, disciplinary action may be needed to ensure that the targets are not undermined or ignored. In the last, the problem may be poor communication or lack of training.

Levels of control

Another choice that you have to make in setting up effective controls is about who should control what. Consider the treatment room in a large general practice (Table 15.1). There will be a number of different levels of control operating.

You will probably be able to identify performance measurements, comparisons and actions from your own experience to add to this example. There may, for example, be a group of staff in your department or section that has its own informal measures and standards.

Table 15.1 Levels of control in the treatment room of a general practice

Staff member	Performance measurement	Comparison with standard	Action
Nurse	Am I seeing an appropriate number of patients in each session?	Is the number changing over time?	Discuss referral patterns and training needs.
Senior nurse	How many patients are seen each week? Are all nurses seeing an appropriate number of patients in each session?	Time keeping; idle time; time spent with individual patients (average and range).	Reorganise duty rosters and/or appointment systems.
Senior receptionist	Is treatment room reception working well? Is paperwork completed by the end of each day and is it accurate?	What are acceptable delays and lapses?	Review organisation and procedures.
Practice manager	What are the costs? What income is generated?	Can efficiency be improved?	Reduce costs or increase income.
GP	Is work being delegated appropriately? Are nurses adequately trained?	How might delegation be improved?	Review referral procedures.
Primary care trust manager	Is the practice employing adequate numbers of nursing staff?	Local and national figures.	Encourage good practice; review staff budget.

There may be another level of management with direct influence over the work of your area. There may be a supervisor who has identified worthwhile monitoring measures that you could also use.

If you are a manager who commissions services, you would find it useful to consider the level of control associated with each of the standards that are set. Identification of these levels, as in Table 15.1, begins to set up a plan for the chain of control that will help those responsible for monitoring performance to take swift corrective action when necessary.

ACTIVITY 15.8

Identify an example of each of the following from your own experience:

■ Control has been exercised solely within the group by the responsible manager.

■ Individuals have successfully exercised control over their own activities.

■ Individuals' control over their own activities has not been successful.

In each of these cases, consider how control could have been put in place differently and more effectively.

For control to be effective, it must be appropriate to the situation and to the staff, as well as being designed to enable measurement of performance against the appropriate standards. If control is delegated to teams and individuals, they may need training so that they understand how to manage the control process. One of the benefits of training staff to understand control is that they can then work with you more effectively to set standards that they believe are worthwhile and achievable.

We have described the process of management control by depicting it as a control loop. Look again at Figure 15.1. Each element in the control loop is an important part of your managerial role and requires considerable skill and judgement. The way in which you exercise control as a manager is at least partly a matter of personal style, although your organisation may expect you to adopt a particular approach. You may feel that imposing control over your staff is unnecessary. This may be appropriate if your staff are willing and able to control their own work to ensure that standards are met. However, meeting standards is increasingly important, and controlling activities to ensure that standards and targets are met is one of the main responsibilities of a manager.

REFERENCES

Balogun, J. and Hope Hailey, V. (2008) *Exploring Strategic Change* (3rd edn), Prentice Hall/Financial Times.

Jones, R. and Murray, N. (2008) *Change, Strategy and Projects at Work*, Butterworth-Heinemann/Elsevier.

Robbins, S.P. and Coulter, M. (2002) *Management* (7th edn), Prentice Hall.

CHAPTER 16

DEVELOPING EFFECTIVE PERFORMANCE

This chapter first looks at team working in health and care and discusses some of the issues that arise when team members come from different professions and different organisations. It goes on to discuss how managers can take a structured approach to training and development of staff, including training needs analysis, development of a training plan and reviewing progress. The final section takes an overview of the manager's responsibilities in dealing with poor performance and the formal procedures that govern grievance and disciplinary processes.

A large part of your work as a manager probably involves collaborating with others in groups or teams. Although the terms are often used interchangeably, it is useful to distinguish between them.

A *group* is any collection of people who interact with one another because they perceive themselves to have a similar purpose or similar interests.

A *team* is something more. It is a group with a sense of a common goal or task, the pursuit of which requires collaboration and the co-ordination of the activities of its members, who have regular and frequent interactions with one another.

The distinction is not clear-cut. It is a matter of degree – a group becomes a team when a similar purpose becomes a common goal and when interaction becomes collaboration and co-ordination.

Most people find that working in a group or team has a significant effect on their behaviour. People in a group may reach decisions and take actions which, as individuals, they would not have had the confidence or aspiration to do. If you consider people only as individuals, you arc ignoring some of the most significant and powerful influences that determine how effectively they will work. Managing groups and teams – including supervising and organising their work so that their talents and resources are deployed efficiently and effectively – is essential to the delivery of health and social care services.

Groups and teams vary greatly in size and complexity. Some managers are responsible for only two or three people. Others are responsible for the work of several hundred or even several thousand. Some managers have no direct line management responsibility for staff but still need to exert influence in the teams of which they are members.

TEAM WORKING IN HEALTH AND SOCIAL CARE

Health and social care teams often have to struggle with issues that dramatically affect people's lives, often at some personal cost to members of the teams. They are usually part of very large organisations which require labour to be organised and controlled, as well as huge sums of money to be accounted for. Teams often work with ambiguous – even contradictory – objectives (for example, 'meet demand and give the best possible care . . . but stay within budget'). They are often organised around a specific task and composed of people from different areas of work who have different concerns and interests (for example, a team of people collaborating to address teenage pregnancy might include social workers, teachers, GPs, health visitors, health promotion specialists and parents).

In some parts of the health and social care sector, developments in information technology have had a significant impact on how groups and teams interact. Where there are electronic communication links within or between organisations, there are more and more 'virtual groups'. Their interaction patterns may be rather different from those of groups that communicate face-to-face – sometimes the culture of communication on electronic nets is free and easy, but some organisations have procedures that require electronic communications to be more formalised.

Managing teams and groups of diverse composition and size requires considerable skills. These include both the conceptual skills of being able to analyse what is going on in the group and the practical skills of dealing with many 'people' issues at once, such as communication skills and influencing skills.

There are a number of reasons why people prefer to work in groups, including for affiliation, to gain a sense of identity, to help each other to make sense of the world, to protect their own interests and to get things done. Many managers say that they get satisfaction from being in a well led work team. Working in such a team, for many, seems to model the sort of inclusive and consultative approach that health and social care services should reflect, and embodies the way they feel they should interact with service users. However, Casey (1985) suggests that genuine team working requires:

> *enormous effort, and quite a large act of faith, on the part of any management group and its leader. It requires a huge effort to . . . say what you mean, express your feelings openly, engage in open warfare, trust your colleagues, speak your mind . . . Most*

British managers have spent their working lives learning the exquisite skills of doing the exact opposite!

He argues that the only justification for that sort of effort would be if it leads to the task being done better. He categorises tasks into three types (Table 16.1), and proposes that the nature of the task is a key determinant of whether a team is needed at all.

Casey does not see the need for any special team skills – other than basic social skills – to solve simple puzzles. 'Typical simple puzzles', he says, 'are technical and inside one member's own technical function – others may need to know but no real sharing is necessary. Often these puzzles arise at a full meeting and then are quickly and properly delegated to the individuals concerned.'

Complex puzzles, on the other hand, involve

work which no individual can do on their own . . . there is a need to share, but only at a level which enables the work to carry on, not at a level of baring of souls. . . . When a group is working well in this mode, members recognise the need for give-and-take, co-operation, negotiation, seeing the other person's point of view and sharing information on a need- to-know basis. . . . We are not talking of teamwork, at least not in the ideal, open, sharing model of teamwork advocated by team builders.

In Casey's view, real teamwork is called for when a genuine problem is faced, because 'nobody knows what to do; no one round the table has the appropriate expertise because nobody knows what expertise is appropriate'. In order to address this sort of problem, people

need to share deeply and personally, because dealing with uncertainty is fearful and you can't do it unless you feel safe. Any suggestions you might make are fragile and tentative and that would leave you vulnerable; you won't do that until you feel supported, liked and valued as a person.

Casey suggests that this is why many groups shy away from addressing genuine problems. Genuine teamwork requires high-level interpersonal

Table 16.1 Types of tasks

Simple puzzles	Complex puzzles	Genuine problems
Solution exists, and can be found by an individual with the right skills.	Solution exists, but requires more diverse skills to analyse and collate the information required to find it.	So difficult that no one knows the answer – sometimes even the problem cannot be understood with clarity.

(Source: Casey, 1985)

skills, especially from the leader, and some real incentive to go through the uncertainty of team building.

Casey's analysis has its merits, in particular in identifying simple puzzles which can often be more quickly and efficiently solved by a single person with the necessary expertise. We are all familiar with situations in which a group wastes time and energy trying to deal with issues like this – often unproductively. However, some people would say that Casey oversimplifies matters, particularly in seeking to make a distinction between complex puzzles and genuine problems. For example, improving the arrangements for discharging older people from hospital is a matter of improving co-ordination between the professionals involved – doctors, nurses, social workers, and managers of home care services and residential homes. Casey would say that this is therefore only a complex puzzle. Yet such a problem can be quite intractable (a genuine problem) from the perspective of any one of the professionals or managers involved, since he or she is responsible for only one of the services that need to be co-ordinated.

Conversely, the following case study suggests that genuine problems can sometimes be reframed as everyday complex puzzles, with the objective of improving collaboration and co-ordination.

Reframing a problem

A psychotherapist contacted one of us on behalf of a multidisciplinary child guidance team based in a hospital. The team comprised psychotherapists, consultant psychiatrists, a social worker, an occupational therapist, a psychologist and two administrators. They were having difficulty working together as a team and had obtained funding for an 'away day' in which to try to sort out their differences with the aid of a facilitator.

The facilitator had difficulty agreeing achievable goals for the day with them, not least because every time he wrote or telephoned he found himself dealing with a different person. He asked every team member to write him a letter explaining what they saw their difficulties to be. When he had read these letters, he wondered what on earth they could do about it all in a few hours.

On the day, he asked them for examples of what they regarded as teams. They said a football team, or the team in an operating theatre. He pointed out all the ways in which they were not like these teams: there was no goal that they were all shooting at; they worked with their clients only singly or in pairs, never all together; they were in different professions with different values and conventions; they all had different bosses; one member, the social worker, was in a different organisation from the rest of them. He asked why they didn't forget about being a team and regard themselves simply as colleagues who met periodically to discuss and co-ordinate their work with children.

The mood shifted during the day. They had seen themselves as failures, unable to live up to their ideal of team working. Now they began to see themselves as achieving a modest but useful level of collaboration in the face of massive obstacles. What is more, they were working together very effectively at that moment, listening to each other, making inventive suggestions and ignoring differences in status.

(McCaughan and Palmer, 1994)

Multidisciplinary and multi-agency teams

An increasingly important aspect of health and social care today is managing teams which include different professions or representatives of different organisations. Bringing together a range of specialisms and expertise offers opportunities to create services that are more effectively integrated for the benefit of patients and service users. Gorman (1998) identifies four features of such teams that require particular attention: their members have different professional perspectives and lines of accountability, work within different legal and statutory frameworks, and carry out work that is funded from different budgets. Let's look briefly at the implications of each of these.

Different *professional perspectives* are based on different sets of values that lead to different interpretations of problems. For example, the medical perspective differs from the social, the managerial from the clinical, the financial from the service provider's. Different professions also bring different experiences: for example, doctors have been through education processes that are didactic and hierarchical in nature; social workers through processes that emphasise the importance of ownership and self-determination of issues by service users and carers. Power relationships may differ, too: a hospital consultant may assume that the influence he or she has in the workplace will be transferred to working in the group, whereas a junior doctor will not have the same expectations.

The whole point of multidisciplinary teams is to bring together a range of different perspectives on the care of people. This purpose needs to be made explicit in the team's objectives and the differences between its members' perspectives need to be explored, not hidden. This necessitates a thorough sharing of background and experience and identifying people's legitimate roles within the group. Gorman says: 'It is your task as a manager to lead your team through the development so that they understand and respect the differences and these differences become a source of strength not a source of weakness.' This is something to which you can contribute even if you are a member rather than the leader of the team.

Many people working in health and social care have dual *lines of accountability*. For example, an occupational therapist may be accountable to the leader of a therapy team, as well as to a senior occupational

The White Paper *Modernising Social Services* (Department of Health, 1998) described the ideal make-up of inspection teams for residential care:

The workforce will consist of people with skills and qualifications from both social care and health care, including nurses. The benefits of combining these two sets of skills and backgrounds will best be realised if there is true integrated working, allowing – for instance – nurses to be involved in inspections of children's homes, and social care professionals to be involved in inspecting social aspects of nursing homes.

therapy professional. When someone is part of a multidisciplinary team, lines of accountability become even more complicated. A GP on a primary care trust's professional executive committee, for instance, will be expected by the other GPs in the area to represent their interests; he or she will also be expected to act corporately, in the primary care trust's interests. The GP may also be responsible for a particular aspect of the committee's work, for example as chair of a working group on a particular aspect of health improvement. In addition to all this, he or she will also have a 'day job', as a GP with particular interests and responsibilities for his or her practice and patients.

Gorman says that, in a situation like this, 'It is important to be as clear as you can so that everyone – you, the staff and your colleagues – are clear what the areas of accountability are and where the boundaries fall between them.' He also argues that it is worthwhile putting in a lot of effort to try to ensure that the people who are engaged in the work of the team have the power to 'own' and implement decisions: 'Although it can take longer in the short term, sometimes a lot longer, the investment of getting all the right people in the room is usually rewarded in the long run. It means that you can ensure that the decision is clear, individual roles are clear and that people will actually deliver on their commitments.'

The health and social care sector operates within a complex array of *legal and statutory frameworks*, and most people have an understanding only of the parts of the law which immediately affect them. In addition to the legal frameworks that govern the professions, the health service has always had a centralised, top-down system of control, with national 'guidance' on practice and procedures issued frequently by the Department of Health, either directly or through strategic health authorities. In addition, each trust has its own frameworks setting out what can and cannot be done by individuals, for example on issues about sharing information. By contrast, until recently, each local authority had its own local system of accountability, with local politics having a considerable impact on day-to-day decision making about social care. In the past decade or so, however, social services departments have became increasingly subject to 'control by government circular'. Gorman points out that, to work effectively within these frameworks, it is necessary to understand them and the impact they have on your colleagues. You need to set feasible objectives in the light of the things you cannot change.

Any cross-boundary activity that involves spending money can raise issues for those with *budgetary responsibilities*. People are usually subject to rules that constrain how their budgets can be spent. Gorman accepts that there may be little that you can do in the short term to change budgetary rules. However, taking advice from someone who thoroughly understands the rules (such as a management accountant or finance director) may give you a clearer idea of the extent to which they are capable of 'interpretation'. You can also make those who set the rules aware of any constraints they may be placing on service

There is a new acronym developing around here – a development of NIMBY (Not In My Back Yard). It's NIMBA – Not In My Budget Allocation.

(Manager of a Mental Health Acute Admissions Unit)

improvements, in the hope that this may lead to changes being made – at least in the longer term.

In all these situations, the time available for team working is a mundane but practical issue for most multidisciplinary and multi-agency teams. It is not easy to work around the busy lives of health and social care professionals to gain the level of commitment that others, with different priorities, expect. The apparently simple task of getting everyone in the same room at the same time can absorb disproportionate amounts of effort. There needs to be a commitment to continuity: multi-agency work can often be undermined by frequent changes in the faces sitting around the table. Even when the same people can meet consistently, decisions often need to be referred back for the agreement of the home agency of each team member. With good planning, however, these challenges can be overcome by anticipating them. The effort is worthwhile if it brings benefits for service users.

Here is an example of effective multi-agency working.

Successful multi-agency working

A mental health NHS trust and a social services department decided to plan and deliver their training programme for community mental health services jointly. To plan the programme, they invited 50 of the key local players with an interest in community mental health services to a one-day conference. Each of the major agencies made a presentation about new initiatives they were planning for the year and the issues they wanted the joint programme to address. This enabled the conference to develop a picture of how community mental health services were likely to change in the coming year and the demands that would be made on staff. The second half of the day was spent identifying and agreeing the main topics that the joint training programme should address. A small inter-agency steering group was formed, with representatives from each of the main players, and given the task of developing the detail of the main topics and agreeing and organising the delivery of the programme. The programme was so successful that the agencies agreed to repeat the process the following year.

(Adapted from Gorman, 1998)

And here is one where things didn't go so well.

Sharing information in multi-agency working

Early on in my experience as a chair of child protection conferences, I had closed a meeting and people were departing. I thought I had concluded the business of collecting evidence of alleged harm or injury to a child, that we had reached consensus about the degree of risk and the actions to be taken, and that we had allocated tasks. But then one of the people involved in the meeting came up to me and gave me some additional information – something she hadn't liked to say in the meeting because she wasn't sure if it was relevant. She related an incident that she had observed between the stepfather and the child which was of very great potential significance. I had to reconvene the meeting. I had learned the hard way that one of the skills I needed as chair of such meetings was to conduct a very formal meeting in order to ensure accuracy of information and objectivity, but that this was only achievable within an atmosphere of trust and with sufficient informality to encourage participation.

ACTIVITY 16.1

Think about a group of which you are a member that includes people from different professions or agencies.

1 How effectively does this group handle issues of different professional perspectives, different lines of accountability, different legal and statutory frameworks and/or different budgets?
2 Is there any special behaviour or support that you – or someone else – could provide that may be helpful to the group?

Groups at work – whether they are formal or informal – can have considerable influence over the way people value what they and others do, and thus their behaviour.

If the present rate of change in health and social care continues, the creation of new groups that work together effectively will continue to be important. Getting people with different perspectives and values to work in collaborative groups will continue to tax the skills of managers. You are now more likely than ever before to work in several teams, in roles that may not be clearly defined. You may be expected to play different roles in different teams, and to contribute to working out what these roles should be. This demands considerable insight into your own style and flexibility, and into that of others.

PLANNING SYSTEMATICALLY TO MEET TRAINING AND DEVELOPMENT NEEDS

Working effectively in groups requires considerable skills, effort and time. However, the potential payback is almost limitless, in terms of improving outcomes for service users. People need training and development to enable them to learn and practise new ways of working – even those who have had extensive professional training prior to taking up posts need support to develop as conditions and requirements change.

Training and development should focus on developing the skills and knowledge that an individual needs to perform effectively in his or her job, as well as on his or her needs for personal growth and career development. It is often categorised into three types:

- *Job-specific training* helps people to acquire and develop the necessary skills and knowledge to do their current jobs effectively and safely, for example induction of new staff, or preparation of staff to enable them to take on delegated tasks or new projects. Staff may also need training to prepare for changes arising from new national requirements (such as new health and safety legislation) or new organisation-wide policies or plans (such as the introduction of a new equal opportunities policy).
- *Continuing professional development* (CPD) is about helping people to keep up to date with the latest research, approaches and techniques within their particular field. This is important for all professionals working in health and social care and is of particular importance in clinical fields where technological developments are continually providing opportunities for improving care. Some professional bodies require individuals to provide formal evidence of CPD for continuing membership and registration to practise.
- *Personal development* provides people with the opportunity to develop a successful career within the organisation and to prepare for a possible career outside. It also recognises that the personal growth of the individual is important in maintaining his or her motivation.

Training needs analysis

An important outcome of appraisal is the identification of training and development needs of all these types for the individuals within your team. This is one source of information for a *training needs analysis*, which pulls together all the individual needs into a summary of the collective training and development needs of the team. But appraisal is not the only source of information for a training needs analysis. You may also wish to gather information from:

- staff questionnaires
- customer surveys
- talking to staff individually or in small groups
- recruitment and induction interviews
- evaluation of training and development events.

ACTIVITY 16.2

Read the case study that follows. It describes how a community health-care trust completed a training needs analysis for the organisation. You may be able to use some of their experiences to develop a process that would work within your department. As you read it, you might like to use a highlighting pen to mark any points that might be useful in undertaking a similar exercise within your own department.

A total training initiative within a community healthcare trust

The aim of our 'total training initiative' was to identify current and future training and development priorities and to make plans to address these. Not untypically, prior to this initiative the trust had no overall approach to link staff training and development to business requirements: it had previously taken a piecemeal approach, dealing with the needs of each professional group separately. The initiative was developed in response to growing demands placed on trusts and their human resource managers to be mindful of cost efficiency and effectiveness at a time when training and development were becoming increasingly important. All the resources directed towards training had to be justified in terms of the trust's service and business needs and priorities. The initiative involved an analysis of all present and future training and development needs to inform the creation of a trust-wide training and development strategy.

We developed a project plan for the work with four key stages.

Stage 1: Work with the senior management team to identify current and future service and business priorities. These were validated with staff at all levels in the organisation during stages 2 and 3.

Stage 2: Work with both the senior management team and service directorate teams to identify organisational and management development priorities to meet the service/business priorities.

Stage 3: Work with the service directorates to identify professional and technical training and development needs.

Stage 4: Work with the trust's Director of Human Resources to review the outcome of stages 1–3 and to produce a five-year training and development strategy.

Stages 2 and 3 involved all staff at all levels in the trust in the training needs analysis in two ways:

■ There were two-hour facilitated workshops with groups of staff from all levels and departments in the trust. A SWOT analysis (strengths, weaknesses, opportunities, threats) was completed in small teams followed by a full discussion of all the SWOTs with the full workshop group.

■ We conducted one-to-one interviews with members of the trust staff drawn from all service directorates and departments. These interviews focused on the individuals' experiences of training within the trust and on current and future training and development needs.

Additional information was provided from the business plans of directorates and departments, job descriptions, personal development plans and reports of exit interviews.

Within the time and resources available, it was not possible to involve every member of staff directly. The training needs analysis involved staff from each directorate and department, ensuring a cross-representation of professional disciplines and roles, level/status, length of service within the trust, age, gender, ethnic origin, shift patterns and perceived capability. The information collected from stages 1–3 was analysed to identify training and development needs within each directorate and department, common needs across the organisation and needs specific to staff groups. The data were also analysed according to training topics. The training needs analysis enabled the organisation:

■ to identify training and development priorities for the next twelve months
■ to produce a timetabled training plan which set out the options available to meet the identified needs, their resource implications, and the advantages and disadvantages of each.

The key factors in the success of this total training initiative were:

■ the establishment of current and future service and business priorities;
■ the involvement of all staff in the process of identifying needs;
■ ensuring all existing information was used (for example, customer surveys, objectives and personal development plans agreed through the appraisal process, staff opinion surveys);
■ the production of a five-year training and development strategy and plan that will receive full support from the senior management team;
■ a realistic and achievable action plan;
■ offering opportunities fairly and equitably to all staff;
■ a review and evaluation mechanism to monitor implementation.

The Project Team kept staff regularly informed of progress through written communication and regular meetings. The process was highly participative, with staff involved in shaping the outcomes through workshops and interviews. When the training plan and programme were published, staff were able to make decisions with their managers about the most effective ways of meeting their individual needs. The senior management team has also used the information gathered by the training needs analysis to help them to develop a range of skills-training packages and to review the appraisal system.

(Sally Cray)

Developing a training plan

As in the case study, a training needs analysis should lead to the development of a training plan to meet all the identified training and development needs of your team. The plan should identify:

- needs that are common to more than one member of the team;
- needs that are unique to individual members of the team;
- how you intend to meet each identified need;
- a timetable for all the training and development activities to be undertaken by the team;
- the resource required to support each training and development activity (time, internal or external expertise, money);
- arrangements for the release of staff, where appropriate;
- arrangements for ensuring that the learning that individuals and the team acquire is brought back to and used in the workplace;
- proposals for monitoring and evaluating all training and development activities;
- proposals for building both the training plan and the outcomes of training and development into your organisation's business planning cycle;
- a way of maintaining records of training and development that individuals have completed, and how this has met identified needs.

The process of developing your training plan is one in which you should involve your whole team. The collective knowledge of the team about development needs will help you to draw up a plan that develops the whole team as well as the individuals within it. You could also involve the team in researching opportunities to meet their needs that exist within and outside the organisation. If you share with the team the process of making decisions about how best to meet identified needs within limited resources, training and development are more likely to be effective in improving performance. Members of the team can help to find ways of sharing their learning with the team, rather than keeping it to themselves.

The work that your team and your department do is likely to change: nothing stands still for very long in the world of health and social care. Your training plan will therefore need to be regularly reviewed and updated to reflect changing work demands and priorities. Even if the team's development needs do not change significantly in the short term, the way in which you choose to meet them may change. For instance, new work demands may create new opportunities for projects to help individuals gain experience in new areas and thus develop their skills. Longer term, as the demands on the team change, new training and development needs will arise to prepare the team to meet new challenges.

Reviewing and evaluating progress

You are likely to spend time and money in training and developing your staff. As a manager, you are responsible for ensuring that this is a worthwhile investment for your organisation. You need to be able to demonstrate tangible benefits as a result of spending that time and money.

Some trainers use course evaluation sheets, but these have become commonly known as 'happy sheets' because they tend to measure how much individuals enjoyed a course rather than tangible benefits. They do not measure the effectiveness of the course in increasing skills and knowledge, or the impact of learning in the workplace. These can only be measured weeks or months after the learning event, when the individual has had an opportunity to put what he or she has learned into practice.

If you are going to be able to measure tangible benefits after a learning event, you must be clear beforehand about the outcomes that you expect from your investment. These may be outcomes for the individual or for your department or both. Here is an example.

Training and development activity

A member of staff will be attending a two-day course on health and safety.

Expected outcomes

The individual will acquire sufficient knowledge and understanding of current health and safety legislation and good practice to develop a health and safety policy for the department.

The outcomes will be measured by:

- meeting with the individual two days after the course and asking him or her to tell me what has been learned
- setting the individual the objective of developing a health and safety policy for the department within six months
- reviewing progress towards this objective at monthly intervals.

ACTIVITY 16.3

1 Think about a training or development activity that one of your staff is due to attend. Identify one or two outcomes that you would like to see as a result of that activity. (These could be outcomes for the individual or for your department or both.)

2 How could you measure the success of the activity in terms of these outcomes?

You can play an active role in helping each member of your team to think about ways of applying and further developing his or her newly acquired skills or knowledge within the workplace. Both during and after the learning activity, you should allocate time to talk to the individual about what he or she has learned and to identify how the learning can be used to improve the individual's own performance and the performance of the department. Your discussions might focus on:

■ what has been learned;
■ whether the learning experience has met the identified development needs;
■ how this learning can be applied in the workplace to achieve improvements;
■ objectives for the individual that will encourage use of the newly acquired knowledge or skills;
■ how the individual can share his or her learning with the rest of the team, so that the team can benefit from the investment in developing the individual.

An equal opportunities perspective

There may be questions to be resolved about who receives development opportunities and who does not. The problem is often one of having to set priorities: the time and money available just will not stretch to everyone. Decisions therefore have to be made about who should be included and for what reasons. Employers are required by law not to discriminate on the grounds of gender, marital status, race, disability or age when making decisions about training opportunities.

Policies on training and development should reflect a desire to maximise the potential of all staff. If a minority group is under-represented in a certain grade or post, or if they have had career opportunities denied to them in the past, it may be possible to design development opportunities with the express purpose of changing this. This is one step that can be taken to promote equal opportunities for minority groups, but all training and development should take special needs into account so that neither direct nor indirect discrimination occurs.

Direct discrimination is when someone is treated less favourably than other people are or would be treated where there is no difference in circumstances.

Examples of this might be:

- refusing someone entry to commercial premises
- refusing to serve someone
- denying someone accommodation.

Indirect discrimination is when your business practices, which are applied equally to everybody, result in a particular group of people being put at a disadvantage

Examples of this might be:

- failing to provide religiously appropriate food when catering, e.g. vegetarian options;
- failing to provide gender-appropriate services, e.g. when delivering personal care;
- offering services only at limited times where this conflicts with religious observance, e.g. a health clinic offered only on Friday afternoons.

However, if as a result of one of your business practices there is a difference in the quality of treatment that some people receive, you might be able to argue that the practice is nevertheless 'objectively justified'. This means that there is a valid reason for you conducting the practice in that particular way despite the effect that it has on some people – this justification is usually based on grounds of health and safety or business efficiency.

(Adapted from Business Link, 2009)

Training and development activities can play several roles in promoting equal opportunities:

- The overall staff development process should address how all members of staff can be developed to their full potential, regardless of gender, marital status, sexual orientation, race, age or disability.
- The equal opportunities dimension should be addressed during in-house or externally arranged courses or workshops on a wide range of topics: decision making, change programmes, personnel selection and interviewing, assertiveness, disciplinary procedures, appraisal interviewing, redundancy, and so on.
- Courses or workshops should provide opportunities for everyone – not just people with equal opportunities concerns – to talk through their views, discuss the practical implications of particular objectives and how implementation difficulties may be overcome, and examine their own practices and prejudices.

- External courses and workshops may provide opportunities for those from disadvantaged groups, who may feel isolated and exposed within their organisation, to support each other, share experiences and pick up new ideas.
- Targeted development opportunities can help individuals who belong to cultural or ethnic groups that are under-represented at particular levels in the organisation to achieve the positions they may aspire to and should rightly hold.

DEALING WITH POOR PERFORMANCE

The ideal way to deal with poor performance is not to let it happen in the first place! However, that is dependent on getting a lot of things right. Motivation theory tells us we have to put many things in place: clear objectives, the resources required, the right skills, clear outcomes and linked rewards, and so on.

In practice, all of us have performed poorly at some stage in our working lives. There is often a fairly stressful period when we first come into a job, while we work out what is wanted from us, and then a further period before we learn how to be effective in the job. Detecting poor performance is not always easy to do for ourselves, let alone for others.

Poor performance is far easier to spot in some jobs than in others. In jobs for which there are clear and objective standards for performance, underperformance is much more easily detected. As we said earlier in this chapter, the aims should be to develop explicit, clear and mutually agreed objectives, to agree appropriate ways of monitoring performance against these objectives, and to address any barriers to effective performance.

In some jobs, however, such as those with job titles including liaison, co-ordination or facilitation, standards of performance often depend to a large extent on the perceptions of other people. It is then necessary to negotiate a shared perspective of what constitutes 'good' and 'not-so-good' performance, and the involvement of other stakeholders may be helpful. Mechanisms such as 360-degree assessment of performance may be helpful both to the stakeholders and to the person in the job.

I find my role very difficult. I have a fairly clear idea of what I ought to do, but my managing group has a mix of different ideas. The trouble is that there isn't any accepted idea of what the job should look like: it's a relatively new role and it's being worked out in all sorts of different ways across the country. I'm not really sure whether I'm doing the right things, and I find it hard to persuade myself at the end of the day that I've done a good job. It requires a degree of arrogance almost – that I'm the best judge of my performance.

(Clinical audit co-ordinator)

ACTIVITY 16.4

If you suspect that an individual is underperforming, it is worth asking yourself some questions. Think of a situation in which you have been or are concerned about the performance of a member of your team or another colleague, and make notes in response to the following questions.

1 Exactly what is it that I am concerned about? If I had to describe this to an outsider, what specific examples or evidence would I present?

2 Do I understand the context in which this is happening? Am I aware of any factors that may be affecting the situation, such as inadequate equipment, stress or incompatible priorities?

3 How important is this problem? What is its impact on patients or service users? Does it harm our collective effectiveness as a team?

4 Are my concerns important enough or legitimate enough to merit intervention? Am I concerned about isolated incidents or small behavioural quirks that may not be important to others?

5 Would another colleague/manager see the problem in the same light? Is there any indication that my concerns are shared (or not shared) by others?

6 Would it be helpful to share my perceptions with the person involved? Would it help him or her to understand how he or she is being seen, and provide an opportunity to clarify some mutual expectations?

The reasons for poor performance usually fit into one of three categories:

- a person doesn't understand what he or she has to do
- he or she is not capable of doing it consistently
- he or she is knowingly not doing what is required.

The first two of these reasons for performance are often described as issues of *capability*. The third, because of the element of 'knowingness', may lead to *disciplinary* procedures if the person is challenging (openly or otherwise) the nature of his or her job. Let's look at each of these two situations separately.

> Our performance problems can be categorised into three: don't understand cooking, can't cook, won't cook. The first is a managerial problem and relates either to poor induction or to poor clarification of role by the manager, the second is a capability problem, the last a disciplinary one.
>
> *(Personnel director)*

Capability issues

The root of a capability problem may not lie with the individual, but with others in the organisation. Perhaps the person was appointed to an inappropriate job in the first place, or perhaps the content or context of the post has changed over time. Perhaps the person's objectives have not been adequately clarified – or perhaps objectives have not been set at all. Perhaps appropriate training has not been provided – either at the stage of induction into the job or at a later stage.

But there may be other factors that *do* lie within the individual. Perhaps the person cannot sustain the necessary level of performance because of physical or mental ill-health. Some health problems, such as stress or substance abuse, may not be immediately obvious.

Dealing with inadequate capability needs to be approached in constructive and supportive ways, with the aim of returning the person to a satisfactory standard of performance. However difficult, it is your responsibility to tackle the problem.

Your first steps in dealing with capability issues will probably be at an informal level, unless the breach of standards of performance is so potentially hazardous as to merit immediate formal action (and if this is the case, you will need to record the details of events as precisely as possible, and involve your personnel department and/or senior management). You should share your concerns about performance, as specifically as possible, with the individual concerned, and encourage the person to state his or her point of view and raise issues that may have a bearing on performance. It is important to be sure that he or she is very clear about the performance standards required in the job and you may find it helpful to refer to job descriptions and appraisal records.

When you have clarified the problem, you will need to establish how best to help the individual, agree the details of that, and set a date for reviewing progress. You should also point out the consequences of not making satisfactory progress: he or she may not be sufficiently aware of the seriousness of the issue – especially if you are being supportive! It is worth making a written record of what has been agreed, so that arrangements are explicit to both parties and you can justify your actions if you need to pursue the issues later.

If you suspect that the person has problems that he or she is unwilling to share with you, it may be beneficial to involve a third party, such as a personnel specialist or counsellor. If you think that health problems may be involved, you may need to refer to sickness and absence records and involve specialist advisers such as occupational health practitioners.

Should your informal intervention fail to produce results, you will need to involve other people, and fully document your concerns and the action you have taken. Your organisation may have a set of procedures for dealing with capability issues.

Disciplinary procedures

Most organisations have rules that govern the behaviour of employees in the workplace. They set out organisational expectations on issues such as:

- time-keeping
- absence
- health and safety
- use of the organisation's facilities
- discrimination
- disclosure of confidential information

- compliance with instructions
- claiming expenses
- accepting gifts or hospitality
- contact with the media.

If these rules are broken, managers may have to take disciplinary action. This may amount to no more than an informal warning: 'I heard you on local radio last night talking about the proposed closure of the resource unit. You must be aware that you are not allowed to make contact with the media to talk about your work without getting approval in advance from me, as your manager. You did not do so. I'm prepared to overlook this breach of the rules this time, but it must not happen again. If it does, I may have to invoke the formal disciplinary procedure.' However, there are some circumstances in which a breach of the rules, such as accepting a bribe, could amount to 'gross misconduct' and result in immediate dismissal.

An organisation's disciplinary rules must be widely known and understood. Employment law places a legal obligation on any employer with 20 or more employees to include, within written terms and conditions of employment, details of:

- any disciplinary rules which apply to the employee;
- the name of the person whom the employee should notify if dissatisfied with any disciplinary decision.

The standard of work produced by an employee can also be a disciplinary matter, rather than an issue of capability, if there is an element of 'knowingness' about non-conformance with performance standards – if the person is familiar with the standards and behaviour expected, but for some reason does not wish to comply.

Failure on the part of an employee to comply with acceptable standards of work performance is often the most difficult area to handle. The key lies in being clear at the outset about what is expected as soon as the employee joins the organisation:

- The standard of work required should be explained to employees clearly so that there is no misunderstanding.
- Job descriptions should accurately convey the main purpose and scope of the job (though the absence of a job description does not preclude disciplinary action if it can be proved that the employee knew what was expected).
- Employees should be made aware of the conditions attached to any probationary period.
- The consequences of not meeting the required standard of work should be explained.
- Where an employee is promoted, the consequences of failing to reach the new standards of performance should be explained.

The Advisory, Conciliation and Arbitration Service produce a number of very useful reference booklets for managers that can be downloaded from their website.

A disciplinary procedure describes the process by which breaches of the disciplinary rules, or other disciplinary matters, should be dealt with. Its purpose is to ensure that an employee who has breached the required standards of behaviour or work performance, but not grossly so, is given a fair opportunity to improve. Although it may eventually lead to the dismissal of the employee, this is not its main purpose. One of the main areas to come under scrutiny, should a case eventually end up at an industrial tribunal, will be the disciplinary procedure itself: whether it was followed properly, and whether the employer's actions and penalties were fair and reasonable.

As a manager, you should know what your organisation's disciplinary procedure is and ensure that you comply with it. However, especially in the health service, the position is complicated by the fact that, in addition to a trust having its own disciplinary procedures, some groups of staff, such as doctors, dentists and nurses, may be governed by their national terms and conditions of service regarding disciplinary matters, so you may need to take advice from expert practitioners in this area. Your human resources department may have experts or, if not, will probably be able to advise you whom to talk to.

Grievance procedures

Grievance procedures exist to deal with problems arising in the workplace which could adversely affect a member of staff's mental or physical well-being, or his or her ability to perform to the standard of work expected. They provide a formal mechanism through which employees – individually or collectively – can bring their concerns or complaints to the attention of their employer and have them addressed. Employment law requires any employer with 20 or more employees to include in written terms and conditions of employment:

■ the name of the person to whom an employee can take a grievance
■ the way in which a grievance will be handled.

An employee can take out a grievance if treated in a way that he or she feels breaks the rules of law, contract, or the 'accepted custom and practice' of the way things are done, and that works to his or her disadvantage.

Fortunately, most managers are rarely involved in formal disciplinary or grievance procedures. In most cases, people wish to perform well and your role is to support them by helping them to improve their performance. There are, however, occasions when staff do not perform well either because – despite training – they are incapable of doing the job, or because they are not willing to do so. Dealing with situations like this is one of the least enjoyable parts of a managerial job, and one that it is very tempting to shirk.

It is, however, part of your role and responsibility as a manager, and 'carrying' someone who is not pulling their weight in the team can have substantial costs, both in terms of its effects on service users and in the stresses and strains it places on colleagues. You may then need to invoke the procedures we have described, and it is important:

- to have a thorough knowledge of the agreed procedures in your organisation;
- to investigate the problem thoroughly;
- to keep comprehensive and accurate records.

It is also important to consider all reasonable courses of action at each stage in the process and to seek help from a more experienced manager or personnel professional if you are not confident about how to manage the process in a way that is fair to all of those involved.

REFERENCES

Advisory, Concilation and Arbitration Service, <http://www.acas.org.uk> (accessed 20/6/2009).

Business Link <http://www.businesslink.gov.uk/bdotg/action/detail?type= RESOURCES&itemId=1082208695> (accessed 23/4/2009).

Casey, D. (1985) 'When is a team not a team?', *Personnel Management*, January, pp. 3–7.

Department of Health (1998) *Modernising Social Services*, The Stationery Office.

Gorman, P. (1998) *Managing Multi-disciplinary Teams in the NHS*, Kogan Page.

McCaughan, N. and Palmer, B. (1994) *Systems Thinking for Harassed Managers*, Karnac Books.

CHAPTER 17

MANAGING CHANGE

Twenty years ago, it may have been sufficient for managers to accept what they found, to keep the organisation moving on its existing tracks, to handle occasional deviations, and eventually, when they moved on, to leave things pretty well as they found them. Today, despite tight resources and ever-increasing demands, the primary task for managers of health and social care, at all levels, is to improve the services they provide to service users. Management is no longer about maintaining the *status quo* (if it ever was); it is about stimulating and implementing change, and encouraging innovation, in order to make improvements.

You may have the task of making a change handed down to you from above, as a result of a decision at a higher level of management. Or you may yourself have identified the need for a change. In either case, taking the lead in bringing about change requires a wide range of management competences. You also need a fair degree of intuition – and some luck. If you can establish an open culture in which you and your colleagues challenge assumptions, test new ideas and share experience, you will be able to learn from your successes – and from the inevitable mistakes. This may be especially important if the change involves working with partners in other organisations, and therefore involves understanding different cultures, structures and patterns of working.

Because management is very much a practical art, the best way of learning from the ideas in this chapter is by experience, in a real situation. Sometimes we suggest that you apply the ideas to a change project of your own, preferably with help from colleagues, especially those who are prepared both to challenge and support you.

ACTIVITY 17.1

Identify an important change that you would like to make at work. You are probably already busy, so don't add unnecessarily to your workload. Choose a problem that you need to tackle in any case – one which matters to you, your manager and your service and is in line with your organisation's aims. It could arise from one of your formal objectives.

You will need to strike a balance between selecting an objective in which there is a fair chance of success and one which exposes you to new, stretching demands from which you can learn; between playing to your strengths and seeking opportunities for personal development.

Decide on who else you will involve. How will you include the rest of your team? Is there someone that you can use as a sounding board to test out ideas and as an adviser when things go astray? This could be your manager or your mentor. It could be a more experienced colleague or even a friend with appropriate experience from outside your organisation.

1 Describe the issue, problem or opportunity as you currently see it. Use the simplest language possible. If you can express it in a single sentence, so much the better. (You may come to see it differently as the work proceeds and you understand more about it: this often happens.)
2 Write down the objective(s) of your planned change as precisely as you can. How will you measure whether you have been successful?
3 Who will be most affected by the change? When will you involve them?

There is an element of risk in taking the lead in bringing about change. You can never be entirely sure in advance what will be required. Change often brings unexpected results – hence the need to be as clear as possible about your objectives from the outset.

DIAGNOSIS

The first step in making a change is diagnosis – answering the question 'What is the issue that requires a change to be made?' or 'What changes are needed in my organisation/department/section to make it function more effectively?' This may seem self-evident. Yet how often do we see changes being made that are unnecessary? And how often do we realise, after a change has been made, that it has failed to address the real issue?

We begin with a diagnostic model, a way of looking at each of the separate elements of an organisation – or part of an organisation – and how they relate to one another, to help you to understand the current situation and what changes may be needed. We then apply the model to a case study in diagnosis.

Don't forget the manager's motto:

Give me strength to change the things that can be changed, the tolerance to accept those that can't and the wisdom to distinguish between them.

Implementing a change will take time and effort. Another aspect of diagnosis is therefore to consider the resources you will need to carry it out. The last part of this section invites you to think about what you personally bring to the change process.

A diagnostic model

Roger's bright idea

Driving into work one day, thinking of the tedious job he had been engaged on for the past three days, Roger suddenly saw the obvious solution. In future, he would not spend the best part of a week every February negotiating the holiday dates with the staff for whom he was responsible. He would simply pin up a chart with a set of rules (no more than two people absent at any one time, no one away in May, the peak season, and no one to split their holidays into more than two sessions) and let them mark in their own holidays.

Unfortunately the logic of his reasoning was not obvious to his staff. 'He's evading his responsibilities.' 'It's his job to decide who is needed when.' 'He's stirring up conflict between us.' 'What happens if I'm away when the list goes up?' 'It's the only time I ever got to talk to him about my own affairs – he's keeping me away from him.'

The next morning Roger's manager wanted to see him. 'I've had a deputation calling on me from your staff,' said the manager. 'They are furious with what they call your uncaring arrogance. What happened?' Roger told her. The manager smiled. 'You'll have to learn', she said, 'that what seems logical to one person often seems devious to someone else. If you are going to try to change a system, make sure that they understand that there's a problem before you give them your solution.'

The diagnostic model in Figure 17.1 is based on the work of Nadler and Tushman (1980). In this model, the organisation is seen as if it were contained by a semi-permeable membrane. Inside the membrane lies the organisation. Outside the membrane, in the environment, there are other systems (collections or sequences of procedures), which influence the organisation and are in turn influenced by it: a process of continuous demand and response.

The organisation can be thought of as a system that has a variety of inputs. It uses these through a process of transformation to create its outputs or outcomes, its products and services.

The inputs consist of the environment, the organisation's resources and its history. The environment consists of constantly changing demands and opportunities that put pressure on the organisation to respond. The organisation's resources are the raw materials that enable it to do its work – its financial and purchasing arrangements, its staff,

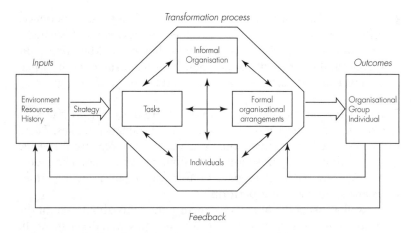

Figure 17.1 The Nadler and Tushman diagnostic model
(Source: amended from Nadler and Tushman, 1980)

their expertise and its alliances. The history of the organisation also contributes to its inputs by showing how its values and beliefs have developed.

The organisation is where the transformational process takes place: it is the inter-related elements of the organisation that enable it to produce its outcomes. Nadler and Tushman (1997) comment that they have been developing this model since 1970 to demonstrate the shift in thinking away from static hierarchical organisational models towards thinking of organisations as dynamic entities adapting in response to changes in the external environment but striving to retain internal balance, or 'congruence'.

The organisation uses its resources through the strategy that sets out how it will achieve its outputs or outcomes. The internal organisation can be thought of as having four components: the tasks, the formal organisational arrangements, the informal organisation and the individuals.

- The *tasks* are the primary part of the system. They consist of the jobs to be done, the characteristics of the work itself, and the quantity and quality of the service provided.
- The *formal organisational arrangements* include lines of account-ability, information systems, monitoring and control mechanisms, job definitions, formal pay and reward arrangements, the structure of meetings, operating policies, and so on. These features of the organisation are relatively easily described, but often become out of date as they fail to keep up with the changing world.
- The *informal organisation* or 'culture' is less tangible and more difficult to alter, but often drives the organisation. It is about 'the way we do things around here', the values, the rites and rituals, the power bases, allegiances, tribalism, beliefs, norms, informal rewards and punishments, the networks, and so on.

■ The *individuals* bring different skills, knowledge and experience, different personalities, values, attitudes and behaviour. They make choices about what they do and how they do it. Matching individuals and their needs to the organisation's formal and informal arrangements is particularly critical at times of rapid change.

The transformation achieved within the organisation produces its outcomes; the services it delivers and/or the products it makes. These can be grouped as organisational outcomes, outcomes from specific groups within the organisation and individual outcomes. The model also shows how feedback loops can inform the organisation in various ways about how well it is performing.

As well as using the model to structure thoughts about each of the separate elements, it is important to consider how well the elements fit together. For example, if the task is very static, a formal organisation that is inherently bureaucratic will make sense. On the other hand, an organisation that has a mix of cultures will work best if managers can adapt their style to suit the different cultures.

The four internal elements of an organisation are in a state of dynamic equilibrium with each other and with their environment. The interdependency of elements within the organisation is very important, because if one element is changed there will be an impact on all of the others. If an organisation is to remain healthy, as one element changes so the others must shift to accommodate.

The way in which the various elements respond to change is often somewhat predictable. For example, the political networks, which are part of the informal culture, respond as they feel their power base shift under them. They will take negative or positive positions depending on how they perceive the change will affect their capacity to make their influence felt.

Those responsible for the formal organisational arrangements will look for more control; bureaucrats become more bureaucratic and call for more of yesterday's information (which, as it was designed for a system which no longer exists, tells them very little). As organisational arrangements as well as tasks and people shift, it becomes increasingly difficult for managers to exercise the necessary degree of control.

Individuals usually fear the unknown. They have established patterns of behaviour for handling and coping with the current arrangements and will be reluctant to develop new ones. For an individual, the change process can be akin to grieving: denial of the change, acceptance of reality and then accommodation to it. Some people pass through these stages in minutes; some never do and suffer increasingly from problems of stress as a result.

When thinking about your change project, Nadler and Tushman's model can be used to help you understand the current situation and how it might respond to your intervention. The model can also be used more proactively, to help you decide on what intervention to make. For example, replacing a conservative, conformist key individual with one who has grown up in, is part of and acceptable to the culture, yet has revolutionary tendencies, can have a powerful effect on the outcome of your initiative.

A case study in diagnosis

A nurse manager from the Marsh Primary Care Trust wanted to provide an efficient, effective, integrated service for people in the town of Dunford, to improve the discharge from hospital and transfer into community care. She wanted to bring together the services of nursing and therapy staff (currently employed by the Marsh Hospital NHS Foundation Trust), the Dunford GPs and the Fenland Local Authority social workers and social care services. Her primary concern was about duplication and waste. To help her understand what changes might be needed to the present arrangements, she spent some time talking to some of the people involved. Here are the notes she made of her conversations.

Dunford: notes from initial discussions

It proved very difficult to make an appointment with any of the five GPs in the town practice. The senior partner found five minutes to explain that co-ordinated primary care was close to his heart. He holds regular monthly meetings with his practice nurse and the health visitor and these enable them to sort out any problem patients. The meetings usually take about half an hour, but they haven't had one for a while: 'We are all rather busy and nobody had anything to put on the agenda – we never deal with anything in depth anyway.'

I eventually got together with two of the other partners over lunch. Most of the time was spent bemoaning the general underfunding of the service, in particular the problems of meeting the ever-increasing demands of an ageing population. The conversation then turned to the proposals for serving a new care village for older people, incorporating a nursing home for those with dementia, that the Fenland Primary Care Trust has commissioned, in collaboration with the Local Authority's Social Services Department and a local housing association. The GPs are worried that this could add significantly to their workload. It was a short step from this to the difficulties of budgeting for older patients and we were soon back into the issues of shortage of cash. They know little about the concept of primary care teams and showed no interest. I also got the impression that they are not keen to be too involved with the other agencies and are very concerned about the enthusiasm of some of their colleagues to work more closely together.

The health visitor who covers the Dunford practice also works in the Marshborough area, which includes a health centre with four GPs as well as one single-handed practice, both in the same Primary Care Trust as the

Dunford practice. Her office is in the Marshborough Health Centre. She shares it with a school nurse, two district nurses, a second health visitor and, occasionally, a community physician employed by the Primary Care Trust, who has a special responsibility for older people. As well as her normal duties, she and the community physician are members of a team which is implementing the transfer of the first patients from the local continuing-care ward to the new nursing home. She is worried about the support needs of the tenants and owner occupiers in the houses and flats in the care village and is not clear who is supposed to be planning to meet them. The four Marshborough GPs, the health visitor, the district nurses and the social worker meet for an hour on the last Friday of the month and, as they work in the same building, there is also a lot of informal contact. However, the health visitor feels that the Marshborough GPs are enthusiasts for team working only if 'they are in charge'. She is supportive of the idea of establishing primary care teams and is interested in what she described as 'better interagency working'. She has reservations about new work with the Dunford practice because:

- she is already overloaded;
- she doesn't rate the chance of success very highly until the senior partner retires – in her view he is one of the old school who just wants the nurses to be at his beck and call;
- along with the other health visitors, she has just been involved in devising a health visitor database – this is producing a lot of paperwork and she can ill afford to spend any more time at meetings.

The social worker made time for a meeting with me, although he expressed some concern that it would probably be more appropriate for me to talk to his area manager. He is normally responsible for the industrial areas of Bindhaven and the market town of Marshborough. In addition, he is currently covering Dunford because his department is understaffed. He knows Dunford well, having worked here before the last reorganisation. He talked about the benefits of integrating the efforts of the three services – health, housing and social services. He would prefer to wait until a full-time worker has been recruited and trained, but this could take a year and he agrees that this is unacceptable. He declined to comment on the people involved in delivering health care in Dunford: he said he doesn't really know any of them well enough to make a sensible judgement. He suggested that I should talk to his area manager, who is apparently one of the lead managers working on the planning for long-term care.

I have yet to meet the district nurse. I know that she is committed to teamwork, and will also be a mine of information.

We can develop a preliminary diagnosis of the Dunford situation using the Nadler and Tushman model.

First, the *inputs*, particularly the *environment*. Restructuring and funding loom large in the minds of the Dunford GPs. What is really worrying them? Can the new arrangements be used in any way to further the cause? What about the shift in emphasis to interagency working and the charter for long-term care? Are the new care village and nursing home an opportunity to progress teamwork? The Marshborough GPs seem to be further down the road towards interprofessional collaboration. Are there any ways in which their experience can be translated for Dunford? What links are there between the practices? How effective is the board of the local primary care trust? To whom, if anyone, do the Dunford GPs listen? The housing association could be an important new player. What is its philosophy? Are there some allies within its ranks?

The service users and their carers have not been mentioned once. What do they think about the current services? What worries them most? Have they been consulted about their needs and how they would like them to be met? Has there been any contact with the Local Involvement Network (LINk)?

Let's look at the *resources* – better collaboration would make it possible to share resources which should enable better use to be made of those that are scarce – but do we have the capacity to carry out and sustain a significant change?

Within the organisation we could look at the *tasks*. What tasks need to be performed and who could best do them? We would want to consider what skills and experience *individuals* need to perform each task – there could be benefits from interprofessional working. Different professional groups tend to have different ways of working and different cultures – different *informal organisation*. This needs to be considered if people are to work closely together and the way in which the *formal organisation* systems are designed will be important.

No one has spoken about the *outcomes* – benefits or otherwise – for service users. Facts are conspicuous by their absence. Are there any data about the social, health and physical needs of Dunford residents, or about the quality, quantity and cost of the services provided, or about the effective use of resources?

We might consider the outcomes in terms of potential outcomes for the organisation, for groups and for individuals. What are the pressing problems? What might be achieved for the customers if the various professionals were to work more as a team – if there was real interagency collaboration? What is there that is currently good and might be put at risk? What do they need to be better at, and what should they stop doing, in order to improve the services they provide? Could they improve their time management and hold structured robust meetings with agendas that detail actions, outcomes and time-scales?

How big an issue is the new care village? Could it be the vehicle for practising a greater degree of teamwork or some interagency working? What is involved in the planning for supported living and long-term care?

ACTIVITY 17.2

Now continue the diagnosis using the headings in the model:

■ inputs (environment, resources, history)
■ formal organisational arrangements
■ informal organisation
■ individuals
■ outcomes (organisation, group, individual).

One way of doing this is to go through the above report, identifying individual issues and writing each on a card. You can then sort the cards into piles which relate to each element of the model in Figure 17.1. Look not only for what is said but also for what may be implied. What is omitted can be very revealing.

How do your conclusions compare with the following?

Inputs

Environment – as we said earlier, there is pressure to change, but the needs and views of service users should be identified before taking any action. The collaboration would not mean that all the resources of all organisations were contributed, but if the ones that are currently used for the services under discussion were used more collaboratively we should avoid duplication and save time, particularly if we can deliver some services at the same time instead of with separate appointments. Some rather negative historical ways of thinking seem to be revealed in the interviews with individuals.

Formal organisational arrangements

The three services – housing, social services and health – have separate management arrangements and, at the operational level, the staff cover different geographical areas. Housing embraces both the local authority and the independent sector. Health includes the primary care trust, the general practices and the hospital trust.

Are there any systems in place which bring the three services together? Has any work been done on a social profile of the area and trends identified? Bearing in mind the power of information, do the three services share any monitoring and control processes? How much work has been done locally on the performance assessment frameworks for both social services and the health service? To what extent, if at all, do these link together?

Informal organisation

Is there one culture, or is there the problem of several separate ones? The GPs seem isolated, and other aspects of the health services seem bureaucratic. Do the social workers have their own culture?

Everyone sounds inordinately busy with no time for lateral thinking. Why is that? Is there just too much work? Do they need to be better organised? Are they busy because they need to be in order to prove something to themselves or to their colleagues? Or are they busy because of the amount of change as a result of the aspirations of central government? Is the busyness a result of reacting against the changes or of working to implement them?

Some of the cultures appear highly 'tribal'. The health visitors have just set up a new database. Did they do this entirely within their profession or did they link in with the monitoring requirements of the performance assessment frameworks (or is there a performance/audit/ data team that could assist)? The older GP preaches a team approach but it doesn't sound as if he practises it (when did he last have an appraisal?). The social worker has worked in the district for a long time but says he doesn't know the other professionals well. Is this really so, or is it a tactic for managing his workload and have his networking skills been considered in his appraisal?

Individuals

Most people seem to be making their own assumptions about the needs of older people, which could well be challenged in any attempt to bring about change. Have they considered holding change management workshops? Does the nurse manager herself really understand the pressure from government for all agencies to work together in the interests of the customers of their services? Do the doctors see themselves as the rightful team leaders? There is a flavour of an historical resentment of this by the health visitor. Does she dislike being seen as the doctor's handmaiden – in the GP's words, being 'his' health visitor? The senior partner thinks in terms of 'sorting out problem patients' rather than in terms of quality.

Are any of the group experienced team/interagency workers? Do they possess the appropriate competences to work collaboratively?

Why is the social worker so cautious? Is it connected in some way with a previous reorganisation or the attitude of the local authority towards using up finite resources?

Outcomes

We have very little information about the outcomes of the service. Presumably there is a problem with co-ordination that has led the nurse manager to propose the idea of trying to improve the service relating to discharge from hospital and prevention through supported living. Will the new home address some of this problem? What about people who need some help but can be supported in their own homes rather than moving? We have not heard anything from the service users yet – their views could be revealing – and so could those of LINk.

Summary

One word, fragmentation, summarises much of the problem. The key task would seem to be integration of the health, social care and housing services for older people in the town of Dunford based on some mutually agreed outcomes.

We will return to this case study to follow the next steps taken by the nurse manager.

Another way of representing the relationships identified by the diagnosis is in the form of Tony Buzan's (1989) 'mind maps'. Figure 17.2 shows the Dunford diagnosis represented in this way.

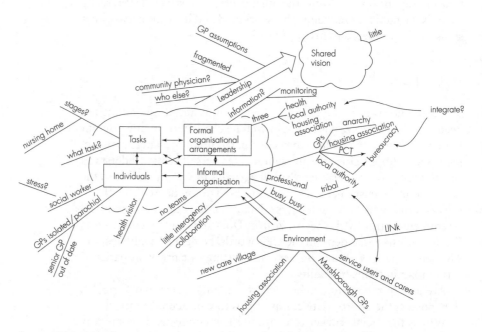

Figure 17.2 A mind map representation of the Dunford diagnosis

ACTIVITY 17.3

Use the Nadler and Tushman model on your own project to:

- improve your understanding of what you already know about the situation;
- identify what you need to know more about;
- plan how you will collect the additional information you need;
- identify those areas where the components of the model do not fit with each other and consider what needs to be done to bring about change.

You may wish to carry out this Activity by making notes under the headings of the model.

You may feel the need to extend this Activity by collecting more information to add to your knowledge of the situation. How you set about this is up to you, but bear in mind that the way in which you tackle it will almost certainly be obvious to those involved. You will send out messages: make sure they are the ones you want to send. Diagnosis is your first intervention in the system. First moves are often remembered.

There is a fairly limited number of ways of collecting diagnostic data: perusal of documents and records, the use of surveys or questionnaires, carrying out interviews, making direct observations and holding diagnostic meetings. All have their advantages and disadvantages.

What you bring to the change process

You stand a better chance of managing change effectively if you understand your own attitude towards change. You will not be able to manage other people through a change if you are unable to handle the emotional and intellectual impact it has on you. Here are some things to think about:

- Keeping in touch with developments in your environment ensures that you and your department or area of work maintain the capacity to make changes when necessary.
- In an era of rapid change, people have to learn new skills in order to cope with changing roles in changing circumstances. How active a learner are you?
- How does change affect you emotionally? How does it feel to be involved in change? Change inevitably produces emotional reactions in those involved. It is therefore important to understand how it affects you, in order to understand better how to help others.

ACTIVITY 17.4

How do you rate your capability to manage your change project? Here are some of the advantages and disadvantages that you might have. Which of them broadly applies to you?

Possible advantages	*Yes*	*No*
You understand your organisation (who has power, how the networks operate, where the barriers are)	☐	☐
You speak your organisation's language (its special jargon, in-jokes, etc.)	☐	☐
You understand the local culture and can act in accordance with its rules	☐	☐
Your mental and/or material well-being depends on your organisation providing effective services	☐	☐
You are a familiar and non-threatening figure to colleagues	☐	☐

Possible disadvantages		
You are too involved with one part of the organisation to see it as a whole or without bias	☐	☐
Your other duties leave you insufficient time and energy to devote to the change role	☐	☐
Your power base is not secure enough to guard you against challenges from your managers or others	☐	☐
Your past successes or failures may prejudice people against you	☐	☐
Other people's expectations of you in your other roles conflict with your efforts to work with them on the change	☐	☐

What implications does this analysis have for your role in your project?

Being aware of the factors that may work to your advantage and those that may work to your disadvantage is an important first step. This will enable you to recognise what kind of support you are going to need and whether you have any urgent development needs.

Stages in the implementation of change

Every change programme involves three states – the current state, the transition state and the desirable future state. All three require managing, and all three compete for resources. It is important to ensure that you have enough resources to cope with the work of managing all three states, or that you have access to someone who can provide them. However, things are not always that simple.

The innovative organisation builds in change as a norm, by encouraging individuals to experiment, to have a go; within reason, it allows a little anarchy. Budgets are not so tightly constrained that the organisation is in a straitjacket. Successful innovations are publicly rewarded, mistakes privately forgotten.

The ice may be broken when an event, often external, and often unplanned, unfreezes the situation: for example, a White Paper is published, there is a change of government, or an institutional horror story breaks.

Out of a number of separate, experimental activities – and possibly one or more ice-breaking events – come successes, whether small or large. If these can be drawn together and shared, it may be possible to bring together a coherent strategy for change. This strategy can then be transformed into action, providing opportunities to do things in ways which are congruent with the emerging future rather than the past. From action comes learning, which in turn informs the development of strategy and thus further action. There are things to be avoided: fragmentation, duplication of effort, too slow a pace, a pace that is unsustainable, fear and rejection of change, and too prescriptive an approach. The things you need to ensure are:

- engagement and commitment from key groups;
- a clear plan with time deadlines for delivery;
- a programme with clear 'milestones' for review;
- managers and staff feeling that transition is being 'managed';
- a pace which is sustainable;
- recognition of success to build confidence;
- a clear communications strategy to ensure that internal messages are clear but that those which come from outside are also heard;
- a cost-effective use of time and resources.

An example of significant change drawing on small experiments and successes occurred in the physiotherapy outpatient department of a general hospital.

Incremental change

One of the physiotherapists found that, in addition to giving instructions verbally, it was helpful to write down instructions for those patients who required a cervical collar. A second physiotherapist had begun to collect a small library of booklets for patients to borrow, such as those produced by the Arthritis and Rheumatism Council. Meanwhile, the receptionist had taken another initiative. A friend had given her a poster for a local support group for arthritis sufferers, which she pinned on the wall in the waiting area.

The senior physiotherapist in charge of outpatients encouraged these staff to share their ideas with each other and with the rest of the staff. A strategy began to be developed to improve the provision of information to patients. Action and learning led to the production of a series of instruction sheets describing exercise regimes. These sheets included titles of relevant booklets which patients could borrow from the departmental library and contact addresses for relevant support groups.

There is much discussion among the staff of ways of improving this information.

The incremental approach to change involves the affected people at all times. It builds on a number of small successes, rather than presenting major hurdles which have to be jumped and which induce resistance. The complexity and freedom of the process, however, require overall direction to ensure that the sum of all this jumble of activity is purposeful. An organisation which operates successfully in this way invariably has three binding forces:

■ clarity about its overall purpose
■ a widely shared vision of a better future
■ a set of beliefs, values and principles which governs the way it operates.

One final thought: it is possible to make mountains out of molehills, to create hurdles when none really exist. The simplest way of bringing about change is just to do it. You may be surprised. Occasionally people will say, 'About time too!' and get on with it. Intuition is a much underrated commodity when judging whether this is possible. But intuition backed by rationality is safer, if less exciting, than intuition alone.

PLANNING FOR CHANGE

Each of the two tools we describe in this section has two functions:

■ to better understand the present situation
■ to plan the next steps you will need to take.

The first tool, *force field analysis*, identifies the forces that are helping to drive your change and those that are opposing it. Having identified the forces, you can then decide which positive forces you can take advantage of and which negative ones you can try to reduce. It is a useful tool to apply to any change project, whether the proposed change is major or minor.

Few change programmes can be successfully implemented by one person. One person rarely understands an organisation well enough to produce an accurate analysis, and is unlikely to have access to all the levers of power. A mix of skills, experiences, personalities and perceptions is usually required to manage a change. Nor is it possible to institutionalise a change – and it is very easy to overturn it – when the ownership is vested in only one person. Successful management of change recognises this by building a network of supporters. These are sometimes referred to as a 'critical mass', borrowing a term from nuclear physics to indicate that their combined energy can be explosive. The second tool described, *commitment planning*, will help you assess the work to be done in building this critical mass of supporters.

Force field analysis

Force field analysis is a tool developed by Kurt Lewin (1947). It is extraordinary how its relevance has stood the test of time. It assumes that in any change situation there are two sets of forces, those driving the change and those which oppose or restrain it. These forces can be written on a chart using arrows to indicate their directions and relative strengths (Figure 17.3). It is important to recognise that they are forces as perceived by the people involved in the change. For example, there may be no intention to make staff redundant, but if the staff believe that the change will make them redundant, the restraining force exists.

If the driving forces for change are stronger than the restraining forces, progress will be made. The list of forces can be developed by brainstorming or by the use of diagnostic tools like the Nadler and Tushman model. It can sometimes be useful to cluster them under

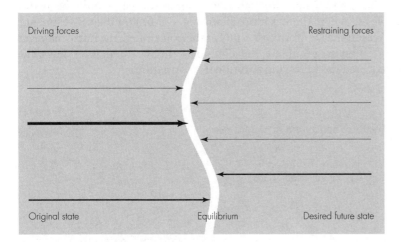

Driving forces   Restraining forces

Original state   Equilibrium   Desired future state

Figure 17.3 Driving and restraining forces

different headings and to use these headings to prompt ideas. Typical clusters would include:

- *personal* (for example, fear of redundancy, loss of competence or loss of pride);
- *interpersonal* (for example, A does not talk to B);
- *intergroup* (for example, home care assistants resent loss of status *vis-à-vis* home care organisers, or surgeons and physicians compete for money to buy new equipment);
- *organisational* (for example, there is an overall shortage of resources or new management structures are being introduced);
- *technological* (for example, records have been computerised or a body scanner has been installed);
- *environmental* (for example, there are more older people or the law on mental health is amended).

Having produced the force field diagram, the first task is to examine it to determine what can be done to reduce the restraining forces rather than increase the driving ones. This seems to be against our natural instincts of pushing change through. However, experience shows that increasing the driving forces produces a quasi-Newtonian effect: for every new force that is introduced, an equal and opposite force tends to arise. If the magnitude of a driving force is increased, the restraining forces often also increase. Some of the restraining forces may even owe their existence to previous attempts to push through change and, paradoxically, the elimination of the appropriate driving force will be helpful overall. You may, however, judge that it is important to maintain some particular driving force and perhaps, with care, increase others.

Completion of the force field analysis may lead to an onset of realism. Once you have a clear view of the forces in play you may decide that your planned change is impossible. Resources are finite. Now may be the time to question whether your resources would be better deployed where there is more chance of a return on their investment.

We left the Dunford case study at the point where the nurse manager was about to complete the diagnosis. In the final interviews she discovered the following additional information.

Dunford: notes from final interviews

The nursing home is a 60-place unit within the care village that will be run by a nationally recognised private provider, which will meet the regulatory requirements in staffing, including employing registered nurses. The sheltered housing in the care village will provide 50 bungalows and flats for people aged 55 and over and will be managed by the housing association and must meet the Care Quality Commission standards. The private provider will be a not-for-profit organisation with a good record for their standards of care. The housing association's managers are entrepreneurs, severely antipathetic to the merest whiff of bureaucracy. It is expected that the residents of the housing scheme will require care and support from a range of services. Routine medical care will therefore fall largely on the Dunford GPs and the therapists currently employed by the Hospital Trust. The community physician carries considerable weight with the Primary Care Trust and the staff of the housing association, because of his excellent work in encouraging the nursing home provider to develop the new scheme.

The district nurse is a mine of information. She says that the social worker is somewhat embittered, having unsuccessfully applied for a team manager's post at the time of the last reorganisation. He has been offered early retirement but, as his wife has recently died, he wishes to keep working to avoid loneliness. He says he is interested in interagency working, but in reality he has little energy or motivation for reform.

His line manager, the team leader for the geographical area which includes Dunford, is new to the local authority. She has come from another county where a successful service for long-term community care has been in place for some time. She is an enthusiast for interagency working.

The Dunford GPs have little contact with their colleagues in Marshborough and even less respect for them. The Dunford GPs are critical of the Primary Care Trust. The Primary Care Trust's new management team is enthusiastic about the concept of integrated primary care and the new care village.

ACTIVITY 17.5

The nurse manager drew up the force field analysis in Figure 17.4.

In the Dunford force field, which restraining forces might usefully be worked on? How might the nurse manager set about reducing them?

There are many possible answers to this Activity. However, you can test your conclusions against the following points:

- The nurse manager's original idea seems to be along the right lines but may have been for the wrong reasons. Her proposals were not supported by facts.
- She could usefully pay more attention to the wider national and local political context.
- She could reflect on the components that would be uniting rather than fragmenting.
- She could redefine and simplify the task.
- She could reflect on how the project might help to reduce existing fears and worries.

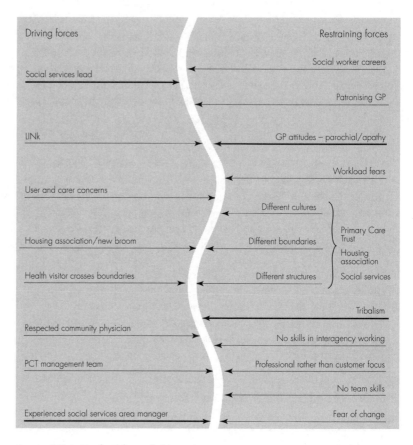

Figure 17.4 Dunford force field analysis

The principles behind reducing the effects of restraining forces are:

■ looking for common ground (for example, common values and common desired outcomes);
■ ascertaining who has influence and respect;
■ seeking to show how achievement of the change will add value elsewhere or help overcome an anxiety or fear.

Commitment planning

The aim of commitment planning is to examine how you can build a critical mass of supporters, ready to explode into action. A commitment plan is a chart (Table 17.1) in which the key people or groups are listed down one side of a sheet of paper. Across the top are four headings which indicate levels of commitment:

Not committed　Likely to oppose the change
Let　　　　　　Will not oppose the initiative but will not actively
　　　　　　　　support it

Help   Will support the change with time and other
               resources, provided someone else will take the lead

Make   Will lead the change process and make it happen.

Each individual is marked on the chart with an 'O' to indicate his or
her current position and an 'X' to indicate the extent of commitment
needed. The difference between the two is a crude measure of the work
to be done in order to build the critical mass. Sometimes it may be
appropriate for the level of commitment to be reduced: perhaps the
leadership should move from one person to another, or perhaps one
person's enthusiasm is preventing others from joining in.

     As an illustration, if we return to Dunford, the key players could well
be:

- the chief executive of the
  primary care trust
- the GPs
- the community physician
- the social worker
- the social services area
  manager
- the board of the Primary
  Care Trust

- the health visitor
- the district nurse
- the therapies manager
- managers from the housing
  association
- the manager of the nursing
  home
- the nurse manager herself.

If we look at each of these using the commitment planning model, we
might map their current positions as set out in Table 17.1.

Table 17.1 A commitment plan for Dunford

Key players	Not committed (oppose)	Let	Help	Make
PCT chief executive		o →→ x		
GP senior partner		x ←——— o		
Junior GP 1	o ————————→ x			
Junior GP 2	o ————→ x			
Community physician		o ————→ x		
Social worker	o ————→ x			
Social services area manager			o —→x	
Board of Primary Care Trust	o ————→ x			
Health visitor		o→ x		
District nurse			o—→x	
Therapies manager			o—→x	
Housing association managers	o ————→ x			
The manager of the nursing home	o ————→ x			
Nurse manager				ox

Dunford: planning for action

The nurse manager realises that her project needs redefinition in the light of what she has found out about the work being done in Fenland on local planning for community support and long-term care. She also realises that the work that needs to be done is potentially enormous and that some realistic boundaries have to be set if she is to achieve any change. Following a useful meeting with the social services area manager, a joint action plan is agreed.

The nurse manager aims to redefine the project and to link it directly with the local agenda associated with the development of the new home. She is going to present it as a pilot project to the supportive key players – the community physician, the therapies manager, the social services area manager and the manager of the new home – with a proposal that they form the core of the project management team. They are to be asked what needs to be done to gain the active support from their chief executives and an action plan can then be drawn up.

In consultation with the community physician, the nurse manager decides to seek to involve one of the younger GPs. She recognises that motivating any of them to become seriously involved is likely to be a major problem because the senior partner's somewhat patronising attitude is hindering the process of change. If he can be persuaded to leave this work to one of the junior partners, there will be more chance of getting the support of the rest of the practice staff. Hence he moves from 'make' to 'let' on the commitment chart.

For the majority of the participants, a substantial amount of work will have to be done to increase their commitment to the project if it is to stand any chance of success. This has more to do with the scale of culture change implied by the establishment of the new home than with any fundamental opposition to its principles and values.

The next stage will be to plan the involvement of service users and carers, probably through the Local Involvement Network (LINk). The aim of the pilot project will be to demonstrate joint working based on clear outcomes. These will reflect local circumstances and the pilot will enable learning to be transferred to a wider base of service provision.

Once you have identified whose commitment is needed, there are a number of ways of gaining it. Here are some suggestions:

- *Use power*. Reward desirable behaviour; ignore or punish inappropriate actions.
- *Treat hurting systems*. Find out what aspects of the current state are hurting the person whose commitment you need, then treat his or her problems. A variation on this is to help people solve problems themselves.
- *Expose the issues*. Find out more about the problems in ways which do not threaten people or force them to adopt stances. For example,

hold a private unstructured meeting to talk about a problem, with no minutes taken and with no outcomes other than a better understanding of the issues.

■ *Educate and develop*. Use the neutrality of a learning situation to encourage open cross-boundary debates.

■ *Role model*. Practise what you preach. As the leader, behave in ways that are in keeping with the desired change.

■ *Use peer pressure*. Use the influence of respected colleagues. This can be particularly helpful in professional cultures.

■ *Encourage sharing*. Expose people to others' successes in ways which enable them to copy useful ideas.

■ *Encourage discussion*. Demonstrate that there are different views of the situation and the potential opportunities and that people involved see the change in different ways.

■ *Horse trade*. 'Do this for me, and I will do that for you.'

A number of methods can be used to understand the issues and identify the work to be done in bringing about change. Two important ideas have been demonstrated:

■ There is a balance of forces in a change situation and reducing constraints is frequently more effective than increasing pressure.

■ Change requires a critical mass of supporters and it is important to build this commitment.

You should now be able to use the diagnostic model and the tools of force field analysis and commitment planning to help you to manage change in your own area of work.

REFERENCES

Buzan, T. (1989) *Use Your Head* (rev. edn), BBC Books.

Lewin, K. (1947) 'Frontiers in group dynamics: Concept, method and reality in social science; social equilibria and social change', *Human Relations*, vol. 1, pp. 5–41.

Nadler, D. A. and Tushman, M. L. (1980) 'A model for diagnosing organizational behavior', *Organizational Dynamics*, Autumn, pp. 35–51.

Nadler, D. and Tushman, M. with Nadler, M. (1997) *Competing by Design: The Power of Organizational Architecture*, Oxford University Press.

CHAPTER 18

PLANNING AND MANAGING PROJECTS

It is one thing to analyse your service delivery processes to identify and design improvements, and quite another to implement them successfully. Implementing change involves applying all your management knowledge and skills in order to complete the project within the required time-scale. Some organisations have established project management procedures and will expect managers to follow the agreed procedure. This chapter outlines the stages that most project management approaches follow.

The key to good project management is keeping three things in balance: time, budget and quality.

A project is something that needs to be done in addition to – and occasionally instead of – the normal day-to-day tasks of managing. It is usually a one-off non-repeated activity that is intended to achieve specified objectives and quality requirements within a time limit. Maylor (1996) defines the characteristics of a project in the following terms:

- It has a clear beginning and end.
- The whole activity is directed towards achieving the defined output or outcome.
- It has a set of constraints that limit and define what can be achieved.
- Its output can be measured in terms of performance against agreed indicators.

A project, almost by definition, involves change. Planning for change involves you, as a manager, working with the impact of the change on all the people involved – service users, carers, staff, service providers with whom you work in partnership and other stakeholders. One of the most important factors in planning a successful project is handling communications and responding to the issues that are raised as a result of communication.

And planning is itself a process. That might seem so self-evident as to be hardly worth stating. But planning is often such a messy, iterative and confusing business that the underlying process may be completely obscured. This chapter focuses on that underlying process in order to help you plan in a systematic way. Planning is rather like preparing for a journey. You need to work out the best way of getting from where you are now to where you want to be.

PLANNING A PROJECT

Jean is the manager of a day centre for adults with learning disabilities. We are going to illustrate the planning process in the context of a project to implement an improvement in her service. At each stage, we describe what she did and invite you to consider how these stages would be similar or different in planning a service improvement in your work setting.

Planning a service improvement

Jean works for a large voluntary organisation providing services for adults with learning disabilities. It has recently received a critical inspection report on its day services, is concerned about the impact of the National Service Framework for Mental Health and is anxious not to lose its contracts with local authorities. A planned major improvement is to extend the 'shared action planning' process to all its service users, and a steering group of managers from each of its day centres has recently agreed a timetable for this. Jean now has the task of implementing this in her centre.

Jean's centre has space for meetings and activities for about 40 people with learning disabilities, ranging from people with physical as well as learning disabilities to people who lead fairly independent lives. Some of them have mental health problems in addition to their learning disability, and some have epilepsy. About half of them live in group homes or hostels, and the rest live at home with their parents or other relatives. The local population includes people from different ethnic minorities, and this is reflected among the 40 service users and the 15 members of staff.

Shared action planning enables the organisation to deploy the skills of its staff to achieve its mission, which is:

To ensure that people with learning disabilities are able to express their wants, needs and concerns, that plans will be made and action taken with them and with their carers to meet those wants, needs and concerns, while due regard is paid to any risks of harm involved, and steps taken to support and protect from harm with the minimum reduction in life chances and choices.

Jean's service has the following features:

- Each service user has a key worker.
- The role of the key worker is to ensure that the service user has the opportunity to express his or her wishes and needs, and to try to make available the life chances he or she hopes for.

- ■ Assessments of need are carried out and updated annually.
- ■ The key worker acts as a focal point for communication, liaising with the people who influence the service user's life – including parents and other relatives, adult education tutors, employers, therapists and health and social services staff.
- ■ The key worker sets up review meetings with relevant parties on a regular basis to ensure that shared action plans are implemented.
- ■ The key worker – together with the service user – keeps records of assessments, review meetings, key events and incidents, and actions taken to implement shared action plans.

At present, only the service users who live in group homes and hostels have a shared action plan. The aim now is for all the service users to have one. This means that the process will have to be introduced to 20 more people and their families, and some staff who have not previously acted as key workers will need to take on this role. There will be more meetings between staff, service users and others, and more records to be kept.

To give herself some time to think about the implications of this change, Jean arranged for one of her deputies to cover for her for a day. She considered shutting herself in her office, but realised that she would have so many interruptions that she would achieve little or nothing, so she found herself a quiet place at home. Her aim for the day was to give enough thought to the major issues to be able to prepare an agenda for a special meeting of her senior team, who would be vital to the successful implementation of the project. She wanted them to think about the issues, and to play a prominent role in planning what needed to be done and in preparing staff, service users and families for the changes to come.

In order to clarify what she needed to do to steer the process, Jean asked herself the following questions, based on what are often described as the seven phases of the planning process:

- ■ Phase 1: What are we trying to do?
- ■ Phase 2: What is the best way of doing it?
- ■ Phase 3: What are we going to have to do?
- ■ Phase 4: In what order should we do things?
- ■ Phase 5: What resources are we going to need?
- ■ Phase 6: Let's review the plan: is it going to work?
- ■ Phase 7: Who is going to do what – and when?

She scanned quickly through the seven phases, making brief notes about each. She realised that she would have to return to all the phases in more detail later, but this first look gave her a sense of what had to be done. Here are her notes.

Phase 1: What are we trying to do?

This is not problematic – shared action planning has been done before and is familiar to staff and service users in the centre. There is no need to develop a new statement of purpose. However, it might be helpful to revisit both the purpose of the centre and the purpose of shared action planning as part of making sure that all staff, service users and families understand what is involved and are prepared for the change.

Phase 2: What is the best way of doing it?

Shared action planning has proved to be an effective means of delivering the centre's purpose, and it will not be necessary to spend much time reconsidering its appropriateness. It can be implemented only if all parties have a good understanding of what it involves and are prepared to play their roles in it. Making sure that everyone is clear about these things is going to be vitally important. Drawing up a plan for clarifying everyone's roles, delegating tasks and putting together a communication strategy need to be items on the agenda for the meeting with senior staff.

Phase 3: What are we going to have to do?

This will be an important item on the agenda. The senior staff's knowledge of their roles and the aspects of the work of the centre for which they are responsible is going to be vital in assessing the current position and making sure that they anticipate what has to be done and what problems may arise. They need to take 'ownership' of the implementation process by setting agreed objectives.

Jean came up with a long list of things to do, grouped under four headings.

Tasks involving everyone

■ Gain the co-operation of staff and service users in extending shared action planning.

■ Review the workings of the existing scheme to ensure that valuable experience is built on and not lost (this may also be a good way of allowing people to say 'goodbye' to the things that they will lose by the change).

■ Understand the anxieties engendered by change and take steps to reduce these where possible.

■ Set up a familiarisation strategy so that everyone involved understands what shared action planning is and the demands it will make on them, whether they are staff, service users, families or partner agencies. It is about co-ordination of all the parties who impact on the life of a person with a learning disability.

■ Anticipate some of the likely changes that will be initiated by service users through the new opportunities they have to express their views about their lives, including the impact on their families.   continued

continued
- Anticipate any risk factors that may emerge.
- Think about the needs of service users and families for whom English is not their first language.

Tasks involving staff

- Discuss anticipated changes in staff roles and working practices with the staff and with the trade union.
- Appraise the new skill requirements of staff and set up any training required.
- Revise staff rotas to take account of changes in working practices.

Tasks I have to do (or delegate)

- Monitor both the implementation of the change and the effectiveness of shared action planning for all clients.
- Plan the timetable for extending shared action planning.
- Develop a reporting strategy to inform the local authorities with which the centre has contracts of plans, progress and anticipated problems.
- Make sure that my own needs for developing new skills are met.

Resources

- Identify the resource implications of introducing new record-keeping systems, changing roles for staff and additional review meetings.
- Calculate the costs of implementation.

Now that Jean has identified the main things that need to be done, let's pause for a moment to explore how you can apply the first three phases of planning to a project in your own workplace.

ACTIVITY 18.1

Think of an improvement that you would like to make in your area of work. Review the first three phases of planning for your project and make notes about what will need to be done under the headings:

- Phase 1: What are we trying to do?
- Phase 2: What is the best way of doing it?
- Phase 3: What are we going to have to do?

(You may wish to keep a project file of your notes on this and subsequent activities in this chapter.)

Now we return to Jean's notes.

Phase 4: In what order should we do things?

At the meeting with senior staff, we'll need to draw a chart showing the sequence of the main activities that will need to take place. We'll also have to consider whether a phased process of introduction would be appropriate. Timing of training for staff and service users will be a key issue and phasing in the new arrangements would avoid having to do all the training at once.

Phase 5: What resources are we going to need?

This will be another item for the senior staff meeting. In addition to freeing up staff time for training and to do new tasks, some new equipment will be needed (including filing cabinets for storing the additional records) and space for more frequent meetings. We'll need to review how space is currently being used in the centre and plan for any necessary changes.

ACTIVITY 18.2

Make brief notes on phases 4 and 5 of your project:

- Phase 4: In what order should we do things?
- Phase 5: What resources are we going to need?

The next step for Jean was to review whether the ideas she had so far would be likely to work in her setting. Here are her notes on the remaining phases of the planning process.

Phase 6: Let's review the plan: is it going to work?

There will be many opportunities for senior staff to review the project as we work together. The shared action planning process includes provision for monitoring progress with individual service users. An overview of progress should be a regular item on our agenda to ensure that key targets are being met and to adjust the plans if it is necessary to make changes.

Phase 7: Who is going to do what – and when?

Delegation is going to be crucial. Appropriate people will need to have delegated authority for each of the activities on the schedule chart. Each person will have to have clear objectives and targets, including dates for continued

continued   the delivery of their parts of the plan. Each person will need to be given the time to undertake their tasks and will also need to have – or have the opportunity for developing – the necessary skills.

By the time Jean had completed her review of the seven phases of planning, she had created the agenda for the first meeting of the senior staff. She now realised that they would need to set up a series of meetings to deal with all the planning issues and to monitor progress.

ACTIVITY 18.3

Complete your project plan by considering phases 6 and 7:

■ Phase 6: Let's review the plan: is it going to work?
■ Phase 7: Who is going to do what – and when?

How easy will it be to make changes?

Stocking (1985) identified a number of factors that assist the rapid diffusion of innovation in a health service, many of which are equally relevant in social care:

■ The existence of identifiable enthusiasts – those who invented or discovered the idea, who are keen to disseminate it, who have reasonable status in their profession or occupational group, and who are prepared to invest considerable time and energy in promoting it – people who will 'champion' the project.
■ The innovation should not be in conflict with current national policies, organisational policies or established climates of opinion among professionals and other groups.
■ It needs to have local appeal to those who have the power to promote change.
■ It has to meet the perceived needs of service users and staff, must 'add value', must not require major role or attitude changes, and should be simple to organise.
■ It should be adaptable to suit local circumstances.
■ Little financial or other resources should be required, unless such requirements can be hidden or increased resources can be made available.

Here are Jean's notes about how closely her plan fits with Stocking's criteria:

The existence of identifiable enthusiasts

I certainly see myself as a 'product champion'. Two of my deputies, several of the other staff and many of the service users are very positive. The cook is particularly keen, as she likes catering for the individual preferences of service users. Some of the parents of service users living in hostels have found shared action planning helpful and campaigned for it to be introduced for all service users.

The innovation should not be in conflict with current policies or established climates of opinion

Shared action planning fits well with national and local policies. Most of the centre's staff have become familiar with it during the five years since it was first introduced, although some find it cumbersome and time-consuming. Some staff are new to it.

It needs to have local appeal to those who have the power to promote change

There might be some difficulty here. Some opinion-formers in the local Mencap group are in favour of shared action planning, but others have campaigned against changes that they see as putting their sons or daughters at risk.

It has to meet perceived needs and add value

Shared action planning is designed to meet the needs of service users, and to enable them to enlarge their horizons. But it can appear threatening to those who think that people with learning disabilities should be protected from the responsibilities and difficulties of life.

It must not require major role or attitude changes

Becoming a key worker is part of the professional ambition of some staff, but for more senior staff it may represent loss of the status they had previously. It requires staff to use their skills wisely, to listen to service users and to recognise that professionals do not always know best.

It should be simple to organise

Shared action planning can lead to substantial reorganisation of activities to accommodate the needs and wants of service users.

It should be adaptable to suit local circumstances

Provided that the principles of good communication, key working and co-ordination are maintained, shared action planning is very appropriate to our local circumstances.

continued

continued   **Little finance or other resource is required**

This depends on how the key worker role is developed. If it is linked to grades and pay, some staff may expect promotion and pay rises, and some may feel that they are losing out. There may also be costs incurred by the service users in taking up new activities.

Jean found this analysis of the centre's situation helpful in identifying the areas on which she and her team would need to concentrate. Judged by Stocking's criteria, they were going to need to pay particular attention to:

- worries of parents and families, especially about perceived risks to service users;
- issues about staff roles and grading;
- the impact of changes in working practices on everyone involved.

ACTIVITY 18.4

Make notes on how the process improvement you were planning in Activities 18.1–18.3 match Stocking's criteria.

Which areas will need special attention when you are implementing your plan?

MANAGING PEOPLE AND CHANGE

Jean is responsible for the use of a building and the physical resources within it, but she knows that the effective implementation of a process such as shared action planning is dependent on the willingness and ability of those who take part in it to make it a success. Their contributions are far more important than the physical resources.

A number of factors influence how people respond to change, and you need to put yourself in the shoes of each of the participants to understand what the change means to them. Some questions to consider are:

1 Who will be active and who will be passive in the process of implementing the project – who are likely to be proactive initiators, passive objects, or victims of the proposed change?
2 For whom will the proposed change lead to a change of identity?
3 What meanings do the *status quo* and the proposed change have for each participant?

4 Who will experience a change in status or image of themselves as a result of the proposed change?
5 How may the proposed change affect their motivation?
6 What will they win or lose?

You will almost certainly find it helpful to discuss the proposed changes with each group of people – or even each individual. This will be a major task, but may well save a lot of time later. Throughout any project, think of the impact on people – people can make the project successful or present obstacles at every stage along the way.

Effective and regular communication is the key to ensuring that everyone involved is informed about progress and it is also the way in which the project manager can be reassured about how things are going or warned if there are things going wrong. Making time to listen to your team and stakeholders is very important as a way of keeping in touch with the impact of the project as it progresses.

The major difference between you and other people is that you know what you are thinking and feeling, whereas other people know only what you look like and how you are behaving. This fundamental difference between you and everyone else in the world makes your behaviour extremely important.

(Honey, 2001)

Effective communication

Jones and Murray (2008) offer a checklist for effective communication in a project:

- Frequent and regular team review meetings with clear and consistent agenda, promptly circulated meeting notes which include specific action points agreed and carried out.
- Working sub-group meetings, where appropriate, to thrash out questions of specific detail.
- Short, regular progress reports to a project's sponsor, customer and other stakeholders.
- Actively managed stakeholder relationships – identifying those whose support for the project is critical and those who may hinder project progress.
- Use of informal as well as formal communication channels to build supporting project-related 'intelligence'.
- Encouragement of frank, honest, but objective reporting with focus on solutions rather than blame when things go wrong.
- Support and feedback to project team members to maintain motivation and commitment.

KEEPING ON TRACK

In this section we focus in rather more detail on two of the phases of planning a project that we described – sequencing activities (phase 4) and scheduling activities (phase 7) – for which a number of techniques are available that you may find useful.

Sequencing activities

Phase 4 of the planning process concentrates on sequencing activities – arranging them in the order in which they need to be done. It is important to identify activities that cannot start until others have been completed. These activities will determine the overall sequence in which you carry out your project because you have no option but to do them in that order. Other activities may be less critical. It may be possible to undertake some of them in parallel: you can do them at the same time. It may be possible for some activities to take place at any time: you can decide when is a suitable point to fit them in.

Two techniques for sequencing activities and representing them in diagrammatic form are *logic diagrams* and *Gantt charts*.

Logic diagrams

One way of sorting out the relationships between a sequence of actions is to use a logic diagram. The name sounds rather daunting, but this is quite a simple technique that can readily be done on the back of an envelope.

A logic diagram is a network of lines that shows the logical sequence of activities and, in particular, which activities must be completed before others can start. For example, in the diagram in Figure 18.1, activity H must be completed before activity I can start. Activity H can be taking place at the same time as activity F, but both must be completed before activity I can start.

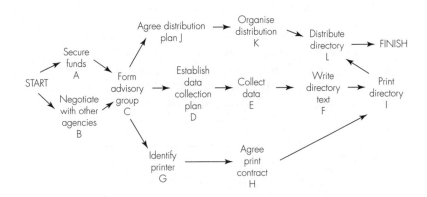

Figure 18.1 Logic diagram for the production of a directory

ACTIVITY 18.5

Sketch a logic diagram for the sequence of activities that you will need to carry out in the project that you have been thinking about.

Logic diagrams are only concerned with showing the sequence of activities. They make no attempt to show the length of time that an activity will take: the lengths of the lines in the diagram do not represent the durations of the activities. To give a more detailed picture of the project – including the time required for each activity – it is helpful to draw a Gantt chart.

Gantt charts

The Gantt chart (named after the man credited with inventing it) is one of the most commonly used techniques for planning a sequence of activities and showing how long each will take. Each activity is drawn as a bar against a time-scale. The length of each bar represents the expected duration of that activity.

A Gantt chart presents the project plan in a visual form that can readily be understood by everyone involved. It can be used at any stage in the planning process, from initial outline planning to the detailed planning of individual tasks. Figure 18.2 is Jean's Gantt chart, showing how she will extend shared action planning.

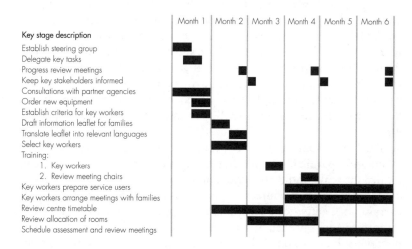

Figure 18.2 Gantt chart for extending 'shared action planning'

You can see from Figure 18.2 that:

■ A Gantt chart shows the sequence and duration of activities and thus reveals any options for changing the sequence.
■ It shows those activities that can be carried out concurrently.
■ Bars need not be continuous.

This technique can be used for planning complex projects as well as simple ones. However, for bigger projects, each bar on the master chart might have to be drawn as a more detailed separate Gantt chart. In Jean's example, the bars dealing with selection, training and the tasks of key workers would have to be planned in more detail, although the overall duration of the activities involved would still need to be completed at the times shown in Figure 18.2.

ACTIVITY 18.6

This is an opportunity to turn the logic diagram that you drafted into a Gantt chart. List all the activities needed to implement your project in sequence in the column on the left. Decide the likely overall duration of the project and head the rest of the columns as days, weeks or months. Draw in the bars to indicate the length of time each activity will take.

A Gantt chart can help you to think about whether you can complete a project on time. You may have started with the first activity and just worked down the list, putting in the time you thought each would take. If so, you will be lucky if the chart shows that you will meet your deadline for completing the project. If you have a deadline, you could start with the final activity and work your way back. If this reveals that you are not able to complete the project on time (or that you should have started it a few months ago!), you can consider how to adjust the plan.

You have a number of choices. It may be possible to carry out several activities in parallel, instead of one after another. You may be able to reduce the scale of the project to eliminate some of the activities. You could increase the resources available (usually the number of people carrying out activities). This might be appropriate if the outcome is important and is needed by a particular deadline. Another option is to negotiate an extension to the deadline to enable all the activities to be completed without increasing resources.

Scheduling activities

Phase 7 of the planning process – deciding who is going to do what, and when – is the final stage before implementation. Up to this point, the plan has been largely hypothetical – working out what you are trying to do, and how you will do it if the necessary resources are available. It is all conditional. But when the conditions have been fulfilled, and the plan has been approved and is about to be put into practice, a further step is needed. You need to specify how the plan will be converted into action. This means being clear about who is to do what and by when, so that all those who will be implementing the project know precisely what is required of them. This also ensures that you, as the manager responsible for it, can co-ordinate and control the often complex range of activities and resources that are needed to implement it.

The specification prepared in this phase goes under various names. It is often referred to as an 'action plan'. Another way of describing this phase is to refer to it as 'scheduling'. The schedules are the part of a plan that sets out the details of who will carry out which parts of the work, and when they are to do it.

Two useful approaches to scheduling activities are *key events planning* and *milestone planning*.

Key events planning

One of the simplest ways of representing a plan in an easily understood way is to list the key events and the date (sometimes even the time) when each event is planned to occur. By 'event', we mean an action or activity that is planned to occur at a particular time. It is different from a 'process', which takes place over a period of time. So 'order publicity material' and 'complete review of publicity material' are events planned for a particular time and could appear on a key events plan, but 'prepare publicity material' is a process rather than an event because the activity would take place over a period of time. 'Key events' are the most important events in the plan; the lesser events cluster around them.

There are two main uses for key events planning:

■ to specify the overall framework of a project so that other people can prepare their detailed plans to fit in with the key events;
■ to identify the target dates in a large project plan that must be met by the people involved in only one part of that plan.

Let's consider an example. A local charity has raised a substantial amount of money to build a hospice. The building is nearing completion and will be opened by a VIP. The commissioning officer is planning the opening ceremony in close consultation with the protocol

Table 18.1 A key events plan for the opening of a hospice

Date	Key events	Other events
2 July	Planning meeting	Receive project status reports Issue detailed plans for each department
6 July	Outline plan of ceremony to VIP	Distribute ceremony plan internally Receive departmental updates Receive building, plant and equipment status report
16 July	Visit of VIP's protocol officer	Receive draft of publicity material Agree press arrangements Confirm catering plans Agree guest list
24 July	Receive comments from protocol officer	Distribute comments Order publicity material Confirm press arrangements Check status of whole project
27 July	Handover of building	Check that equipment installation complete Test equipment
30 July	Planning meeting	Review handover Receive final lists of problems from departments
2 August	Rehearsal	
6 August	Final planning meeting	Review publicity material Review status of any problems
13 August	VIP visit	

officer (the VIP's representative) and has drawn up the key events plan shown in Table 18.1.

This is not a comprehensive list of everything that must take place to achieve a successful opening ceremony. Its purpose is to highlight the dates on which key events are planned to occur and by which the activities contributing to those events must be complete. It enables the people responsible for the different aspects of the ceremony (publicity, catering, finishing the hospice, etc.) to adjust their own plans to fit in with the dates of the key events and to identify any possible problems in meeting them.

By the addition of an extra column to Table 18.1, it would be possible to indicate who is responsible for ensuring that each event occurs as scheduled. Each of these people could then produce more detailed schedules of who was going to do what and by when.

Milestone planning

Milestone planning is very similar to key events planning. The difference is that, whereas a key events schedule lists the main events irrespective of the time intervals between them, a milestone schedule lists a series of dates at fixed intervals (the milestones). It shows the stage that each of the main activities is expected to have reached by those dates.

Milestone planning is often used to monitor and control events to ensure that they remain on course. The manager calls for progress reports to be submitted at the fixed dates, so that he or she can check whether everything is going according to plan. The technique is illustrated in Table 18.2.

PROBLEMS WITH PLANNING

The seven phases of planning a project that we have described are an idealised and rational sequence. Planning starts at phase 1 and moves smoothly forward. If managerial life were as simple as that, planning would be merely a matter of moving steadily through the phases to the point when implementation begins. Thereafter, the manager would cease planning and start controlling – ensuring that everything was going according to plan.

But life is often not as simple as this. Countless complexities may conspire to make the planning process more like a game of snakes and ladders than the neat linear process that we have depicted. Nevertheless, even a game of snakes and ladders has an underlying logic: the aim is to progress in a particular direction, despite the hazards and despite having to visit old ground time and again. Similarly, planning has an underlying logic, with the aim of progressing in a particular direction. But in the hazards of real life, there is a risk of losing that sense of direction. Our aim in spelling out the phases has been to give you a 'map' to help you keep on track throughout the planning process.

All sorts of things make planning a good deal more complex – and less rational. Let's look at two common problems: you can find yourself going round in circles, and your objectives may be vague. We then conclude the chapter by looking at a solution – making contingency plans.

Table 18.2 Part of a milestone plan

Milestone	Main activities	Other activities
30 June	Building complete Services 90% complete	Computer installation commenced
31 July	Services complete Planning starts for moving medical records	Budgets complete Staff informed of individual tasks

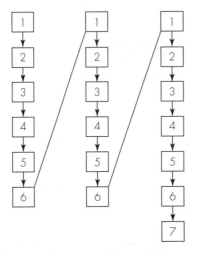

Figure 18.3 Multistage approach

Going round in circles

You may have to go back over the same ground several times, refining and modifying as you go. One way of describing this inevitable revisiting of old ground is to refer to it as *multistage planning* (Figure 18.3), implying that you go through the whole process once, and then again, and then again, until your plan is sufficiently refined to be put into action.

Multistage planning is likely to be a necessary part of implementing a project within your own service or department. It is likely to be even more necessary when developing major plans at the corporate level. Here is how one planner working in the health service described the process.

First stage

This would be the production of a plan in general terms, outlining the overall aims and objectives, a rough estimate of the costs and the time required. This would be an outline plan that would be in sufficient detail to show that there would be a reasonable likelihood that it could be carried out.

Second stage

A plan would then be produced which would still be fairly broad, based on rough estimates. All the people involved in the project would contribute to the plan and identify the activities required of them to achieve it. A number of options would be developed, listing the alternative ways and means of meeting the aims and objectives. These would be considered by the participants and a preferred option should emerge once everyone has ascertained the feasibility of achieving their respective contributions. A consolidated plan would be produced.

Third stage

If the second stage plan seemed feasible, a final plan would be produced. This would be more detailed than the previous plans and would provide an action plan for implementation.

In this illustration, the terms 'first stage', 'second stage' and 'third stage' are used to emphasise that planning is a multistage process rather than a single pass as implied in the 'rational' seven-phase approach. These terms are not generally used, but the principle of multistage planning is widely practised.

An alternative way of viewing this multistage process is to regard it as being *cyclical*. Each cycle takes you through all the seven phases (Figure 18.4). At the very least, you will need to go round the loop two or three times as you refine your plan. The first time round you will probably do little more than identify and resolve some of the major problems, finishing up with the broad outline of a plan. The second time round (if all is going well) you will be able to add more detail and begin to make decisions. The third time round (if you are lucky) you might finish up with something that could be put into effect with a reasonable chance of success. It is little wonder that you often feel that you are going round in circles when you are planning – you *are* going round in circles, but you are gathering more information and refining the details as you do so.

In real life, you are rarely likely to be able to maintain forward progress round the circle for very long. You will often need to drop back a couple of phases, just as in snakes and ladders, before you can make further progress. So the process is better described as iterative rather

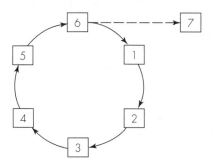

Figure 18.4 Cyclical approach

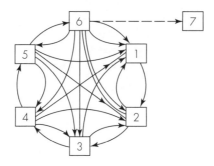

Figure 18.5 Iterative approach

than cyclical, acknowledging the fact that your forward progress may be interrupted by having to return and adjust something that you have just settled. The idea of planning as an iterative process is illustrated in Figure 18.5, which demonstrates why planning can seem such a confused and confusing process.

However you look at it, planning is rarely a straightforward process. It is usually necessary to go over the same ground several times, refining the plan and adding more detail as the route becomes clearer.

Vague objectives

How often, when you are planning, have you sat down and carefully worked out precisely what you are trying to achieve? Unless you know what you are supposed to be achieving, it is very difficult to plan to achieve it.

It may be difficult to describe clear and precise objectives because the situation or task is unclear. Sometimes, however, we are our own worst enemies and we describe objectives in vague terms even though we have all the ingredients we need for precision. One way of avoiding this problem is to check that your objectives are SMART (specific, measurable, agreed, realistic and time-bounded).

The objective 'Go on holiday in the summer' is definitely not SMART (but it may be a goal). The objective 'Take a walking holiday for two in the Black Forest in the middle two weeks of June at a cost not exceeding £600' is very SMART and you can see the difference at a glance.

When you apply the SMART test to your objectives, you may find they are not sufficiently precise. The action that is then needed may be as simple as adding in more detail (which was available but you had forgotten to include it). Alternatively, you may realise that more work is needed before you can improve the wording of an objective (which may take you into the iterative approach illustrated in Figure 18.5).

Contingency plans

We have focused on some of the factors that make planning hazardous. We all know that events have a remarkably perverse way of evolving in unexpected directions. It is not surprising, therefore, that plans often appear to 'go wrong'. In fact, they don't go wrong. They just don't quite fit the reality that finally emerges, and they need to be adjusted if they are to remain operable. It is often possible to make the necessary adjustments so that the plan is still workable, and it is one of the tasks of managers to keep plans continuously under review and to adjust them as circumstances demand. Flexibility is therefore one of the most important characteristics of any plan – and of any planner.

But circumstances can sometimes change quickly and dramatically so that the original plan is no longer operable. Suppose a key member of staff were to leave Jean's team just as her project is to be implemented? She would need a contingency plan. Perhaps she could train another member of staff to cover the same tasks. Perhaps someone could be seconded to Jean's team from elsewhere in the organisation or from another organisation. Perhaps the plan could be rescheduled or partially implemented.

Throughout the planning process, you should keep on asking, 'What if this goes wrong? What if that goes wrong?' If the answer is that it doesn't matter, a contingency plan may not be necessary. But if it does matter, a contingency plan is essential. You should be constantly on the look-out for contingencies that could have significant consequences, and prepare contingency plans to deal with them if they do occur.

Planning is not a simple process. Even when planning quite a modest project, it is often necessary to go round in circles, revisiting old ground repeatedly and adjusting as you go. However, it is helpful to use a structured approach – to keep the seven phases of planning in mind to ensure that you include all the important elements. You need to maintain some order within the chaos in order to make progress towards improving services.

Managing more complex projects

Large and complex projects, particularly ones that involve several partner agencies or specialist contractors, are managed using a framework that is focused on effective use of resources to achieve a business improvement. Many public service organisations in the UK use a project management method called PRINCE2, which has been developed and refined over years of use by project managers in many different contexts. Colin Bentley (2007) sets out the main advantages:

PRINCE2 gives:

■ *Controlled management of change by the business in terms of its investment and return on investment*

■ *Active involvement of the users of the final product through-out its development to ensure the business product will meet the functional, environmental, service and management requirements of the users*
■ *More efficient control of development resources.*

The focus is on the rationale for the project, set out as a business case. The method is structured to take users through the process of managing a project, introducing appropriate techniques at each stage and placing particular importance on delivering what is required by the business case. It is more elaborate than the seven-stage plan described in this chapter but follows a similar sequence of stages and some organisations prefer their project managers to use it. It is designed to be suitable for use in any type of project, large or small and is available for use in the public domain from the Office of Government Commerce (OGC, 2009). PRINCE2 is a framework that enables a manager to structure and organise a project, but does not include a very wide range of project management techniques or guidance on the leadership and people management skills necessary to achieve project outcomes successfully.

REFERENCES

Bentley, C. (2007) *PRINCE2: A Practical Handbook*, 2nd edn, Butterworth Heinemann.

Honey, P. (2001) *Improve Your People Skills*, 2nd edn, Chartered Institute of Personnel and Development.

Jones, R. and Murray, N. (2008) *Change, Strategy and Projects at Work*, Open University/Butterworth Heinemann.

Maylor, H. (1996) *Project Management*, Pitman Publishing.

OGC (2009) *Prince 2*, <http://www.ogc.gov.uk/methods_prince_2.asp> (accessed 27/12/2009).

Stocking, B. (1985) *Initiative and Inertia: Case Studies in the NHS*, Nuffield Provincial Hospital Trust.

INDEX

Note: *italic* page numbers denote references to figures/tables.

access to services 158, *159*, 162–3, *240*, 258, *260*, 266
accountability 74–6, 143, 212–18, 319; clinical governance 213–15; managerial 215–17; multidisciplinary teams 299–300; NHS 78; personal 217; professional 218
accountants 199, *199*, *200*, 203, 205–6
Adair, J. 37, 39
adaptive systems 125
aims 28, 190–1, 252
Alban-Metcalfe, R. 42
Aleszewski, A. 219
Alimo-Metcalfe, B. 42
Allison, M. 45
assessment 130, 178, 212, 274
audit 214, 270–2
Audit Commission 165, 213, 271
authority 55–6, 212, 217

Balogun, J. 287
Bennis, W. 40
Bentley, C. 357–8
Berry, L. 158–9, 241
best value 143, 213–14
Blake, R.R. 48
Blanchard, K.H. 38
boundaries 117–19, 171, *172*, 184, 208–9; working across 157–66
British Association of Social Workers 75
budgets 9, 14, 15, 27, 190–206, 287; financial risk 222; incremental budgeting 197, 198; input and output 194–7; multidisciplinary teams 300–1; negotiating 201–4; purpose of 192–3; reports 204, 205; statements *191*, *195*; targets 205; timetabling 198–201, *199*, *200*; zero-based budgeting 197, 198

bureaucratic model 136, *136*, 137
business planning 207, 209–12
Buzan, T. 326

Cancer Plan (NHS) 155–6
capability issues 311–12
Care and Social Services Inspectorate 213
care plans 150–1, 258, 275
Care Quality Commission 122, 213, 253, 332
carers 93–4
Carr, S. 135
Carruthers, I. 238
Casey, D. 296–8
cause and effect (fishbone) diagrams 242–6, *244*
cervical cytology screening programme *260–1*
change 18, 247, 287, 316–37; case study 321–6, *326*, 332–4; commitment planning 331, 334–7, *335*; diagnostic model 317–21, *319*, 322–6, 327; force field analysis 330, 331–4, *331*, *334*; implementation of 328–30; projects 338, 341–2, 345, 346–7; resistance to 9
Chapman, C. 250
Child and Adolescent Mental Health Service (CAMHS) 107
children 85, 102, 120, 156, *267*; child-centred services 87–8; disabilities resource centre 13–16; feedback from service users 107–8; multi-agency working 301–2; occupational therapy *263–4*
choice 73, 79, 133, 135
citizenship 73, 79, 111, 134
clinical governance 143, 213–15, 265, 266

commissioners 122, 136, *136*, *137*, 234, *234*
commitment planning 331, 334–7, *335*
communication 53, 98, 158, *159*, 163, 164–5; budgets 192, 205; change management 329, 347; electronic 296; outsourcing 118; projects 338
community care services 146, 150
community meals services 95, 98–9, 153
competence 42, 75, *159*
competitors 123
complaints 111–14, 145–6, 147, 215, 243, 258
concurrent (steering) control 288
confidentiality 215, 312
consultants 129–30, 186, 299
consultation 109, 134, *135*, 139, 186; attitudes to 143–4; data collection 144–52; Local Area Agreements 208; planning 140–4, 152; quality control loop 144–5, *144*
consultative management style 50–1, *56*
consumerist view of services 133
contingency plans 357
continuing professional development (CPD) 214, 218, 303
continuous improvement 230, 231
contracts 190, 192
control loop 274, 275–7, 278, 294
co-ordination 192–3
costs 118, 130, 131, *196*, 205; input/output budgets 194–7; process cost analysis 183; quality issues 228, 229–30, 235, 237–8, *239*; savings 184, 202, 203–4, 238; *see also* budgets
Coulter, M. 280
courtesy *159*
credibility *159*
critical mass 331, 334, 337
Crosby, P.B. 228, 229
customers 93–6, 119, 121; assessment of quality 158, *159*; chains 99–102, *100*, *101*; internal 95, 104, 138, 231, 233; non-care 122; quality chain 231–3, *232*; roles 96–9; *see also* service users
cyclical planning 355, *355*

data collection 138–9, 140, 144–52, 157; diagnostic data 327; focus groups 148–9; interviews 148, 149; postal surveys 146–7, 149; questions 149–51
Davis, S.B. 230
decision-making 56, 134, 300
defensiveness 151
delegation 38, 55–6, 190, 283, 294, 343–4
demands 124–5, 126, 127, 253
democratic view of services 133–4
demographic structure 126–7

Department of Health 77–8, 96, 172, 213, 230–1, 232, 240, 265–6, 299, 300
Department of Trade and Industry 237
deprivation gap 156
diabetes 266
Dickinson, H. 165
dignity 75, 77, 79, 82, 240
directive management style 50–1, 56
disability 13–16, 82, *135*; *see also* learning disabilities
disciplinary procedures 292, 311, 312–14
discrimination 67–8, 308–9, 312
dispositions 42–3
diversity 67–9, 82, 84
Donabedian, A. 259

effectiveness 20–34; definition of 21; identifying needs 24–5, 26; planning 23–4; service quality 240, 258; SMART objectives 28–30; standards *260–1*, 265
efficiency 29, 79, 182, *240*, 258, *261*
elapsed time analysis 182, 183
eligibility 131
employment law 308, 313, 314
empowerment 42, 59, 158–9, 163; partnerships 73; quality improvement 236–7; service relationships 136–8, *137*
environmental issues 76
environmental risks 220
equal opportunities 308–10
equality 82, 84
equity 78, 79, *240*, 258
Everett, T. 268
Every Child Matters (2003) 85, 102, 156
evidence 133, 138–52; accountability 212; authentic 139–40; current 140; focus groups 148–9; interviews 148, 149; postal surveys 146–7, 149; quality control loop 144–5, *144*; questions 149–51; sufficient 139; valid 140
evidence-based practice 214
expectancy theory 64–5, *64*
expectations 65, 106–7, 229, 236, 241, 247
expenditure 191, 194, *195*, 210, 211, 222

far environment 115, 116, *116*, 120, 131
feedback 107–10, 143, 144–52, 171, 181, 185; management control 288; project teams 347; quality control loop 144–5, *144*; standards 258; systems thinking 278, *278*
feedforward control 287–8
Fiedler, F.E. 38
financial risk 222
fishbone diagrams 242–6, *242*, *244*
fitness for purpose 228, 229
focus groups 10, 108, 148–9

force field analysis 330, 331–4, *331, 334*
formal organisational arrangements 319, *319*, 320, 323, 324, *326*

Gantt charts 349–50, *349*
General Medical Council 76, 77
general practitioners (GPs) 12, 93, 128, 129, 299, 300; chain of specification 102; Dunford case study 321–3, 325, 333, *335*; incentives 67; organisational boundaries 117; terminal illness case study 160, 161; values 76, 77
Glasby, J. 165
goals 84, 86; *see also* objectives
Groetsch, D.I. 230
Gorman, P. 299–300
governance 111, 143, 213–15, 265, 266
grievance procedures 314–15
Griffiths, R. 348
Grint, K. 40, 43
Groocock, J.M. 228, 229
group, definition of 295; *see also* teams

Hales, C. 17, 18
handover analysis 182, 183
Handy, C. 45–6
Hartley, J.F. 45
Haywood-Farmer, J. 241
health and safety 218, 220, 307, 312
health insurance 122, 127
health services 100, 102, 171–2, 207, 208; accountability 212–13; clinical governance 213, 214; commissioners 122; customer-supplier relationships 94–5; needs and demands 126–7, 128–30; outcomes 154; partnerships 22–3, 125; social model of health 73, 79; standards *260–1*, 265–8, *267*; terminal illness case study 158–65; values 73, 77–80; vulnerable clients 221; *see also* National Health Service
Hersey, P. 38
Herzberg, F. 63–4
hierarchy of needs 62–3, *62*
Holland, P. 238
home care services 117, 125, 130
honesty 74, 75, 76
Honey, P. 347
Hope Hailey, V. 287
Horizon House 96, 97
hospitals 95, 129–30, *270*, 329–30
Hunter, D. 31
Hutton, M. 237
'hygiene' factors 63, *63*

illness 127, 128–9; terminal 158–65
image 52–3
incentives 66–7

income 191, 210, 211
infection control 232, *267*
influence 54–5, 171
informal organisation 319, *319*, 320, 323, 325, *326*
information 18, 134, *135*, 181, 186, 278; *see also* data collection
in-house services 117–19, *118*
innovation, diffusion of 344–6
inputs: diagnostic model 318, *319*, 322–3, 324; fishbone diagram 244, *244*; systems view 277, *277*, *278*, *279*, *279*
inspections 208, 213, 299
Institute for Public Policy Research 79
Institute of Healthcare Management 1, 75–6
integration of services 9–10, 79, 125, 127, 153, 172; commissioners 122; integrated care pathways 208–9; outcomes 165–6; quality chain 231; values 80, 83, 118; working across boundaries 157, 158–9, 163, 165; *see also* partnerships
integrity 37, 43, 74, 75
internal environment 115, 116, *116*, 131
International Standards Organisation 228
interviews 107–8, 109, 148, 149
iterative planning 355–6, *356*

jargon 110, 150
job demands 17–19, 22
job descriptions 217, 312, 313
job satisfaction 63–4, 67, 166, 237, 274
job-specific training 303
Johnson, A. 230–1
Jones, R. 281, 347
judgement 84, 253
Juran, J.M. 228

key activities 32
key events planning 351–2, *352*
Koch, H. 253, 262, 268
Kotter, J. 36
Kouzes, J.M. 44

labour market 123
ladder approach to objectives 26–7, *26*
leadership 18, 35–57, 86, 166; behavioural theories 37–8, 39–40; contingency theories 38–40; management relationship 35–6, *35*; Nolan Committee principles 74, 75; as social process 43–5; styles of 37–8, 45–51; transformational 40–3
learning 40, 307, 308
learning disabilities 83, 262, 339–46
legal and statutory frameworks 300
legislation 116, 120, 154

Lewin, K. 331
lifelong learning 214, 215, 218
Liverpool Children and Young People's
  Participation Unit 107–8
Local Area Agreements (LAAs) 208
local authorities 117, 122, 130, 154, 208;
  accountability 300; clinical governance
  213–14; risk registers 223
logic diagrams 348–9, *348*

management control 193, 212, 273–94;
  control loop 274, 275–7, 278, 294;
  corrective action 275–6, 276, 278–9,
  291–2; informal versus formal 288–9;
  levels of 292–4, *293*; management by
  exception 283–4; measuring and
  comparing 275–6, 276, 279–83;
  monitoring 275–6, 276; people factors
  286–7; procedures and systems 284–6;
  qualitative versus quantitative 289–90;
  systems view 277–9; timing 287–8
Management Education Scheme by Open
  Learning (MESOL) 1–2
Management Grid 48, *49*
management style 45–57; image 52–3;
  influencing others 54–5; personal
  authority 55–6; personal values 50;
  self-confidence 53; setting an example
  52
managers 7–19, 124, 171, 185–6;
  accountability 212, 215–17; activities
  and skills 7–17, 22, 23; aspiring
  managers programme 68–9; budgets
  199; complaints procedures 111, 112;
  disabilities resource centre 13–16;
  intermediate care services 8–11;
  leadership role 36, 41; managing
  upwards 54–5; nature of job 17–19;
  practice 11–13; risk management 218;
  service relationships 136, *136*, *137*; *see
  also* management control
Manthorpe, J. 219
Maslow, A. 62–3
Maxwell, R. 239–40, 258
Maylor, H. 338
McSherry,R. 266
measurement 21, 145, 156–7, 208;
  management control 275–6, *276*,
  279–83, *293*; standards 250, 251, 256,
  271–2
meetings 9–10, 12, 347
mental health services 80–1, 82, 96, 97,
  154, 259–62, 301
mental models 40, 42
mentoring 68
milestone planning 353, *353*
mind maps 326, *326*
monitoring 268–70, *268*, *270*, 275–6, *276*

morale 15, 60, 232
morbidity 127
Morgan, J. 268
Morris, B. 233
mortality rates 127
motivation 41, 58–70, 286; budgets 193,
  205; definition of 59; diversity 67–9;
  emotional motivators 61; expectancy
  theory 64–5, *64*; external initiatives
  66–7; Herzberg's theory 63–4, *63*;
  Maslow's hierarchy of needs 62–3, *62*;
  psychological contract 65–6
Mouton, J.S. 48
multidisciplinary teams 25, 157, 176, 298,
  299–302
multistage planning 354–5, *354*
Murray, N. 281, 347

Nadler, D. 318–20
National Health Service (NHS) 1, 230–1,
  239–40, 258–9; Cancer Plan 155–6;
  clinical governance 213, 214;
  leadership 41–2; processes 176;
  standards 249; values 77–9; *see also*
  health services
National Institute for Health and Clinical
  Excellence (NICE) 172, 213, 253, *267*
National Service Frameworks (NSFs) 154,
  172, 252–3, 339
near environment 115, 116, *116*, 120,
  121–6, 131
needs 24–5, 26, 39, 104, 126–31;
  Maslow's hierarchy of 62–3, *62*; service
  quality 228, 229, *240*, 258; SMART
  objectives 29–30; training 303–5, 306
Nolan Committee 73–5

Oakland, J. 229
objectives 19, 20, 26–8, 31–3, 98, 310,
  317; budgets *199*, 201; business
  planning 210, 211; capability issues
  311; information gathering 151;
  long-term and short-term 30–1;
  management control 273; measuring
  and comparing 281–3; quality of 21;
  review and evaluation 21, 24, 32;
  SMART 28–30, 33, 356; vague 356;
  vision 86
objectivity 74, 75
occupational therapy services *200*, 263–4,
  269, 299–300
older people 82, 153, 172, 229, 321–2,
  332–3
openness 74, 75, 76, 201, 215
organisational culture 18, 22, 45; informal
  319, *319*, 320, 323, 325, *326*
outcomes 104, 153–7, 165–6, 178, 179;
  diagnostic model 320, 323, 325–6;

Local Area Agreements 208; measurement of 250; quality issues 240, *261*; standards 259–62, *263–4*; training 307

outputs 154, 178, 179, 195; diagnostic model 318, *319*, 325–6; systems view 277–8, *277*, *278*, *279*

outsourcing 117–19, *118*

Oxleas NHS Foundation Trust 96, 97, *97*

Parsloe, P. 219

partnerships 23, 73, 87–8, 125, 157–65; consultation 142; Local Area Agreements 208; NHS 78, 79; outcome measurement 165–6; outsourcing 118; service user participation 134, *135*; stakeholders 122; values 86–7; *see also* integration of services

pathways: integrated care 208–9; process mapping 172, 173, 176, *177*, 179, 181–4

patients 12, 93, 129–30, 275–6; long-term and short-term objectives 31; standards *261*, 266, *267*; surgery 175–6, *177*, 181; *see also* service users

Pearce, P. 266

performance: assessment frameworks 212, 258–9; budgets 193, 205; business planning 209–10; clinical governance 214; expectancy theory 64; measurement of 21, 145, 156–7, 208, 256, 271–2, 279–83, *293*; poor 310–15; procedures 285

personal authority 55–6

personal development 41, 303

personal mastery 40

personality traits 37, 77

Pfeffer, J. 124

physical safety 158, 162–3

pilot projects 287–8, 336

planning 23–4, 98, 207, 208–12; budgets 192, 198–201; business planning 207, 209–12; commitment 331, 334–7, *335*; consultation 140–4, 152; contingency 357; cyclical 355, *355*; force field analysis 330, 331–4, *331*, *334*; guidance 208–9; iterative 355–6, *356*; multistage 354–5, *354*; problems with 353–6; projects 338, 339–46, 347–57; quality control loop *144*, 145; scheduling activities 351–3; sequencing activities 348–50

policy 207, 208, 345

politics 125

Posner, B.Z. 44

postal surveys 146–7, 149

power 55, 299, 336

prejudice 84–5

PRINCE2 method 357–8

priorities 30–1, 98, 126, 144, 208, 348

private sector 122

probity 76

procedures 284–6

process cost analysis 183

processes 45, 134, 171–89, 241; definition of 173; fishbone diagram *244*, 245; flow 174–6; identification of weaknesses 180–3; mapping 172–85; service improvement 179–80, 183–8; standards 259–62, *263–4*; systems view 277, *277*, *278*, *279*, *279*

professional bodies 120, 123, 218, 253

professional development 214, 215, 218, 303, 309–10; *see also* training

projects 8–9, 18, 338–58; change management 346–7; complex 357–8; contingency plans 357; diffusion of innovation 344–6; planning 338, 339–46, 347–57; problems with planning 353–6; scheduling activities 351–3; sequencing activities 348–50

provident associations 122

psychological contract 65–6

psychological safety 158, 162–3

public services 73–4, 79, 118, 208, 212, 230

purpose 45, 153–4, 210, 280–1, 330

puzzles 297, *297*, 298

quality 11, 66–7, 119, 227–48, 258–9; accountability 212; auditing 271; clinical governance 213, 214, 215; customer assessment of 158, *159*; definitions of 227–30, 233; dimensions of 239–41, 258–9; effectiveness 21–2; importance of 236–8; perceptions and expectations 241; problems 238–9, *239*, 242–7; quality chain 231–3, *232*; quality control loop 144–5, *144*, 149; *see also* standards

Quality and Outcomes Framework (QOF) 66, 67, 129

questions 147, 149–51

Qureshi, H. 146

recruitment 15, 77

regulators 122

reliability *159*

reputational risk 222

requirements 94, 103–7, 228, 229, 235–6, 247

residential care 94, 130–1, 142, 229, 230; children with disabilities 13; complaints 243; Dunford case study 332–3; inspection teams 299; organisational boundaries 117

resources 22, 251–2, 342, 343; budgets 202; diagnostic model 318–19, *319*, 323, 324; force field analysis 332; resource dependence 124–5
respect 76, 77, 82
responsibilities 73, 79, 82, 199, 239; accountability 212, 217; budgetary 300–1; risk management 219, 220
responsive model 136, *136*, 137
responsiveness 19, 158, *159*, 162–3, 210, 266
review and evaluation 21, 24, 32, 307–8, 343
rewards 59, 64, 66–7, 286
Reynolds, J. 45
rights 73, 79, 80, 82–3, 84, 134
risk 27, 218–23; definition of 219; register 222–3; risk assessment 14, 208, 219; risk management 214, 218, 219, 222; types of 220–3
Robbins, S.P. 280
Rogers, A. 45
Royal College of Nursing 213

safety 158, 162–3, 218, 220, 221, 240; monitoring *270*; standards 265, 266, *267*
Salancik, G.R. 124
scheduling activities 351–3
Schmidt, W.H. 37–8
security 158, *159*
self-confidence 53
selflessness 74, *75*
Senge, P. 40
sequencing activities 348–50
service environment 115–32; components of 115–16; needs and demands 126–31; organisational boundaries 117–19; stakeholders 119–24
service users 1, 93–114, 121; chain of specification 102; complaints 111–14, 145–6, 147, 258; consultation with 140–4; different types of 93–6; expectations 106–7; feedback from 107–10, 143, 144–52, 171, 181, 185, 258; influencing 54; involvement of 10, 44, 105, 110, 150, 240, 358; learning disability services 339–40; mental health services 80–1; needs 24–5, 29–30, 104, 126–31; participation of 133–8, 143; partnerships 73; pathways 172, 176, *177*, 179, 181–4, 208–9; perceptions of quality 227–8, 233, *234*, 235, 236, *239*, 241; process mapping 173–4; quality chain 231–3; relationships 135–8; requirements 94, 103–7, 228, 229, 235–6, 247;

standards 254, 255, 257–8; *see also* customers; patients
shared action planning 339–44, 345–6, *349*
Shaw, C. 270–1
SMART objectives 28–30, 33, 356
social acceptability *240*, 258
social care services 171–2, 207, 208; accountability 212–13, 217; clinical governance 213–14; commissioners 122; complaints 145–6; feedback from service users 108–9; multi-agency working 301; needs and demands 127, 130–1; outcomes 154; partnerships 22–3, 125; values 73, 82; vulnerable clients 221
social class 128
social justice 75, 78, 79, 111
social model of health 73, 79
social work 75, 108–9, 299
societal values 72–7, *72*
stakeholders 42, 119–24, 131; business planning 209; communication with 347; partnerships 165; process mapping 180; *see also* service users
standards 122, 142, 145–6, 229, 249–72; audit 270–2; business planning 209, 210; core 266, *267*; definition of 250–2; developmental 266, *267*; failure to comply with 313; frameworks 252–4, 265–8; inspections 213; management control 277, 278, 279, 293–4, *293*; monitoring 251, 268–70, *268*; output 278; procedures 285; professional bodies 218; resetting 291–2; service design 188; service user feedback 151; structure, process and outcome 259–62, *263–4*
stepped care model 184
Stocking, B. 344
stress 15, 50, 114, 311
structure 259–62, *263–4*
supervision 14, 217
suppliers 105, 106, 117–19, 123, 205, *232*
support services 137, 140
surgery 175–6, *177*, 181, 185–6
surveys 145, 146–7, 149, 185, 255, 288
'symptom iceberg' 128
systems 173, 285
systems thinking 40, 125, 277–9

Tannenbaum, R. 37–8
targets 21, 212, 286, 290–1; budgetary 193, 205; business planning 209–10, 211; Local Area Agreements 208; partnerships 23; quality control loop 145; standards 258; time 255, 256, 259

tasks 32–3, 39, 297, *297*; diagnostic model 319, *319*, 323, *326*; shared action planning 341–2, 343–4; task-oriented leadership 49–50
teams 295–302; leadership 36, 39, 40, 45, 47–8; motivation 59–60; multidisciplinary 25, 157, 176, 298, 299–302; objectives 31–2, 33; process 187, 188; project 8, 347; training plans 306; values 72, 80–3
Thompson, K. 184
time management 19, *55*, 183–4
trade unions 123
training 294, 302–10, 343; capability issues 311; equal opportunities 308–10; job-specific 303; multi-agency working 301; needs analysis 303–5; plans 281, 306; review and evaluation 307–8
trait theory 37
transformation process 174, *174*
transformational leadership 40–3

trust 54, 87, 143
Tushman, M.L. 318–20

user-led services 134, *135*
utilisation rates 127

value for money 78, 79, 209, 234
value-added analysis 182
values 43, 71–88, 134, 252, 330; group 72, 80–3; individual 72, 83–6; management style 50; organisational 72, 77–80, 319; societal 72
Vanu Som, C. 265
vision 40, 41, 43, 71, 86–8, 330; business planning 210, 211; mind map *326*
volunteers 59, 65–6, 282
Vroom, V.H. 64–5

Webb, S.A. 134
Wedderburn Tate, C. 44
Women's Royal Voluntary Service 153
workload outputs 195